An Epidemic of Uncertainty

An Epidemic of Uncertainty

Navigating HIV and Young Adulthood in Malawi

JENNY TRINITAPOLI

The University of Chicago Press
Chicago and London

The University of Chicago Press, Chicago 60637
The University of Chicago Press, Ltd., London
© 2023 by The University of Chicago
Published 2023
Printed in the United States of America

32 31 30 29 28 27 26 25 24 23   1 2 3 4 5

ISBN-13: 978-0-226-82554-0 (cloth)
ISBN-13: 978-0-226-82571-7 (paper)
ISBN-13: 978-0-226-82570-0 (e-book)
DOI: https://doi.org/10.7208/chicago/9780226825700.001.0001

Library of Congress Cataloging-in-Publication Data

Names: Trinitapoli, Jenny Ann, author.
Title: An epidemic of uncertainty : navigating HIV and young adulthood in Malawi /
    Jenny Trinitapoli.
Other titles: Navigating HIV and young adulthood in Malawi
Description: Chicago ; London : The University of Chicago Press, 2023. | Includes
    bibliographical references and index.
Identifiers: LCCN 2022061283 | ISBN 9780226825540 (cloth) | ISBN 9780226825717
    (paperback) | ISBN 9780226825700 (ebook)
Subjects: LCSH: AIDS (Disease)—Social aspects—Malawi—Balaka. | Risk—Socio-
    logical aspects. | Population—Health aspects. | Balaka (Malawi)—Population. |
    Balaka (Malawi)—Social conditions—21st century. | BISAC: SOCIAL SCIENCE /
    Ethnic Studies / African Studies | SOCIAL SCIENCE / Methodology
Classification: LCC RA643.86.M32 B35 2023 | DDC 362.19697/920096897—dc23/
    eng/20230106
LC record available at https://lccn.loc.gov/2022061283

Contents

Abbreviations

ABC	abstain, be faithful, and use condoms
AHI	acute HIV infection
AIDS	acquired immune deficiency syndrome (the medical condition caused by HIV)
ANC	antenatal care
ART	antiretroviral therapy
ARVs	antiretroviral medicines (colloquial)
CD4	cluster of differentiation 4 (a type of white blood cells, also called T-cells, targeted by HIV)
CLS	consequential lightning strikes
CRVS	civil registration and vital statistics
DHS	Demographic and Health Surveys
DSS	demographic surveillance system
ELISA	enzyme-linked immunosorbent assay
HBM	health belief model
HIV	human immunodeficiency virus
HSA	health surveillance assistant
HTC	HIV testing and counseling
ICTs	information and communication technologies
IFS	ideal family size
IPV	intimate partner violence
MDFRA	Marriage, Divorce and Family Relations Act
MDICP	Malawi Diffusion and Ideational Change Project
NGO	nongovernmental organization
NICHD	National Institute of Child Health and Human Development
PLWHA	people living with HIV/AIDS
PMTCT	prevention of mother-to-child transmission

PrEP	pre-exposure prophylaxis
PSLE	Primary School Leaving Exam
RBF4MNH	Results-Based Financing for Maternal and Neonatal Health
SRH	sexual and reproductive health
STI	sexually transmitted infection
TCA	theory of conjunctural action
TLT	Tsogolo La Thanzi
UNAIDS	Joint United Nations Programme on HIV/AIDS
UPE	universal primary education
UTT	universal test and treat
VCT	voluntary counseling and testing (see also HTC)
WHO	World Health Organization

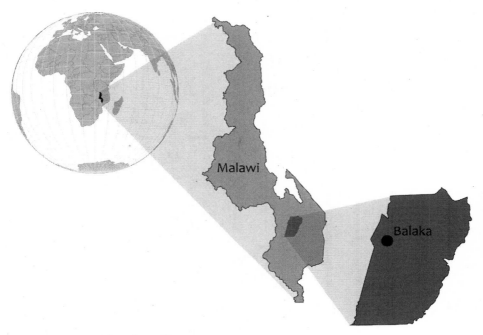

Map situating Balaka in the world

1

Introduction
Surveying the Shadows of Uncertainty

In early August 2019, one of our research team's most talented interviewers poked her head into the data room and motioned that she needed me for something. Usually serious and stately, Caroline was choking with laughter and wiping tears with an ivory handkerchief; from down the hallway, I could hear the respondent laughing as well. Over the course of a decade, our longitudinal study of relationships, childbearing, contraception, and HIV risk only occasionally produced such visceral comedy. "Jenny, this respondent is clever," Caroline said. "She is open about her life, and, wow, she is good at telling stories. We are just enjoying talking with one another, but I need some paper because my notes will not fit on this small line for 'other reason,' and we need your help deciding what to put down for her marital status."

Marital status is not among the items survey researchers typically consider a complex construct. The choices are straightforward: never married, currently married, cohabiting, divorced, separated, or widowed. However, Patuma's marriage was indeed an "it's complicated" situation, and her vivid narration took me on a journey from uncertainty to certainty and back again.[1]

My husband and I have three children together. The first one? That was unplanned; I was only 15. But we stayed together and got married two years after the first one was born. All of my children are with this man, and all of his children are with me. We have been happy together since 2006. But as of late, I have been doubting him. For example, one night he did not come home, which is something he had never done before. And then, about a week later, another night. Maybe if he was a security guard, but my husband is a welder, and welders don't work at night. I talked with him about it; I told him about my suspicions. I even called our *ankhoswe* [traditional marriage mediators], but they didn't help, they just said, "Well, after all, he is a man, and that's how men sometimes behave. You just have to accept it. There's no need for you to end the marriage over some doubts." But I was not ready to accept that. Not with this disease. My mother died from it when I was one year old; my father had already run away to Nsanje district. I was raised by my granny, but since I myself am an orphan, my own children don't have grandparents who could raise them.

From there, I started hearing rumors about his behavior—hearing that he has another partner. My friend called me and told me she was standing at Mavuto Lodge watching my husband enter that area with a woman. And she advised me; she said to me, "Patuma, you have to catch him red-handed." So I started paying very close attention to where he was going and when, even following him from time to time. I usually just stay at home farming while he goes to work in town, but I started moving around to find out more about what he is really doing. Last week I followed him to a certain place, near where my friend had seen him; indeed, he was meeting a woman there. The two of them went into the bush. You know . . . where people sometimes go to have sex. So I was right to have those doubts. Still, I didn't say anything to him. I just went home.

The next day, I went to the bush in the late afternoon, and I hid there for hours. I was so scared; I was scared of the bush buffalo trampling me, I was scared of being bitten by snakes, and I was cold. After waiting for hours, probably six hours, I went home in the dark, shivering. I was a mess. My husband was there at home, and I told him that I had been visiting our friend who was at the hospital.

I paid attention to how he was behaving, and I decided to go again to the bush. I hid on the ground in those grasses, a bit far away from the road. I had not eaten anything since the morning, so I was hungry and worried about snakes. But I had dressed more warmly the second time. I had prepared well to hide in the bush, like an animal or like a mad person. Then I started thinking, "What am I doing? I am going to get killed! Trampled by bush buffalo or murdered by another mad person hiding in the bush." Just then, my husband appeared with that same woman. The woman was carrying a *jumbo* [a plastic bag] with something he had given her. I stayed quiet, and they took off their clothes and started doing sex. I moved closer, and when I saw that they were, you know, *very busy*, I crept near to pick up the trousers of my husband and a wrapper of the lady, and I crept to another spot to grab the jumbo. I wasn't close enough to get the underpants. I left those, and I snuck away. I returned to my home, very late, in the dark; and I was not happy, but I was proud of myself. In the jumbo he had brought her four eggs, some tomatoes, and a small bottle of cooking oil.

In the morning I did my chores as usual. I washed his trousers and that wrapper along with all the other clothes. I hung everything out to dry. When the laundry had dried, I took down my own clothes and the children's clothes, but I left his trousers and that wrapper hanging outside the house. Later in the day my husband came home; I welcomed him and asked him if he would like to eat, and he said that he would. So I brought out the jumbo he had given to that lady, and I slowly took out the tomatoes and the eggs to start preparing the food. We were sitting in the front of the house. I got my knife and started chopping the tomatoes, and I was looking at him but staying quiet. Then I asked him, "Please bring me some more charcoal for the stove, so that I can fry these eggs in this oil." He went around to where we keep the charcoal, and from there he could see his trousers and her wrapper hanging on our clothesline.

So now we are discussing whether to end the relationship. We are still staying in the house together. Naturally, my husband has called the ankhoswe to come to the house for mediation. They will be here either tomorrow or the next day. Today your project has asked me a lot of questions, including about my marital status, but the truth is that today I don't know whether I am married or whether this marriage has ended.[2]

"Don't know" answers in survey research are typically regarded as a problem: a research anomaly, a violation of the assumption of "perfect information," a source of missing data, a nuisance to analysts. Consider, instead, that *don't know* answers are a portal to understanding the social world more deeply and that they can be studied deliberately, in an empirical framework. Patuma's difficulty answering a supposedly straightforward question about a basic demographic trait speaks volumes about the force of uncertainty in everyday life. It raises questions about what uncertainty about a marriage means to her, how prevalent this state is for others in this community, and what consequences this uncertainty has for how Patuma moves about in the world—how all of us move about in the world.

For the purpose of completing the questionnaire, we categorized Patuma as married; her answers to other, adjacent questions—the suspicion of other partners, a question mark on whether the marriage will still be intact a year from now, a recent call to the ankhoswe—would indicate to analysts concerned with relationship quality that this marriage is in a fragile state. The uncertain relationship is linked to another salient uncertainty: a question about her HIV status. Patuma had been tested for HIV three times in the past year, twice during antenatal care (ANC) and once when she started suspecting her husband of having other partners. She indicated in our survey that she has friends who are HIV positive and doing well thanks to antiretroviral therapy (ART), that if she tested positive she believes she would probably get the treatment she needed to live a long life, and that she does not know her HIV status. Even on receiving a negative result from the testing services offered within our study's protocol, Patuma still articulated doubts about her HIV status. Like thousands of other women in Balaka, Patuma is uncertain. In fact, she is navigating an epidemic of uncertainty.

When I call HIV/AIDS an *epidemic of uncertainty*, I am referring to an epidemic that has been ongoing for more than thirty years in sub-Saharan Africa and in Balaka, Malawi, the setting of this study. Because HIV is an established disease, the uncertainty that accompanies it cannot be attributed to novelty—things not yet known that with support from the scientific community and time will become known in due course.[3] The AIDS-related uncertainty that characterizes Balaka today has become a stable fixture of social life—a feature, not a bug. Across the globe, young adults navigate the terrain of family formation without a reliable map or a lifetime of experience to guide them. In AIDS-endemic contexts, young adults face the looming threat of HIV infection at every turn, which elevates the stakes of the decisions they have to make. Daily life involves navigating a uniquely treacherous landscape, whether taking small and mundane steps (like getting dressed for a funeral) or big, consequential leaps (like deciding to marry or leave a spouse).

In this book I take readers on a decade-long tour of the HIV-related uncertainty that permeates one corner of southeastern Africa. In doing so, I produce new empirical parameters for tracking the region's ongoing epidemic—measures of uncertainty that capture the full reach of HIV in the whole population, not just among the infected. I show that HIV-related uncertainties in Balaka are consequential and linked to other contingencies and conjunctures, many of which are concentrated in adolescence and early adulthood.[4] Building on these key empirical contributions, I also provide a framework for thinking more clearly about other kinds of uncertainties that characterize the transition to adulthood: livelihood and economic uncertainty; romance and relationship uncertainty; fertility and the reproductive realm.

As a general approach, the investigation of uncertainty from a demographic perspective provides a template for how scholars might render an empirical account that grapples both with a concrete object of inquiry and with the uncertainty that object generates. The shift involved in centering the uncertainty, rather than the phenomenon, in the analysis may advance understandings of other social problems that are, fundamentally, dilemmas of uncertainty. I approach this task with a diverse set of methodological tools to engage both the microanalytic facts of uncertainty (as a psychosocial phenomenon, it is experienced and felt by individuals) and the macro-level features of uncertainty as a population-level phenomenon (it is not reducible to individual-level experiences and, though invisible, shares some of the properties of material aggregates). My goal is to show that in the aggregate uncertainties have a force similar to other macro-level population-related structural contexts and processes, that these uncertainties can be measured, and that their effects on behavior and related outcomes can be analyzed.

Research at Three Intersections

The arguments I advance in this book are situated at three intersections: geographic, substantive, and intellectual. First, the literal, geographic intersection (depicted in fig. 1.1): Balaka is both a growing district capital and a quintessential hinterland. Balaka Boma sits just alongside Malawi's main road,[5] which bisects the country north to south, and the Trans-Zambezia Railway, which connects Mozambique's Indian Ocean ports to Zambia on the west. Located at the crossroads of these two thoroughfares, Balaka Boma is perhaps best characterized by *movement*, a place where people come and go, doing business of various sorts; by its *market*, which operates every day of the week; and by its *marriage* patterns. The boma is densely populated, home to a district hospital, a government clinic, two private hospitals, at least a dozen secondary schools, a five-thousand-acre commercial farm, a Chinese-owned

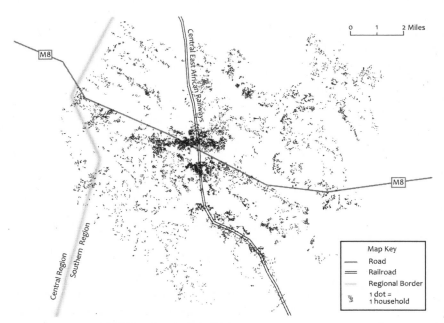

FIGURE 1.1 Map of the TLT catchment area in Balaka

Source: TLT Household Listing, 2019.

cotton ginnery, a limestone factory, and a large Italian-run Catholic mission. The boma is surrounded by rural communities, villages, where most families rely on subsistence agriculture. The movement that characterizes the boma cultivates diversity (religious and ethnic), through both labor migration and marriage. Southern Malawi is predominantly matrilocal; upon marriage a husband typically moves into his new wife's community, and, correspondingly, upon divorce a man leaves his wife's home.[6]

The substantive intersection concerns the relationship between HIV and fertility. Both HIV prevalence and fertility are higher in Malawi's southern region than in the country's other two regions; further, the median age both at first marriage and at first birth is significantly lower in Balaka than in the country's major cities.[7] It is not just the high levels of HIV and fertility that matter here; it is the relationship between the two that motivates a careful examination of young adulthood, especially the project of family formation and its perils. HIV in Malawi, as in the rest of sub-Saharan Africa, is primarily transmitted through heterosexual sex. So the risks of contracting HIV and of becoming pregnant are synchronized. Behaviors that affect one—like abstinence, coital frequency, and condom use—necessarily affect the other, and individuals' attitudes to each have consequences for both. This reality creates a set of critical dilemmas for young adults who want children but also worry about infection from a partner. Navigating healthy childbearing while avoiding HIV is a labyrinth of trade-offs.[8] As shown in figure 1.2, young Malawians are subject to peak levels of HIV infection (where prevalence rises starkly) during the "busiest" time of their reproductive lives (when age-specific fertility rates peak). Put simply: How do young adults negotiate relationships, sex, and childbearing in the context of a severe AIDS epidemic?

The third intersection involves two intellectual traditions in the social sciences—one quantitative and demographic, the other ethnographic and theoretical. Writing about the relationship between demography and social history, Daniel Scott Smith characterized demography as "relentlessly and routinely analytical" and dryly praised the important work of enumerating the size and structure of human populations, writing, "while getting the numbers right may not seem to be much, it is better than getting them wrong."[9] The Tsogolo La Thanzi study (described in more detail in chapter 2) was designed to sit at the intersection of interpretive approaches that privilege the experiential realm and the empirical relentlessness demographers are well known for. The approach fits with Veronique Petit's agenda for *comprehensive demography*, an intellectual pursuit that emphasizes the "absolute necessity of anchoring demographic analyses in their specific contexts," maintains that "data are only meaningful if demographers use appropriate theoretical re-

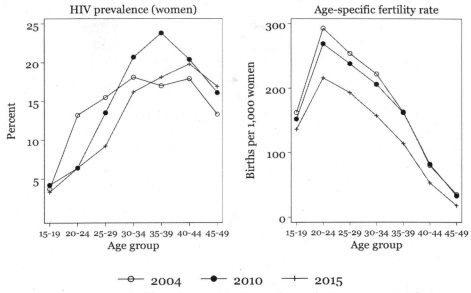

FIGURE 1.2 Age-specific HIV prevalences and fertility rates for reproductive-age women in Malawi

Source: MDHS 2004/2005, 2015.

sources to provide an interpretive model," and insists on the inseparability of *counting* and *understanding*, putting "measurement and interpretation on the same plane."[10]

Ordinary people do not view the world the same way professional demographers do. At the same time, ordinary people perceive and interpret all kinds of things about their surroundings, including demographic processes. Their perceptions may be closely aligned with the "reality" determined by experts or, for a variety of reasons, may be contradictory. Jane Schneider and Peter Schneider powerfully linked process and perceptions in their study of the ideological consequences of demographic change in Sicily: "The underlying challenge is one of connection: how to move, analytically, from a global transformation in the dynamics of mortality, fertility, and migration, to the day-to-day experience of deaths and births and departures in a local setting, then to local attributions of meaning to these events, and back to the ways we think about population processes in general."[11] By making popular perceptions of demographic processes central, rather than peripheral, to demographic research, the connections between counting and understanding become intellectually generative, with implications for a variety of substantive concerns. Take, for example, a society in which infant mortality is higher among unmarried mothers than among married mothers, and those differences in survival probabilities are perceived by the population experiencing those rates. That mortality differential becomes relevant for religious notions of divine justice, beliefs about stigma and honor, and the rituals governing food preparation and sexual behavior.[12] In this book I aim to connect the known and shifting patterns of an established epidemic to the sense people make of it and show that both the patterns and the understandings have real consequences for social life. In so doing, I hope to erode some of the barriers that often separate these two traditions and dissolve long-standing assumptions about what kinds of methodological and substantive pairings "go together."

Demographic Concepts for Understanding Uncertainty

This book situates both HIV and young adulthood within two core substantive concerns of demography: fertility and mortality. The links between HIV and mortality are quite clear and well established in the literature. HIV and fertility, on the other hand, are typically studied as entirely separate processes by distinct groups of scholars; I treat the two as inextricably linked. I also connect HIV and fertility to important topics at the periphery of demography: marriage, divorce, family structure, income, poverty, and livelihoods. Philip Hauser and Otis Dudley Duncan famously described the field of population studies as "at least as broad as that of the determinants and consequences of population trends,"[13] and I take an expansive approach to identifying and elaborating both the determinants and the consequences of uncertainty as important population trends.

The demographic nature of my methods relates closely to the materials. My primary materials are cross-sectional and longitudinal sample surveys, but I also invoke a multivocal trove of marginalia associated with these surveys, including excerpts from my own fieldnotes, memos from project supervisors and interviewers, and passages from survey-embedded ethnography. I follow a single cohort over an extended period and link this cohort's collective experience to the period-specific influences they experience by virtue of moving through history together. I model the experience of this cohort with a focus on the population at risk. This work is rooted in a quantitative tradition that treats a probability as a property of the external world and leverages parameters to make sound comparisons between groups (e.g., men and women) under the assumption that this activity can reveal something true about the world that is worth knowing—for example, that HIV prevalence is higher among women ages 15–19 than among men the same ages. Demographic research is committed to carefully defining the population at risk of exposure to the potential occurrence of a vital event, whether a death, a pregnancy, a

birth, an HIV infection, or a marriage. While the total population is, defini-
tionally, at risk of death, once married, a woman is no longer at risk of getting
married. A population lens refines the view by moving away from "all people"
to focus on a more carefully defined "at risk" group. This shift improves accuracy, and the demographer's habit of disciplined denominators reflects the
underlying commitment (in Smith's words) to "getting the numbers right."[14]

To illustrate the practical stakes of counting well with respect to HIV, recall
that as recently as fifteen years ago HIV prevalence estimates for sub-Saharan
Africa were derived from nonrepresentative samples of women attending
antenatal clinics: pregnant women, young, mostly urban, with resources to
access transportation and clinics. During this period, experts overestimated
HIV prevalence by between 50 and 300 percent, and when those estimates
were finally corrected using population-based samples, some members of the
international community breathed a sigh of relief after learning that prevalence was closer to 15 percent than to 30. When processing the corrections
in Malawi, some of us panicked, realizing that the crushing adult-mortality
burden we thought was a consequence of 30 percent HIV prevalence was
actually the consequence of an epidemic about half that prevalent and far
more severe.[15] Non-population-based sampling misled the scholarly community's work of tracking subsequent declines in prevalence[16] and reductions
in incidence, underestimating the effectiveness of real-time behavior change,
guided by local sensibilities and solutions.[17] So while it may not seem like
much, the ordinary work of counting well to generate sound estimates of basic quantities is indispensable for making any kind of inference or interpretation. One key lesson from forty years of HIV epidemiology is that even the
most complex mathematical models will not compensate for the weaknesses
of unsuitable data.

I rely on demographic theories and models to transform an abundance
of data (i.e., the aforementioned materials) into accounts of *how population
processes work* and *what they mean* to the people living in an epidemic. Those
who equate demography with the "bean-counting" stereotypes of census taking, projection making, and actuarial estimation may be surprised to encounter the theoretical depth of this tradition. As Rupert Vance pointed out more
than seventy years ago, "In theory, demography remains relatively unstructured. It lacks, shall we say, a 'binder' for its diverse findings."[18] I agree with
Vance that the concepts, insights, and findings from demography and population studies are too varied to ever coalesce into a singular theory that binds
them all together. But demographers have cultivated an abundance of valuable concepts, and I have arranged this book around four that I regularly rely
on to identify and answer key analytic puzzles about uncertainty in social life.

Think of these concepts as stage lights in a theater production. Some do the important work of shedding light on aspects of social life that are easy to miss; they illuminate the character and the action. Other lights guide the viewer's line of sight; they show us where to look. Still others set the mood, enhance the music, and capture the passage of time. The lighting is never the star of any play, but it would be difficult if not impossible to see anything without it. The four concepts are as follows:

- Norman Ryder's cohort—an aggregate of individuals, defined in spatial and temporal terms, that shares the experience of period-specific conditions and stimuli at particular ages—and an accompanying model that emphasizes the cohort as a crucial analytic unit for studying social change.[19]
- Susan Watkins's link between gossip—which simultaneously provides narrative, explanation, and judgment—and demographic behavior, with an emphasis on the importance of socially salient "others" for understanding the intimate sphere and its connections to large-scale demographic change.[20]
- A theory of conjunctural action (TCA), which places an emphasis on the eventfulness of life. As Jennifer Johnson-Hanks and colleagues write, "Conjunctures are where stuff happens—people get pregnant, married, divorced; they convert to a new religion, go back to school, or move across the country." TCA embraces a traditional demographic view, which poses a radical contrast to methodological individualism. "We argue," they continue, "that social demography should focus on the distribution of contexts in which events might occur, rather than on the characteristics of individuals: More Keyfitz, less Becker."[21]
- The puzzle of population processes occurring simultaneously at two scales—micro and macro, individual and aggregate—and ongoing debates about whether and how to integrate these scales analytically. Human beings die, whereas a population aggregate does not; individuals enter, replacing those who exit, and even though each individual is different and their circumstances unique, population-level patterns are often stable. How is this possible?[22]

While featuring these quintessentially demographic insights, analyzing HIV as an epidemic of uncertainty requires taking a deliberately sociological stance, emphasizing the experiences of individuals. I lay out the demographic patterns according to the standards of the field and pair these with analogous analyses of how young adults in Balaka perceive their world, taking their accounts of vital events (and near-misses) seriously without taking them literally. The foundations for such an approach are widespread across the social sciences, but the basic insight of Dorothy Swaine Thomas and W. I. Thomas's famous theorem makes the point clearly: "If men define situations as real, they are real in their consequences."[23] Applying the theorem to HIV, I am just as interested in what a woman believes her HIV status is as I am in the result of the HIV biomarker obtained from a finger prick. To the extent that HIV has become less deadly now that antiretroviral drugs are widely available, that fact will be manifest one way in the life of a man who believes that those drugs exist, that they work, and that he could access them if he ever needed to, and another way in the life of his hypothetical counterpart who perceives no such decline in mortality and fundamentally mistrusts biomedicine.

Relatedly, ordinary people perceive changes to the fertility, mortality, and migration rates they contribute to and are affected by. They do not analyze these processes in the same way demographers do, but they notice when many men migrate to South Africa to find work, they know when they have attended more funerals in one year compared to the last, and they recognize pressures on land in terms of both availability and suitability for farming. While a young woman may not have a working theory of how men's migration alters the economic conditions of her village, her marriage prospects, and her risk of contracting HIV, the explanations she gives for each of these phenomena are important in their own right. From a sociological perspective, perceptions of demographic processes and fluctuations are interesting, important, and consequential *regardless of their accuracy* because (in an accumulating fashion) these perceptions motivate actions that produce vital events that constitute demographic rates that are, in turn, consequential for a host of other population-level and individual-level phenomena.[24]

Demography, Narrated from the Inside

Let me offer an example of how demographic phenomena are narrated from the inside, in connection with each other, with a true story that links HIV to fertility, child mortality, and divorce with an emphasis on the uncertain and the unknown. This passage comes from fieldnotes I wrote in 2010, in conjunction with Alice, an interviewer and close friend.

> Regarding respondent [name] (age 23) who was seven months pregnant and HIV positive at her first interview.[25] A few months later, she hasn't returned to be reinterviewed. Alice recruited and interviewed the respondent, so she knows the entire reproductive and marital history, including HIV status: respondent and husband both knew they were positive when the study started and were taking antiretroviral drugs. Alice travels to the respondent's home to see if everything is OK. At the compound, there are two houses with people living in them and three houses that have no people. Alice finds the respondent at home, but there is no baby. The baby has died, and the husband has left.

Before saying anything about the husband and baby, the respondent ac-
knowledges the conspicuous emptiness of the compound: "We were many
people at our compound, but most of them died because of AIDS. One of
them is my mother. She died of AIDS, and her husband died from it too. We
have three houses that have no people to live in. My mum and my two aunts
have all died of AIDS. I don't know why we all die of the same disease." She
goes on to explain the death of a child as a result of her HIV infection: "If I
have unprotected sex, I can become pregnant at any time. If I get pregnant
I will be pregnant, but that child will not survive. Believe me or not, HIV is
dangerous. My best friend, she stays at [name of village], she started having a
problem of ulcers. She and her husband were tested and found with the virus,
but fortunately, they have two children already. After this one died, my husband left me on that same day and went back to his home."[26]

Respondent tells Alice that her husband left her because she is not bearing
children. He told her that he cannot stay without children. What he said, specifically, was, "I don't think you're failing to have children because of the HIV.
Don't you see all around us? There are many HIV-positive women who go to
clinics. You see them at the hospital receiving ARVs [antiretroviral drugs].
They go to antenatal, they are still bearing children, and those children are
surviving. This is not like the old days. HIV-positive women today are having
babies without any problems at all. HIV is not your problem. There's something else going on. This is the second baby you've lost. My family members
are saying that you've been bewitched, and I can't help you with that."

Respondent: "I need to hear the truth from you. What are your plans? Are
you divorcing me, or what? You have already said that you cannot afford to
have two wives at the same time because you are poor. That much I understand, plus I would not stand for a co-wife. If you had told me that you would
like to marry another woman who will be your second wife, I would tell you
to just go ahead with her. Now tell me what you want. Just be straightforward."

Husband: "You were my first wife in my life, and the two children that
I lost with you were the only children I had in my life. Since this problem is
not mine but it is yours, I will leave you here and look for another woman to
marry. I don't mean the HIV problem. You have some other problem, which is
why I have decided to leave you."

Alice, who is HIV positive (disclosing this explicitly to me for the first
time as we write up these notes) tells the respondent: "Sister, I didn't tell you
this when we met last time, but I have HIV too. And since I've had it, I've had
two healthy babies and no miscarriages and neither of my children has it." So
I think your husband is right. There is something else going on with you, and
you are going to need to figure out what that is.

A lot happens in this brief passage: we bear witness to an infant's death and
a divorce, preceded by a previous death and HIV infections and diagnoses.

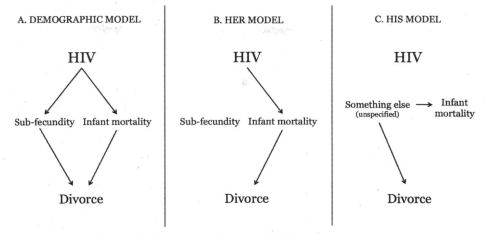

FIGURE 1.3 Three models for explaining Alice's respondent's divorce

Viewing this story from the perspective of academic demography, presuming each element is time stamped with perfect accuracy, I would draw a mini-model with causal arrows from HIV status to subfecundity (difficulty conceiving) and infant mortality (child survival) through to relationship quality and stability (fig. 1.3, panel A). The scholarly literature supports such a model—*a model of* HIV, childbearing, and marriage—and the hypothesized relationships would be borne out quantitatively by suitable, longitudinal, sample-survey data.

For the people living through it, births, deaths, marriages, and bouts of illnesses are not items on a checklist of vital events but crucial stakes in a larger framework of meaning related to ultimate concerns. We stand here at the edge of the material world of viruses, which all three actors in the exchange acknowledge and understand well from a knowledge perspective, and the supernatural world—an apparent curse on this poor young woman who has had to bury two children and many close relatives. Daniel Scott Smith pinpointed one of the paradoxes of our discipline when he wrote that "when demographers deal with 'sex and death' . . . they characteristically eliminate the pleasure from the former (hiding it under the category 'fecundability') and the terror from the latter (death tables being euphemistically called 'life' tables)."[27] Indeed, the vocabulary of academic demography often attempts to be laughably neutral. With an emphasis on rates, demographers invoke phrases like union formation, coital frequency, union dissolution, and excess mortality; as the protagonists of our very own lives, however, we experience love, sex, breakups, death, and grief.

This husband and wife understand the world with different models. Their interpretations are colored by disparate perceptions of demographic phenomena—specifically, the broader landscape of fertility and mortality and HIV's role in it. Theirs are *models for* how to act within a particular reality.[28] Both invoke demographic phenomena in their accounts—and the result is not a singular, coherent, "local" perspective but a pair of incompatible interpretations. In our respondent's model of the world (fig. 1.3, panel B), HIV begets death. She resides in a compound that has been hollowed out by AIDS, and the absence of her female relatives is still palpable. She attributes the death of two children to her own HIV status; this is basically a pessimistic, overdetermined version of the demographic model, save the fact that she has no trouble conceiving. Because of her status, her children will not survive; she doesn't want to repeat the experience again. She plans to have a tubal ligation and either live alone or find a man who, unlike her husband, does not need children.

The husband has lived through these same events—diagnosis, pregnancies, and deaths—but his perception of the population phenomena that surround them is totally distinct. Engaged with clinicians in HIV care, he sees HIV-positive women living normal lives and having healthy children. He draws no connection between HIV and his own losses. It is precisely this *lack* of a clear, causal arrow that begs for alternate explanations, a void that his family has filled with a narrative of witchcraft but that he leaves more open-ended. If his words are to be believed, it is this mysterious "other problem"— not HIV—that drives him from the marriage (fig. 1.3, panel C). Regardless of its accuracy, his model defines the course of this relationship; he is the one who leaves. The mere suggestion of witchcraft may startle some readers, but it is worth pointing out that Alice—a trained HIV counselor who has been living positively with HIV for almost two decades and is intimately familiar with treatment regimens, family planning recommendations, and the unique challenges of having children as an HIV-positive woman—likewise articulates a model that emphasizes the "something else." When a woman who is receiving ART loses two children, something else is not right. Here, again, it is not HIV itself but the uncertainty surrounding it that has consequences for this marriage. Note that when elaborated algebraically, his model would include an unnamed error term.

Population Chatter as Vernacular Theory

Taking the standard academic labels, the three substantive concerns of demography—fertility, mortality, and migration—do not obviously constitute strong fodder for everyday conversation. When one listens carefully, however, conversations about fertility, mortality, and migration are everywhere. Undergraduates complaining to each other about the hassles of contraceptive side-effects are engaging in population chatter;[29] the wisdoms they share with each other about the sources of free condoms and which sexual and reproductive health (SRH) clinics are least unpleasant fall into the category too. A woman confiding to her cousin that she is putting off responding to her roommate about renewing their lease because she really hopes her long-distance boyfriend will ask her to move in with him is, in a fundamental way, having a conversation about marriage and migration. And a mother-in-law who makes passive-aggressive remarks about how all her friends are busy with their grandchildren is playing a role in sustaining the birth rate.

In addition to narrating and responding to the demographic phenomena that pertain to their own lives, people also *perceive* the fertility, mortality, and migration conditions around them. In everyday conversation, perceptions of demographic phenomena are manifest in comments about the value of immigrants to the US economy (e.g., "So entrepreneurial!"), wondering aloud about whether the COVID-19 mortality rates published in the major newspapers are trustworthy, or passing judgment on a couple traversing an airport with a gaggle of, say, five unruly children.

Again, ordinary people don't talk about population phenomena in the same way academic demographers do, but ordinary people talk about population phenomena quite a bit, and their chatter often takes the form of gossip. Watkins's research on the demographic transition in nineteenth-century Europe linked the grist of the intimate sphere to large-scale social change with an epic account of fertility decline that centers gossip as a driver of demographic convergence.[30]

> Gossip has often been scorned as idle and malicious talk, particularly associated with women. Gossip is certainly a form of social control: some behaviors are condemned, others praised. But the "best kind of women's gossip" provides narrative, explanation, and judgement: in the stories of others, the talker narrates a sequence of events that implies an explanation, and talker and listeners alike speculate on the meaning of the events, reach a common point of view, and reassure themselves of what they share.[31]

Population chatter is especially pertinent to our goal of understanding demographic behavior when it renders visible the importance of salient "others" in the intimate realm. That impatient mother-in-law isn't just there; theoretically and empirically, her judgments matter for the reproductive decisions of a particular couple and for the aggregate-level patterns.

In her study of population dynamics in Mali, the anthropological demographer Sara Randall relied on population chatter to solve a fascinating
puzzle:[32] Why would concerns about sterility and subfecundity be widespread
in a society wherein most women bear five or six children each? Both demographers and people on the inside understand that fertility concerns are
not absolute but relative. In Randall's case, nomadic Kel Tamasheq families
compared themselves to the Bambara, a neighboring ethnic group, in which
women were typically bearing eight or nine children. Kel Tamasheq women
were not ignorant of demography but acutely aware of the same fertility
trends demographers were interrogating. On this basic fact both demographers and women agreed: Kel Tamasheq fertility may not have been low by
any standard, but it was *lower*. From here their explanations diverged. Demographers identified a unique marital pattern—monogamy, late first marriage, less than universal marriage for women, and slow rates of remarriage.
For us, these features of the marital pattern were totally sufficient for explaining the observed differences in lifetime fertility for two ethnic groups. Population chatter, on the other hand, revealed that Kel Tamasheq women blamed
biological constraints for their subfertility; they were deeply concerned about
a well-specified gynecological disease called *tessumde*. Specialized herbalists
treat tessumde, large swaths of the population understand themselves to be
afflicted by this disease, and healthy women still fear it today.

In some circumstances, population chatter is remarkably compatible
with demographic accounts. If traditional, rate-based demographic explanation is a crude line drawing, then population chatter adds color and shade—
explanation—and turns the simple sketch into a detailed image. Watkins
shows us the full picture when she instructs us to think about French women
gossiping while washing clothes as a process of knowledge dissemination.
Over long periods conversing with others like them, these women explain
and judge strategies for avoiding pregnancy (and the acceptability of these
strategies) with husbands, kin, and neighbors. The account truly takes us all
the way from the wash house to a new understanding of macro-level fertility decline. Sometimes population chatter reveals a series of variations on a
general model of demographic behavior. This is evident in the example of Alice's respondent's and her husband's differing explanations for their marriage's
inevitable end. Occasionally, as in the Kel Tamasheq example, population
chatter completely contradicts the demographic explanations. Where local
perceptions and demographic realities diverge, how do we determine which
one is "correct"? It is my view that we should refrain from trying to adjudi-
cate between them. A fully emic approach to understanding Kel Tamasheq
fertility through population chatter would have us testing for rare sexually

transmitted infections (STIs) and overprescribing antibiotics to treat something that sounds a lot like pelvic inflammatory disease. And if we listened only to the demographic explanation that links economic structures to a particular marriage pattern with consequences for fertility, we would miss the fact that women in this population actually live with—and in fear of—a specific disease that has a major influence on their understanding of health, their health-seeking behaviors, and their marriages. We need both the population chatter and the high-quality, population-based estimates to understand demographic phenomena.

Social scientists have much to learn from listening carefully (and systematically) to population chatter in everyday conversation. As a bonus, when reading or listening to a person who has developed a good ear for population chatter, the material can be riveting. Whether it is gossip, self-disclosure, or an early observation about population trends, population chatter shares the elements of the very best gossip.[33] Unlike the characteristic even-handed (or laughably neutral) tendency of academic demography, as interpreters of their own lives, people instinctively moralize the demographic sphere. For this reason, I propose we treat population chatter as a kind of vernacular theory: vernacular, because our focus rests on everyday language and conversation rather than on formal speech and policies; and theory, because when people engage in population chatter they are not trying (and failing) to generate good estimates. They are constructing—with their interlocutors—theories about how the world around them works, how it is changing, and how they are to understand it.

This Book

This account of HIV as an epidemic of uncertainty is the result of nearly two decades of research on HIV and fertility in Malawi. Uncertainty is an immodest topic; it poses dilemmas that are simultaneously philosophical, statistical, and social scientific. The researcher's habit is to assess what is unknown and then find that thing out. What we don't know constitutes a research question; in parallel, what our respondents don't know constitutes a missing data problem. But how might we, as social scientists, integrate known unknowns in our models of human behavior? How do we distinguish known unknowns from the unknowns that are fundamentally unknowable? How do we wrap our minds around that crucial "something else"? And what can we learn by studying how people make these distinctions in their own worlds? In our everyday lives, we use facts, knowledge, perceptions, heuristics, ignorance, assessments, and intuition to navigate our respective worlds. In that sense, this book is only nominally about HIV and AIDS; the more general purpose is to connect the uncertainties people experience to the concrete phenomena that cause them and use that connection to think seriously about the role uncertainty plays in social life.

The metaphor of uncertainty as a shadow cast onto a landscape allows us to view social life with greater clarity. The shadows of uncertainty are consequential, not because of their own weight or force (after all, they have none), but because, when traversing a landscape, we organize our movements around both the terrain itself and the shadows. Shadows can be cold and ominous; people sometimes take the long road in order to avoid the accompanying sensations. If I find myself standing within one of these scary shadows, I might engage in deliberate actions to navigate back into the sun. For example, I might end an uncertain relationship that brings me more confusion than joy. In other circumstances, however, shadows offer a pleasant shade that people deliberately move into, for example, when starting a new relationship, a new business venture, or migrating to town from the village to pursue better educational opportunities. Throughout our lives, we find ourselves in ominous shadows and pleasant shade for long and short periods. We might stand in the shadows of uncertainty alone, travel through it in the company of others, or sit for a while to rest while contemplating the next destination.

In AIDS-endemic contexts, HIV casts an especially prominent shadow. The projection of an extremely large mass—a thirty-year epidemic that has killed over one million Malawians since the early 1990s—the shadow of HIV in Balaka provides a powerful example of uncertainty exerting a unique, independent force on the social world. Beyond the specific example of HIV, I show that relationship instability and mortality perceptions also project onto Balaka's social landscape sizable and consequential shadows that pattern this society in concrete, measurable ways. Here the interplay between the micro-level actions of individuals and the macro-structural view of uncertainty as a population-level phenomenon is evident: when an uncertainty looms large enough, it may be utterly impossible to escape.

Chapter 2 outlines the main contours of population change in Balaka between 2009 and 2019. This includes rapid population growth, urbanization, the introduction and proliferation of mobile phones, the expansion of education, the arrival of new technologies for treating HIV, and a series of three distinct policies for rationing treatment in an environment of high demand and limited resources. This is a decade of significant social transformation, and uncertainty is a predictable accompaniment of change. Yet patterns of HIV prevalence and fertility remain remarkably consistent, presenting some genuine puzzles of continuity and change. This chapter also introduces the

Tsogolo La Thanzi (TLT) study: its origins, design, procedures, epistemological underpinnings, and limitations. I describe the challenges of longitudinal studies, including the perennial problem of disentangling age and time. Using the TLT survey data, I show that HIV prevalence among women triples over the study period and discuss the drivers of the epidemic as an interaction of social and biological processes, including migration, mortality, marriage, divorce, pregnancy, and fertility.

Chapter 3 sketches the parameters of an intellectual program I call uncertainty demography: the empirical study of known unknowns using the perspectives and tools of demography and population studies. Not to be confused with demographic uncertainty (the errors in our forecasts of future populations), something along the lines of uncertainty demography has been afoot for a decade or more but has not previously been unified within any kind of framework. After introducing what distinguishes uncertainty demography from other approaches in the social sciences, I summarize some especially admirable demographic contributions to the study of uncertainty as a force in the world and as an object of inquiry. Drawing on examples related to mortality, fertility, and family formation in four distinct modes of inquiry, I suggest that an empirically grounded demography of uncertainty is useful for the social sciences because it transcends some stalled debates in the field (i.e., positivism vs. interpretivism, choice vs. constraint), emphasizes the interplay between macro and micro social phenomena, and provides unique clarity on how the unknown and unpredictable are manifest in individual lives and in persistent social structures. In contrast to purely theoretical approaches, the term "uncertainty demography" serves two purposes: it captures the growing consideration of uncertainty as a topic in demography, and it suggests the value of bringing to bear demographic tools to understand the role of uncertainty in social life, broadly.

Chapter 4 advances an empirical examination of uncertainty as a measurable phenomenon that should be treated as an object of study in its own right. Embracing the condescending caricature of the demographer as "bean counter," I advance a method for measuring personal uncertainty that uses literal beans to solicit subjective probabilities in an interactive format. Using HIV as the emblematic case, I then show that uncertainty is a pervasive and patterned feature of Balaka's epidemic and that it characterizes HIV-endemic populations more generally. Put in the perspective of simple proportions, the TLT study shows that Balaka's generalized HIV epidemic with an infection rate of 12 percent generates an epidemic of uncertainty that reaches 60 percent. Not only is HIV uncertainty pervasive; it is consequential, manifest clearly in the extremely corporal domains of fertility and health.

Although tools for early diagnosis and treatment have improved over the past two decades, AIDS-related uncertainty seems almost impervious to biomedical solutions. That is because the epidemic of uncertainty is simultaneously contemporaneous and prospective: it is also about the future. Chapter 5 shows that uncertainty is prevalent even among those who were recently tested for HIV and uses qualitative data to show why this is the case. Modern medicine provides individuals with test results that assess their viral load and a diagnosis that is fundamentally retrospective; that is, it reflects a set of past-tense behaviors, exposures, and events. When we use demographic tools to view uncertainty as a relational and existential condition—and not primarily as a medical issue—we begin to understand it as a consequence of risks and vulnerabilities that are inseparable from romantic relationships.

Chapter 6 starts with the assertion that sexual relationships always convey a certain amount of risk and vulnerability. This fact is made especially visible when young adults navigate romantic relationships and the sexual realm in the midst of a generalized HIV epidemic. In Balaka trust is costly and even casual infidelities can have fatal consequences. In this high-stakes setting, relationships are forged, moralized, and managed very deliberately, with high levels of gossip and suspicion characterizing the entire community. At the individual level, relationship formation and relationship dissolution are strategies for staying safe. At the population level, these strategies produce a pattern of rapid relationship churning that facilitates the spread of HIV. For both men and women, rumor and gossip are pillars of decision making in the romantic realm, underscoring uncertainty's rightful position among the pantheon of social forces.

Chapter 7 further examines relationship uncertainty by looking outside the couple, at the role of socially salient others (people and things) for structuring the observable patterns of relationship stability and uncertainty. In the era of AIDS, traditional marriage guardians have become increasingly relevant for raising and settling intimate disputes but are becoming less present in the marriages of young adults today. A new technology, the mobile phone, has become a tool of relationship maintenance, surveillance, and sabotage. And when it comes to relationship uncertainty, female friends represent a double-edged sword, relaying information that sometimes reduces relationship uncertainty and sometimes exacerbates it. Phones and friends have measurable effects on relationship uncertainty and dissolution, while marriage guardians (ankhoswe) represent a stabilizing force. As these major social transformations play out, with phones becoming more prevalent and ankhoswe less, young adults are left increasingly uncertain in their relationships and more perpetually uncertain about HIV.

Chapter 8 leverages a core concern of demography and a vocabulary of net risks to illuminate the paradox of HIV: high deadliness and low urgency (given its long latent period) make HIV simultaneously an exceptional disease and a footnote in the complicated lives most young adults lead. I connect the mortality transition as understood from the expert demographer's view to the mortality experiences and perceptions that characterize the TLT cohort's experience navigating the epidemic from the inside. I leverage ethnographic and survey data to show that HIV risk and HIV-related uncertainty are among the many mortal vulnerabilities that characterize daily life. For decades HIV dominated the international community's agenda for allocating resources, but HIV frequently ranks as the third or fourth most pressing concern for infected individuals and their affected families.[34] In light of massive, macro-level declines in mortality rates and available antiretroviral treatment, HIV is a distinctive, acute, often-deadly condition that is simultaneously seen as no big deal—just one of many hassles people worry about and manage in a milieu of perpetual scarcity and uncertainty.

The concluding chapter chronicles the events in one woman's life over a four-month period to show how several varieties of uncertainty intersect, constituting an epidemic of uncertainty that includes but expands far beyond HIV itself.

2

Ten Years in Balaka
The Excellent and Imperfect Data of Longitudinal Studies

Tsogolo La Thanzi

Tsogolo La Thanzi means "healthy futures" in Chichewa, Malawi's most widely spoken language. Designed in 2007 and initiated in 2009, the Tsogolo La Thanzi study emerged from a set of unanswered questions, a constellation of friendships and collaborations, and some happy accidents in the realms of funding and practical support. My colleague Sara Yeatman had been writing about childbearing and HIV for years.[1] I had been writing about the role of religion in Malawi's AIDS epidemic.[2] In the process, I had become increasingly interested in young adulthood—specifically, how young people who had been hearing about HIV since they could walk and were now "of that age" were making decisions about marriage and childbearing, from flirting and dating to contraceptive choice and child spacing. For almost two decades, the prevention campaigns saturating anglophone sub-Saharan Africa were anchored in the message "ABC": abstain, be faithful, use condoms. But our age-mates in Malawi wanted children; A and C were off the table, and anyone who has ever been in a relationship knows that the full scope of B is never completely within one's control.

The conversations between Sara and me took place at this intersection: How are these risks synchronized? How were epidemiologists and public health scholars modeling them? And how did young people living through the epidemic make sense of the risks themselves? Imagine a woman who wants to have four children (the average ideal family size for Malawi in 2009), and imagine this woman adheres perfectly to every recommendation espoused by the global health community, including condom use. Under the current conditions of Malawi's epidemic, how much risk would she be taking on just to have four wanted children? How risky does that feel to her? How would *you* navigate the trade-off between having the kids you wanted to have and protecting yourself from a disease that was cutting short the lives and relationships you saw around you? I was a new mother, with a second kid on the way; Sara was in the early years of an exciting relationship, wading, as young adults everywhere do, through questions about what the future may hold in terms of partners, career, and family. These were exciting, eventful, and uncertain times for us. How much harder would it be if we were juggling, simultaneously, the weight of a generalized HIV epidemic looming over it all?[3]

Thanks to the training we received at the Population Research Center at the University of Texas at Austin, we disciplined our curiosity into a set of research questions that could be addressed empirically, and we planned to write a pair of empirical papers together: HIV and fertility; fertility and HIV. But as the project evolved, we started running into dead ends. High-quality fertility surveys had begun to ask about HIV-related issues and featured the twin strengths of large sample size and national representativeness. But these studies were cross-sectional, making it impossible to examine the issues of process that had grabbed our attention in the first place. Using data from one of the demographic surveillance system (DSS) sites in sub-Saharan Africa could get us close.[4] We could calculate trends over time for the sites themselves and for subpopulations (e.g., age groups, wealth quintiles) within them. But most DSSs follow places, not people. The best trends we could estimate would reflect the composition of an always changing population and, at best, allow us to generate true trajectories for a highly selective (i.e., nonrepresentative) group of stayers. Though incredibly valuable in their own right, DSS data could not answer our questions.

A few of the best longitudinal studies in the region (e.g., the Malawi Diffusion and Ideational Change Project [MDICP]) were following young adults with an intersurvey period of between two and three years.[5] When we started carefully analyzing these data we found that nearly everything we were interested in happened during the intersurvey period. The 16-year-old schoolgirl who had never had a boyfriend and was not at all worried about HIV was, when reinterviewed at age 18, nursing a 1-year-old, divorced from the baby's father (who never really provided for them), and infected. Her account and recollections would be interesting and instructive, but they could only tell us so much. Prospective data on fertility were collected from women who had been diagnosed as HIV positive and enrolled in prevention of mother-to-child transmission (PMTCT) programs. Their health, including pregnancies and child-health outcomes, had been carefully documented. But these studies captured the experience of a highly selective group of women (educated, urban, positive, clinic going) who shared precisely the characteristic of interest.

Our path became clear. To really understand the challenges involved in navigating young adulthood amid a generalized AIDS epidemic, we would need a large enough representative sample of women. We would need to catch them before or just as they entered the most epidemiologically perilous stage of their lives. We would need to follow up with them at close intervals to capture changes as they were taking place—engagements, pregnancies, divorces, introductions of new partners. And we would need to be just as interested in these women's subjective experiences as we were in their serostatus. (Serostatus is the *state* of having, or not having, detectable antibodies against a specific antigen, as measured by a blood test.) Seasoned in the art and unpredictability of household interviews, we knew that frank conversations about sex, contentment, worry, hope, and hardship would be impossible if husbands were nearby or sisters were washing clothes within earshot. We would need a dedicated research space to ensure both privacy and consistent conditions for our interviews; the women would need to come to us. In an ideal world, we would gather men's perspectives too and link their data to the women's trajectories to understand how couples navigate the complexity of this stage of life together. We would need to set a study like this in just the right location. Necessary conditions were a serious HIV epidemic, high fertility, and matrilocality.[6] And we would need real resources to field something like this.

Together Sara and I designed a longitudinal survey of young adulthood that could be leveraged to answer questions about the strategies young adults use to navigate the competing goals of having children they want to have and avoiding HIV infection. It would be expensive and difficult to execute, and we realized there was a high probability we would never actually get to field it. But the exercise invoked by the question, "What would we need to know in order to be able to answer X?," was instructive, clarifying, and, for us, great fun to work out. With support from Malawian colleagues in nursing, demography, and economics, we submitted our proposal to the National Institute of Child Health and Human Development (NICHD) and crossed our fingers. Months later, we received an email from our program officer: "Go ahead and buy yourselves some cheap champagne. I suggest Bulgarian." Our proposal had received a top score and was funded through a special initiative to advance understandings of HIV and fertility. It was time to put these plans into action.

The TLT study was originally designed to run from 2009 through 2011; subsequently, the project was renewed twice. I refer to the component parts as TLT-1 (2009–11), TLT-2 (2015), and TLT-3 (2019) and sketch the overall timeline in figure 2.1. In April 2009, we conducted a complete household listing of all residences within a seven-kilometer radius of Balaka's main market.

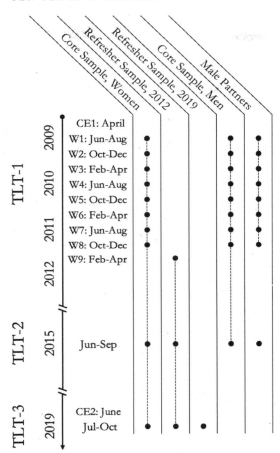

FIGURE 2.1 Timeline of TLT study components

Note: Each dot represents a wave of survey data collected from five distinct samples during the decade-long study period. W stands for wave. CE stands for full catchment enumeration exercises.

Immediately thereafter, we drew a representative sample of 1,500 women and 600 men between the ages of 15 and 25 and recruited them to participate in the panel study. These respondents participated in eight waves of interviews spaced out over four-month intervals (ending when the respondents were ages 18 to 28). The life course events we wanted to analyze are concentrated in these early ages: in 2010 the median age at first marriage for women in Malawi was 18, the median age at first birth was 19, the age-specific fertility rate peaked between ages 20 and 24, and new HIV infections also peaked at ages 20–24 and 25–29. We reinterviewed male and female respondents in 2015 (TLT-2) when they were between the ages of 21 and 31. Then in 2019 we again reinterviewed the full sample of women, now ages 25 to 35, totaling ten interviews over the course of a full decade of their lives. We refreshed the women's sample twice to compensate for attrition: once in 2012 and again in 2019. During their first interview (and at all subsequent interviews up to 2015), women who reported any ongoing romantic or sexual partnerships were given tokens with unique identifiers and asked to share these tokens with their male partners (husbands and boyfriends), who could then enroll themselves in the study. This nonrandom, representative sample of male partners was designed to facilitate dyadic (i.e., couple-based) analyses and makes it possible to compare the traits of women to the traits of the men with whom they make decisions.

The TLT study is unlike any other study we know of in three important ways. First, it is an intensive, HIV-focused longitudinal study of a cohort-specific, population-based sample. Most HIV research uses clinic-based populations, which typically exclude HIV-positive individuals who do not know their status or seek care and do not engage HIV-negative individuals in that population. These exclusions mean that clinic-based data aren't suitable for answering questions about how people living with HIV/AIDS (PLWHA) might be different from others. Most demographic research on HIV in Africa relies on Demographic and Health Surveys (DHS) data, which despite their many strengths, suffer the limitations of all cross-sectional data. The TLT study fills a unique need in providing detailed data, from a population-based, representative sample, over time. Second, during its first phase, TLT advanced an experimental approach to HIV testing and collected biomarkers for HIV status. Together this allowed us to document HIV status and incidence over time and, simultaneously, generate an account of young adulthood that emphasizes experiences—how people perceive and anticipate the very processes demographers study as aggregate rates. Third, in addition to population-representative samples of men and women, TLT took a dyadic approach to analyzing HIV risk and infections, romantic relationships, and fertility preferences, behaviors, and outcomes. Once enrolled in the study, women referred the men in their lives to participate too. We linked the responses of husbands and boyfriends to our female respondents. Detailed dyadic data of this type are rare and almost never follow couples over time and beyond the end of their relationships (male partners stayed in the TLT-1 sample through wave 8 even if their relationship with a female TLT respondent ended).[7]

Setting the Stage

Before turning to uncertainty as its own phenomenon, I map Malawi's demographic, epidemiological, and sociopolitical terrain and drop a few con-

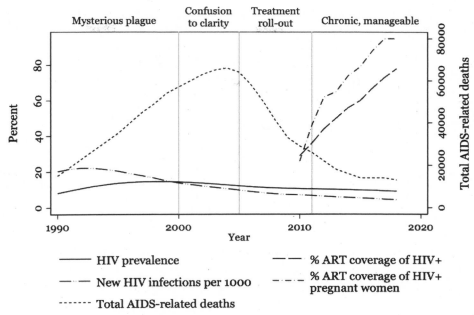

FIGURE 2.2 Four eras of HIV in Malawi

Source: UNAIDS.

Note: Periodization by author.

ceptual anchors to situate the TLT cohort in this broader context. UNAIDS and the World Bank publish key indicators related to health and development annually; four key metrics—HIV prevalence, HIV incidence, AIDS-related mortality, and ART coverage—are presented in figure 2.2 on a thirty-year timeline. I start the clock in 1990, when the fact that there was an AIDS crisis in Africa was just becoming clear. Although adult HIV prevalence in Malawi (calculated as a percentage of adults 15–49) had already far exceeded the threshold of a "generalized epidemic" and the incidence rate (new infections; a measure of spread) was high, AIDS-related mortality had just started its ascent. In both urban and rural areas, young adults had begun to die from mysterious conditions, their deaths often prefaced by symptoms like sudden and severe weight loss and grotesque sores.

To follow the course of Malawi's AIDS epidemic, one must keep an eye on all four metrics simultaneously while bearing in mind that the only metric people can truly perceive in real time is AIDS-related mortality. Furthermore, while estimates of AIDS deaths per thousand constitute a key metric from a demographic perspective, in experiential terms, this metric is not experienced in deaths per thousand but in personal loss: "I helped dig three graves last week"; "I sang at ten funerals in September"; "Those years were difficult for me: I buried two of my brothers in 1994, then my father in 1996, and a sister in 1997." To those living amid an epidemic, incidence is completely invisible and prevalence detectable only in terms of the symptomatic population; at any given point in time, the sick constitute just a small fraction of those living with HIV. Beyond the experience of mortality attributable to AIDS (either explicitly or euphemistically), the toll of HIV is also lived through the caregiving burden healthy adults bear as they provide for sick friends and family members and is experienced, not through viral load, but in terms of care visits made, kilometers walked, meals prepared, trips to the hospital made, and blankets washed.

Figure 2.2 demarcates four eras during this period. This is my own, unofficial periodization based on a close reading of annual reports produced by Malawi's Ministry of Health and the National AIDS Commission, high-quality survey data from the MDICP and the DHS Program, global HIV statistics generated by UNAIDS, a corpus of demographic and ethnographic studies set in and around Malawi during this period, and the benefits of hindsight.

1990–1999: MYSTERIOUS NEW PLAGUE

During the early years of Malawi's epidemic, HIV was spreading rapidly, but most of the people living with the disease were asymptomatic. Scientific consensus about how a virus becomes a syndrome had been established in the global community, but the facts were not yet widely known worldwide.[8] Given HIV's long latent period, the deaths that took place in the early 1990s were shrouded in mystery; they were the consequence of infections that had taken place almost a decade earlier, and it is precisely this quality of the long latent period that allowed HIV to spread so widely.[9]

When the mysterious wasting illness began to appear in Malawi (primarily among prime-age adults, though infant mortality also spiked at this time, for unspecified reasons), discussions about the resulting deaths were characterized by a sense of confusion.[10] Are men more susceptible? Are women? Does it help to drink a lot of alcohol? The epidemiologist Adamson Muula notes that there were many local names for HIV, including *mtengano* (dying in twos), since it quickly became clear that the death of one partner would soon be followed by the death of the other.[11] These illnesses and deaths climbed steadily over the decade, first in urban centers and later in rural villages. Moreover, the disease was a constant topic of conversation across the country—among the educated elite as well as the subsistence farmers in rural areas. By 2000 the entire country was affected, and the new disease was openly addressed in news-papers, radio programs, schools, and religious communities. This is the con-text into which the TLT cohort was born (between 1984 and 1994). They are the first cohort never to have known a world without AIDS, and these were the epidemic patterns that constituted their "normal" as young children.

2000–2004: FROM CONFUSION TO CLARITY

Writing in 2004, Susan Watkins identified 2001 as a turning point in Ma-lawi's epidemic—the moment in which most rural people understood cor-rectly that this disease was fatal, that it was sexually transmitted, and that it could be prevented.[12] In 2001 rural Malawian adults were attending three or four burials per month. By 2005 that number had risen to eight, and religious leaders of large congregations reported that they were officiating about twelve funerals monthly.[13] The fact that this would be the worst of it could not be known at that moment, but HIV prevalence had already begun to decline—a function of high AIDS-related mortality and the decline in new infections, which began as early as 1999. Scholars now attribute the decline in incidence to an eclectic bundle of behavioral changes that became manifest during this previous period of chaos, confusion, and climbing mortality. Once people understood that the primary mode of transmission was sex, the decline in incidence was swift. Scholars documented widespread changes, including later age at first sex, fewer extramarital partners, strategies for selecting safer partners, rising divorce rates, and lower levels of remarriage and noted that these changes preceded all the major international and national prevention campaigns.[14] Although the specific changes named here (e.g., marital strate-gies, partner reduction) are imperfectly aligned with the official ABC mes-sage that saturated anglophone sub-Saharan Africa, they nonetheless reduced the spread of HIV. This marked the shift from confusion to clarity: AIDS was devastating communities, but its causes and consequences had become clear. Men and women now had some tools with which they could collectively nav-igate the epidemic.

In 2003 Malawi's National AIDS Commission began to mandate routine (i.e., opt-out) HIV testing of pregnant women as a dimension of antenatal care. Outside of antenatal care (ANC), the testing apparatus was clumsy, primarily provider-initiated at the clinician's discretion, with limited labora-tory capacity, and results typically taking days—sometimes weeks—to pro-cess.[15] Although antiretroviral drugs were available to HIV patients in the United States and other high-income countries, they were extremely scarce in Malawi. In 2004 almost a million Malawians were infected with HIV, but only three thousand patients were receiving treatment.[16] The distribution of these lifesaving drugs was completely unstructured: there were no national systems for monitoring, recording, and reporting distribution, and the health care workers distributing these drugs had little to no training.[17] In this environment, only the very lucky few got any drugs.

When HIV mortality peaked, around 2004, the TLT respondents were between 10 and 20 years old. So the high AIDS-related death rates that characterized Malawi from 2000 to 2008 are the death rates that ravaged their parents' and grandparents' generations. Their mothers (born between 1939 and 1979) were sexually active adults during the late 1980s and early 1990s, while HIV was circulating in the population, brand-new to scientists, and still invisible to community members. The TLT cohort is marked by having experienced some of the highest rates of orphanhood documented in modern times. Nearly 20 percent of our respondents were maternal orphans when the study began, and 32 percent had already lost their biological fathers. A mortality burden of about one funeral per week characterized their experience of early childhood and adolescence.

2005–2010: TREATMENT ROLL-OUT AND EXPANSION

While the period 2000–2004 was defined by excruciating mortality and behavior change, that of 2005–10 was marked by technological innovations, national policy shifts, international recognition of the AIDS crisis, and the mobilization of resources through the global health community. After mortality rates peaked, the epidemic began to stabilize. Mortality fell more rapidly than it had risen. Incidence kept declining. Treatment became a reality. And prevalence plateaued because HIV-positive individuals were living with HIV rather than dying from it.[18]

During the ART roll-out period, both diagnostic tools and treatment options improved considerably. Inexpensive, rapid tests that produced results within 30 minutes became widely available, and their availability facilitated a spate of creative government and research-sponsored initiatives promoting voluntary counseling and testing (VCT) and experimenting with uptake using home-based and mobile clinic approaches.[19] More than seventy VCT sites for client-initiated (i.e., self-selected) HIV testing were established across Malawi, and the "know your status" campaigns began. Even the data got better: prevalence estimates themselves improved now that population-based testing had become a reality.

Although ARVs were still scarce in 2005–6, the treatment landscape took on an entirely new shape—that of a comprehensive national HIV policy and universal ARV program.[20] The new program established clear criteria for allocating ARVs (those at WHO clinical stage 3 or 4 were eligible), put in place a national reporting system, and moved the responsibility of distributing ART from urban hospitals to local clinics across the country. For those who were eligible to receive them, ARVs were either free through government hospitals or low-cost though private clinics.[21] ART coverage remained low (under 30 percent), but it was real, and people began to understand the strange distinction between treatment and cure. Single-dose nevirapine became universal policy in 2006, dramatically reducing the probability of mother-to-child transmission and interrupting the cycle of vertical transmission that had defined earlier birth cohorts.

The epidemiological context of 2009, when the TLT study began, was the point at which much of the policy world began to declare victory in the fight against AIDS; the rate of new infections had declined to the lowest point on record since the disease was first identified, HIV prevalence fell to about 11 percent, and AIDS-related mortality had begun to plateau. Testing procedures remained fairly consistent, but the testing lingo shifted from VCT (emphasis on the voluntary and the testing) to HIV testing and counseling (HTC, emphasis on the counseling); testing rates had risen from 7 percent and 15 percent of women and men, respectively, having ever been tested in 2004 to 73 percent of women and 52 percent of men in 2009.[22] As they moved into adulthood, TLT respondents were familiar with testing, optimistic about treatment options, and attending fewer funerals. They saw sick friends and neighbors recover upon initiating ART, and they watched women living with HIV give birth to perfectly healthy babies thanks to a cheap and simple one-dose pill.

2011–PRESENT: AVAILABLE ART AND THE TRANSFORMATION OF HIV FROM DEATH SENTENCE TO CHRONIC, MANAGEABLE CONDITION

Before 2011 infected individuals had to be very sick to begin treatment, and many did not recover.[23] Because of limited access to cluster of differentiation 4 (CD4) count, machines, and the myriad challenges of managing PMTCT when women are frequently pregnant and breastfeeding for extended periods, Malawi's Ministry of Health developed and adopted a new approach to ARV distribution called "Option B+." Option B+ built on the mandatory testing embedded in ANC protocols since 2003 and began to enroll all pregnant, HIV-positive women attending ANC on lifelong ART.[24] Implemented in 2012, Option B+ kicked off a dramatic increase in HIV treatment; the number of Malawians on ART increased from approximately 200,000 in 2009 to nearly 900,000 in 2015[25]—during which time adult HIV prevalence held steady at about 11 percent. Not surprisingly given the design of the program, ART coverage increased sharply among women but did not expand for men.[26] Option B+ set a new precedent in the policy world and was adopted by twenty-one countries in Africa by 2012.[27] But the policy was never widely communicated to the general public in Malawi; residents had the sense that women were being prioritized over men but may not have understood exactly why.

After five years of Option B+, Malawi began to phase in a test-and-treat policy designed to be truly universal. The universal test and treat (UTT) approach introduced in 2016 combines a proactive approach to testing with a robust referral system and a commitment to initiating those who test positive for HIV on ART immediately (i.e., the same day), regardless of sex, pregnancy status, age, WHO clinical stage (i.e., severity of symptoms), CD4 count, or ability to pay. UTT reduces morbidity and mortality; it lowers infection rates by reducing both horizontal transmission to uninfected partners and vertical transmission (mother to child) and has been more successful at retaining patients than any other previous approach. In recent years, progress toward total coverage of the HIV-positive population may have slowed but has not stalled. "Universal" treatment articulates the policy's aspiration, not a description of the fact. Under UTT, Malawi has moved beyond the logics of rationing that characterized earlier eras and now distributes ART freely to all of those in need. Malawi almost achieved a wildly ambitious goal set by UNAIDS that 90 percent of all people with a diagnosed HIV infection be receiving sustained antiretroviral therapy by the end of 2020. Today an estimated 80 percent of the HIV-positive population receives ART, and ART coverage for ANC-attending pregnant women in Malawi is almost perfect (over 95 percent). Distributional challenges persist but are reasonably well managed by both clinicians and patients.

Overall, the expansion of ART in Malawi has been more miracle than failure. In the 1990s ARVs were a pipe dream; in the early 2000s they were reserved for the dying and the lucky few. Since 2015 the general public knows that these drugs exist, personally knows someone who has recovered upon receiving them, believes that treatment works, and is optimistic that should they ever need ART themselves they can get it.[28] In a period of thirty years, HIV has been transformed from a mysterious plague that was killing dozens of community members each month and seemed almost unavoidable to a stable feature of the epidemiological landscape—treatable, chronic, and manageable.

THUMBNAIL SKETCH OF THE POLITICAL
AND POLICY BACKDROP

Although HIV prevalence in Malawi has remained relatively stable from 1990 to today, within their lifetimes, the TLT cohort experienced the transformation of HIV from a mysterious, deadly plague to a chronic and manageable condition. To illustrate, the Lexis diagram rendered in figure 2.3 pins this cohort's experience and the TLT study's focal period to a few key plot points that constitute the broader political and policy backdrop. The diagonal lines represent the lives of the youngest and oldest members of the TLT study from their births in 1984 or 1994 to today. On the life lines, I have overlaid three types of events: (1) national political transformations (dotted lines, labeled at the bottom); (2) a selection of important HIV-related moments discussed in the section above (dotted, labeled at the top); and (3) four policy shifts salient

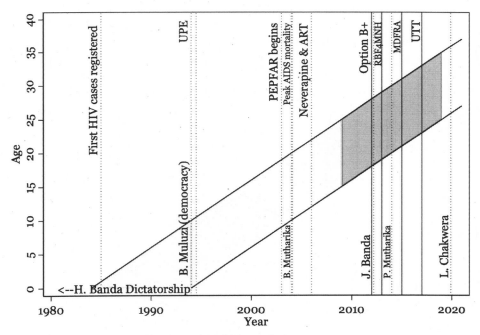

FIGURE 2.3 Major events in Malawi and TLT life lines in Lexis space

Note: In Lexis space, we are interested in the intersection of individuals' lives with the broader context, such as having observed peak AIDS-related mortality at age 11 or the shift to universal test and treat policies at age 21. The diagonal lines represent the life lines of the youngest and oldest TLT respondents, and the darkly shaded area represents the TLT observation period. Political transitions are marked at the bottom of the dotted vertical lines; major policy shifts and landmark moments in the HIV crisis are labeled at the top of vertical lines. PEPFAR is the US President's Emergency Plan for AIDS Relief.

to young adulthood (solid lines). The intersection of the life lines (diagonal) with the (vertical) "event" lines shows the age at which TLT respondents experienced X event or policy, the dark-shaded area represents the swath of the life course (that combined area of age and time) that the TLT study captured in real time, and the lightly shaded area in between identifies this cohort's experience since birth and what we can know about their lives from retrospective reports.

When Malawi gained independence after nearly one hundred years of British colonial rule, Dr. Hastings Kamuzu Banda ruled the country for twenty-seven years, his presidency and regime meeting the definition of a legal dictatorship. The year 1994 marked the transition to democracy, when President Bakili Muluzi took power in the nation's first multiparty election and held office for ten years.[29] There is no empirical link to make between the onset of HIV and the transition to democracy in Malawi, but their co-occurrence is salient to those who lived through these changes. HIV and democracy often were—and still are—discussed jointly and interpreted as part of the same shift. Older Malawians remember life before HIV as life under one-party rule and view the high mortality and the behavioral changes the AIDS epidemic catalyzed as features of this new, democratic era.

Bingu Mutharika took office in 2004, during the height of the HIV crisis and a devastating drought. Mutharika steered the country through torrid waters: he harnessed the international community's support to fund the fight against HIV while battling these same foreign donors against structural adjustment policies that would have suffocated the agrarian economy and starved millions. Life expectancy rose from 46 when Mutharika took office in 2004 to 58 when he died in office in 2012 at the age of 78, at which time Vice President Joyce Banda assumed executive powers for two years. Banda lost her 2014 election bid to Peter Mutharika (brother to her predecessor), who was unseated in 2020 after the legitimacy of his 2018 reelection came into question.[30] On its face, the pace of political transitions may seem tangential to the task of understanding uncertainty and HIV for young adults. It should be noted, however, that after a combined one hundred years of colonial rule and thirty years of dictatorship, Malawi's political landscape has been characterized by nearly constant change. TLT respondents born in 1993 experienced six presidents in their first twenty-two years, whereas their parents experienced one or maybe two in their entire lives. Although neither the British nor Banda were good leaders for Malawi, those regimes were nothing if not stable. The shift from stable authoritarianism to eventful democracy, accompanied by a new disease that has become a permanent fixture, marked an era of perpetual change and uncertainty.

The vertical lines denoting the major shifts in HIV (e.g., first cases, peak mortality, and treatment availability) have been discussed already, as have two of the policy shifts that intersected with the TLT study period: Option B+ (2012) and UTT (2016). I want to briefly note three other policy shifts with major implications for this group of young adults. These pertain to the domains of education, marriage, and maternal health.

Access to primary education started expanding in Malawi during the 1980s, and Universal Primary Education (UPE) became official policy in 1994, when primary-school fees were categorically abolished. The expansion of mass education has been noted as a transformative force across sub-Saharan Africa, with implications for public health, democratic nation building, fertility, and economic development.[31] Malawi is, without doubt, one of the most successful cases of UPE, achieving 90 percent net enrollment as of 2019.[32] Among the younger cohort, it is difficult to find anyone who has never attended school; however, it is also true that not everyone finishes primary education and ascends the social ladder. For one thing, UPE is not as free as we might think. Schools still require parents to pay considerable sums—occasionally, free labor as well—to supplement teachers' salaries and fund-raise for new construction projects. Schools also require uniforms and supplies, and it is not uncommon for students to miss school for lack of soap needed to wash their uniforms.[33] Poor quality of instruction and high competition to pass the Primary School Leaving Exam (PSLE) discourage many from finishing the "mandatory" eight years of primary education. Grade repetition—several years at the same level or even demotion to a lower grade—is both common and demoralizing for students. Those who beat the odds and proceed to secondary school now face the real challenge of affording their education: secondary schools are not free. Affordable, public institutions are highly selective—reserved for the best-performing students. To meet the rising demands for education, private schools charge crushing fees and boarding expenses are hefty. In the wake of UPE, school remains a major concern for young adults, both for themselves and with respect to their children's well-being.

In February 2015, Malawi passed the Marriage, Divorce and Family Relations Act (MDFRA). In the eyes of the international community, the major implication of the MDFRA was to set the minimum age of marriage at 18 and reduce Malawi's position on the list of countries ranked by child marriage prevalence.[34] However, it was the more mundane implications of the MDFRA that resonated across the nation and within the TLT sample. It expanded regulation of all marriage: civil, customary, and religious, marriages by repute, and permanent cohabitation. This required new bureaucratic structures, including a new marriage certificate. Prior to the MDFRA, the vast majority of marriages had been informal. Civil Registration and Vital Statistics (CRVS) coverage estimated that less than 2 percent of marriages had been registered with the government. The 2015 MDFRA established the present requirement that religious and traditional marriages be registered at the village level, creating a new regulatory role for traditional authorities (i.e., village chiefs), who became responsible for recording and reporting customary marriage.[35] Frankly speaking, the added administrative burden on chiefs was minimal; marriages, like births and burials, were already recorded in most village record books and had been for many years if not decades. With the MDFRA, the ministry began providing each traditional authority with a special logbook for recording marriages, and the shift authorized chiefs to solicit a fee when registering each marriage.[36] These fees to register a marriage with the chief are not high—between US$3 and US$5—but they are new and noteworthy.

The marriage registration fees became a big topic of conversation in 2015, when the act was first introduced, and appear in narratives of relationship formation, both retrospectively when young adults recount their courtship trajectories ("And then we went to pay the chief") and prospectively as they start planning for a marriage ("He loves me; he's saving to pay the chief"). Chiefs can impose fines on residents who fail to register their marriages, and while these fines may be minimal, the looming threats of carrying unpaid debts to one's village are stunningly harsh: one's land may be reallocated or one may be refused burial in the village, which imposes a major financial burden on one's family and represents eternal, existential separation from one's family and group. Other implications of this law have been emphasized from a human rights perspective: the new act defines parents' minimal financial obligations to children (i.e., child support), provides stronger protections for married women in the event of divorce (especially land claims), and establishes Family Counseling Panels designed to intervene in cases of abuse, neglect, or abandonment. These topics are seldom discussed in Balaka's public sphere. Fees and fines with respect to marriage are the hot topic, and it is worth mentioning a few of the salient ones here: fines for polygamy (up to 100,000 MK, or US$125), fines for marrying under a false name, and fines for making false declarations about marriage (not disclosing a spouse).[37] In chapter 6 I show how the policy details relate to trust and uncertainty in romantic relationships.

Around the same time that Option B+ was being designed, announced, and introduced with much fanfare a different policy was more quietly introduced in four districts, including Balaka. Designed and funded by a partnership between the Norwegian and German governments, the Results-Based Financing for Maternal and Neonatal Health (RBF4MNH) initiative would invest more than US$10 million in the maternal and child health system between 2011 and 2014. The program was designed in response to the observation that institutional delivery rates had risen sharply in the preceding years— from 38 percent in 2004 to 70 percent in 2010—while the stubborn maternal mortality ratio had barely declined over the same period. RBF4MNH took a two-pronged, carrot-and-stick approach to improving health outcomes for mothers and babies, intervening at both the individual and organizational levels (see table 2.1). The carrot included incentives to hospitals for supply-side performance agreements and demand-side cash transfers to pregnant women. The stick involved fines to women for nonhospital deliveries and other failures to comply with maternal health recommendations. Evaluations of the program by the global health research community on two- and four-year time horizons provide little to no evidence that RBF4MNH meaningfully increased uptake of antenatal care and hospital births or that it improved birth outcomes for babies or mothers.[38] The supply-side changes were widely discussed in policy circles and national newspapers but largely invisible to

TABLE 2.1 Published Dedza District by-laws promoting health-seeking behavior for maternal and neonatal care

Action	Punishment
Woman not attending antenatal clinic	Pay one chicken per missed ANC visit per trimester
Woman attending antenatal care not accompanied by her husband	Bring a letter from the chief explaining why the husband is absent or pay two chickens per missed ANC visit
Home delivery	The woman pays one goat, the man pays one goat, and the people who assisted in the delivery pay one goat each (after thorough investigation of the circumstances leading to the involvement of the assistants)
Traditional birth attendant (TBA) delivery	The woman pays one goat, the TBA pays a goat and two chickens, and the husband pays a goat
Woman delivers on the way to the hospital	See Home delivery
Not seeking medical care following home/TBA delivery or delivery on the way to health facility	The woman pays three chickens in addition to the payments listed under "Home delivery"
Not going for postnatal check at one week	The mother pays three chickens

Note: Rather than write its own by-laws, Balaka District adapted the Dedza program whole cloth. The fines can be paid in terms of the items charged or money equivalent to the same as follows: chicken = 2,500 MK (US$6); goat = 12,000 MK (US$30).

most Balaka residents. The demand-side changes, on the other hand, were a constant topic of conversation and consternation. Writing about the rumblings about this policy during its earliest days in Mudzi Village, the anthropologist Janneke Verheijen paints the picture: "Indeed, the first Mudzi woman to give birth after the reward was introduced, decided to deliver at home out of fear for sinister practices such as blood or organ stealing at the clinic. The chief's fine for non-hospital deliveries then pushed the next Mudzi woman to deliver in the clinic despite her fears. She returned safely and with the promised money, after which the initial distrust disappeared and all women delivered at the clinic again."[39]

The Lexis surface in figure 2.3 allows us to locate these moments of political transition, epidemiological change, and policy shifts with respect to life lines that represent the experiences of actual people who age over time. For older generations, the onset of HIV is a plot point that marks a clear "before" and "after" in their lives. Across the literature on AIDS in Africa, adults who have lived through the AIDS epidemic consistently use phrases like "the nowadays disease" or "before HIV came along."[40] Born between 1984 and 1994, the TLT cohort is the first in Malawi to have been born into the context of endemic HIV. They were never instructed to *change* their behavior; in terms of their social, sexual, and moral development, this cohort was always navigating AIDS. Their formative years were marked by a major mortality transition from extremely high to very much improved, though still among the highest in the world. They witnessed the eventfulness of democracy in terms of political leadership. They have been subjects of a series of major policy shifts designed by the international community, and they experienced both the intended impact and the unintended reverberations these policies inflicted on local communities. Their lives so far have been very much defined by two forces: AIDS and sociopolitical change. Both forces are central to my empirical investigation of uncertainty.

Gertrude, Resident Ethnographer

As already shown, policies on testing and the distribution of ARVs were changing over the study period, as were a set of policies designed to promote maternal and child health. Balaka is filled with competing kinds of information about who has authority over what in terms of marriage, property disputes, paternity questions, and domestic violence. Interested in how these policies were being thought about, discussed, and implemented in our research site, we collected a number of different types of data during this period, including clinic records, documents from chiefs' courts, in-depth interviews with health workers, and what I refer to here as survey-embedded ethnography.

The ethnographic data in this book come from fieldnotes written by an extraordinary research assistant named Gertrude. In 2011, just as Option B+ policy was being implemented, Sara and I read a remarkable article that skewered tropes of female victimhood and transactional sex as drivers of HIV in sub-Saharan Africa and offered instead a portrait of small-scale businesswomen with earning potential, sexual agents with their own desires, thoughtful contributors to debates about how love, lust, risk, and material exchange actually work in the world.[41] The ethnographic material was gripping and unrefined, free of that veneer of propriety that often colors the data researchers gather about women's romantic lives. The author, Janneke Verheijen, and her research assistant, Gertrude Finyiza, spent their time farming, knitting, playing bao, and drinking tea in a village they called "Mudzi."[42] Unbeknownst to us when we first encountered this research, this village turned out to be located at the outer edge of the TLT catchment area. Indeed, at least three TLT respondents moved into Mudzi from their natal villages within the catchment area.

Janneke and Gertrude's portrait of village life captured the eventful chaos of young adulthood in Balaka. Yes, destitute Mudzi women sometimes initiated sexual relationships with men who could provide them with food, clothes, soaps, and lotions. But they just as often loved men who could not provide economically at all. Many had children with multiple men, each time hoping that the father would stick around. One Mudzi adolescent tricked a suitor into supporting her by helping her build mud bricks to complete her family's home. Nearly every day for four months straight, the besotted young man labored beside her, and when her family's small home was finally complete, she ran away to live with other relatives in a faraway town, victorious in her attempt to postpone the responsibilities of marriage and childbearing. Written in the tradition of thick description, these researchers showed how the relationships between men and women in Mudzi could not be reduced to either their economic or emotional components. They specified big concepts like "poverty," "family," "marriage," and "support" with care and sophistication. Their elaborations of "love" and "risk," in particular, were extremely relevant to the big-picture goal of the TLT project: to generate a meticulous empirical account of young adulthood that seriously engaged both the unique experiences of individuals and the persistent properties of aggregates.[43]

In 2014, while preparing for the 2015 survey wave, Sara and I approached Janneke about a possible collaboration, and because Janneke was between jobs, our timing was fortuitous. Together Janneke and Gertrude returned to

Mudzi. Their charge was specific but open: to document the everyday conversations women were having about love, marriage, family, and fertility, with
an eye to understanding what women understood about the changing policy
landscape and extra attention to the views and experiences of women in their
late teens and early twenties. We were especially interested in whether and
how residents perceived the changes to the logic of ART distribution that
Option B+ would be imposing on district hospitals and local clinics. After
a month of writing jointly about the aforementioned topics, Janneke returned to Europe, and Gertrude remained in Mudzi and wrote for three more
months, sending her fieldnotes in weekly batches.[44]

These fieldnotes were critical for understanding how HIV policy roll-outs
were being perceived: they directly informed our approach to measuring perceived fairness in drug rationing and helped us design new survey questions
to capture how young people define a good relationship. Because the degree
program Gertrude was about to enroll in didn't begin until 2016 and because
we simply relished reading her fieldnotes each week, Gertrude's ethnographic
eye took on a more central role throughout 2015. In April Gertrude moved
from Mudzi to Balaka Boma, where she wrote about her conversations and
interactions for a period of five months—two leading up to the 2015 survey
and three coterminous with it. Having grown up in a different region and
lived most recently in Mudzi, she learned about Balaka from its residents by
being new in town. How do things work around here? Your marriage customs
are not clear to me; how do you arrange things? What's better, life in the boma
or life in the village? Who helps when you have problems at home? Where
can I get contraception around here? Who offers testing services? Just curious, but what do girls around here do if they need an abortion? How do you
know if a man is really trustworthy?

Gertrude's interlocutors run the gamut in terms of life experience. She
rents a house in Stella's parents' compound.[45] The extended family is rife with
conflict, the descriptions of which illuminate questions about the resources
people draw on to navigate different kinds of trouble. Gertrude is pursued by
men her age and by much older men. Older women offer her plenty of advice. She makes friends with vegetable sellers at the market. A woman named
Tiyamike becomes a good friend. Tiyamike's married boyfriend is the topic of
many illuminating stories about marriage and romance, and the boyfriend's
suspicious wife appears frequently in the fieldnotes. Gertrude and Tiyamike
spend long stretches of time at New Styles hair salon in the main market,
where they chat with customers and occasionally assist Enid, the owner, with
her clients. Gertrude captures stories from bicycle taxi drivers while rid-
ing across town to visit friends; she chats with women who have been TLT

respondents and with men who have cheated their way into our study. She writes in solitude at the end of every evening. Her memory is excellent, and her descriptions are vivid. She uses minimal punctuation and irregular spelling and occasionally makes mistakes with pronouns (common, as Chichewa pronouns are not gendered). I have edited the excerpts used throughout this book for clarity and verified them with Gertrude for accuracy.

In addition to the salon, the setting of all my favorite vignettes, Gertrude has a few regular spots for conversation and amusement. One of them is a tailoring shop, owned by a man about 40 years old who employs two male apprentices. Their clients are men and women who bring fabric, make requests, and pass time chatting while the tailors measure, cut, and sew. The following fieldnote describes Gertrude's first encounter with the trio at the tailoring shop. Written during her second week in the boma when she was still learning her way around, it is typical of Gertrude's interactions. The "I" in the ethnographic data is always Gertrude.

While making my way, I saw three men in the tailoring shop sewing clothes. I decided to stop because they didn't have customers. I asked them, "How much is it to make a nice dress?" One of the men said, "It depends on the material that you have." Then I said, "You all look happy. That must mean life is good with you." And the men said, "There is no need for us to be angry. If we were angry, customers would be afraid to come here."

Then I said, "Where do you prefer to stay, the village or town?"

They all agreed that town was better. I asked why.

Man 1: In town, all the people look healthy, even if they are HIV positive, because of the nice food they eat here. And the people always look strong compared to the ones who stay in the village.

Man 2: In town there's a lot of casual labor someone can do in order to find food and soap. You can do things like washing people's clothes, selling someone's things at the shop, bicycle hire. And people are also friendly here.

Man 3, interjecting: Especially those who drink beer, they are more friendly, and you will find that people buy beer for each other here. Village people don't do that.

Then I asked, "What happens here if someone wants to get married?"

One of the men said, "You go to the chief and pay money; it's now 3,000 MK. And if you also quarrel with your friend about witchcraft, the chief asks you to pay money. And if you don't go to attend funerals, the chief asks you to pay three chickens. And if you deliver at home, the chief will ask you to pay. And if you have complications when giving birth at home and you want to go to the hospital, at the hospital they also ask you to pay money. Nowadays, if you deliver at hospital you receive some money, like my wife gave birth in December and she received 5,000 MK, and I was happy. At that time I didn't have money to buy some of the things that my wife wanted, and she was able to buy because of the money that she received at the hospital. She was able to buy maize flour, soap, sugar. That program of giving money is good because not all people at the hospital have the necessities."

The other man added, "But I heard that those women who deliver through scissor don't get the money, and I don't know why that is."[46]

I asked, "Have you ever heard about TLT?"

One of the men said, "Yes, they were here in 2009, but now they left. People were receiving money there, but I was not involved in TLT."

Then the other man said, "I was involved in TLT, my friend gave me a token to go because he didn't like the questions that they were asking. And after answering many, many questions we would receive 500 MK. They were questions like, how many times did you sleep with your wife this week? People were cheating, they were mentioning ten to fifteen times, when that is not true."

We all laughed.

"I have been married for nine years now, and my wife has become rude. I think I will chase her away so that I can marry you."

I laughed and replied, "How can you marry me when you don't even know me? And you didn't propose to me."

The other men laughed and said, "This is Balaka; you will get married here. When people come here, they find things they like and they want to stay." I asked, "What kinds of things?" He said, "It's easy to find a job, business works, and people have got money."

Gertrude's method is chatting and listening. She raises general questions about town versus village, marriage, family conflict, and mediation and asks what if anything people think about TLT. She herself never raises the topic of HIV, and she keeps people talking, often in small groups. As exemplified in this exchange, Gertrude chats with people when she can see they're not busy. Her other strategies for chatting are accompaniment and help. She accompanies friends as they travel on foot to a destination such as the borehole, the clinic, a friend's house, or an errand. She helps her interlocutors while they engage in repetitive, time-consuming labor: shelling peas, pounding flour, fetching water, braiding hair, washing clothes, sometimes for hours at a time. She becomes known as good company—helpful and respectful, a good tenant, cooperative—but also as an educated, independent woman who may not be taking her search for a husband seriously enough. When Gertrude and Tiyamike are together, older women deride them for being too talkative and too loud. Most people are delighted when Gertrude pays them a visit; they share a lot about their lives, including dark details stated in matter-of-fact (rather than emotional) ways.

Some key methodological points are obvious but still worth stating explicitly: our survey data are imperfect. The fieldnote above points to two different types of errors I factor into my analysis of the TLT survey data and the interpretations I draw. One is bias and mischief in people's responses to our survey items. This can operate in different directions, such as the boastful reports of coital frequency these men joke about or underreports due to social desirability bias, which has been widely documented in the literature.[47] The other type of error concerns the sample itself, raising questions about TLT's enrollment processes and procedures for tracking respondents over time. Our research team labored tirelessly to verify the identities of randomly sampled respondents at the time of enrollment and to confirm the identities of these respondents when they returned to the research center for subsequent interviews. We verified identities using photos and questions, asking, for example, about details from previously reported relationship and birth histories. Each month we caught a few imposters. The most common variant was a female respondent's sister presenting at the research center for an interview, sometimes preempting the respondent's appointment time without her knowledge in order to claim the incentive and sometimes sent by a busy respondent as her proxy. We may not have caught every single imposter, but most imposters were identified before the interview was conducted and sent home, usually with a jovial exchange about their failed attempt to sneak into the study. In other cases, imposters were interviewed and it was only later that this came to light—for example, when the actual respondent came to the research center or during data processing when we discovered highly incompatible birth histories. We dropped those questionnaires from our data sets. No longitudinal study is immune to these concerns. We worked diligently to guard against the imposter problem and deal with it by dropping entire surveys when evidence of imposters came to our attention.

It is worth noting that the token process for enrolling male partners makes this sample vulnerable to fraudulent enrollment. On occasion, women gave tokens to a brother rather than to the intended boyfriend, expecting that the brother would give her a cut of his incentive. We verified the identity of the male partners at the research center when they arrived to enroll, but it is important to acknowledge that the male partners do not constitute a truly random sample and have to be used very cautiously when leveraged in combination with women's responses as dyadic data.

I maintain that our survey data are both excellent and imperfect. Throughout this book I attempt uncomfortable levels of transparency regarding the weaknesses of measurement, empirically unsolvable estimation dilemmas, and possible ambiguity in my own interpretations of key findings.

Many different substantive points could be taken from Gertrude's conversation with the tailors, but I highlight here the fact that Balaka residents are constantly and casually discussing the things that cast shadows of uncertainty over their lives. The question of how to navigate life in the boma has everything to do with livelihoods and money: jobs, prices, markets, fines. People in Balaka talk about money a lot, and they talk about food a lot.[48] The challenge of securing daily necessities (maize, water, relish, medicine) and small luxuries (soap and sugar for the postpartum wife) is a constant rather than a variable for most of the population. Some people do have savings and cash for maize, but most are managing the balance of household production and consumption on a daily or forty-eight-hour time frame. This tailor will start and finish making a dress for Gertrude on the same day she brings him the fabric. She will pay him a small deposit, with which he will buy the requisite zippers, which he does not have "in stock," and a small vial of lubricant to oil his sewing machine. When she claims and pays for her dress the next day, he will close the shop early and return home with charcoal for cooking and fish for his family's dinner that evening.

The realm of health care and fertility is another topic of easy and ongoing chatter and much uncertainty. How healthy or sick people look is observed and discussed in relation to caloric demand, in relation to fertility, and in relation to HIV. Balaka is a high-fertility context in which contact—primary or by proxy—with antenatal and delivery services is dense. It is also a context characterized by a heavy disease burden that includes malaria, meningitis, and cholera, in addition to HIV-related maladies like pneumonia and thrush. Two of the men in this exchange are particularly knowledgeable about the logistics of childbearing and antenatal care: they know the details of these institutions just as they know the prices for vegetables, petrol, and beer. Others know far less, and this tends to correlate with their proximity to direct experience with these institutions. Not surprisingly, the reproductive health–related chatter is more robust in Gertrude's conversations with her female interlocutors, but the domain is not exclusive to women, nor are these conversations restricted to a "separate spheres" gender divide some scholars describe as characteristic of "Africa."

HIV also comes up a lot in everyday conversation, even among people who don't know one another well. The topic is not particularly sensitive. It is treated casually, often with humor and judgments some may cringe at as "inappropriate." This is how people in Balaka speak about HIV, its associated maladies, its causes (bad luck, stupidity, promiscuity), and its consequences (wasting, bad complexion, stupidity). Some excerpts contain things I would not ever say out loud and phrases I would sternly chide my American children for saying. This is Balaka: a context in which **gossip and kindness are not necessarily antithetical**. Is the neighbor pregnant or just gaining weight? Will the father of that pregnancy stick around? Do you think she's taking ARVs?

Finally, men are men, and in the romance department, Gertrude has options galore. So do her female friends. Faithfulness—in relationships and in marriage—is widely stated as an ideal but is not necessarily held as a true expectation. We can estimate the typical shelf life of romantic relationships and the prevalence of extramarital partners in Balaka using our survey data. Gertrude's observations of her friends and neighbors add to these understandings and sometimes complicate them. There is a soap-operatic quality to the constellation of romance, betrayal, conflict, and reconciliation Gertrude observes in her network. She is simultaneously an observer of and a true friend to the men and women she writes about. These are not characters or caricatures but real people, with flaws and feelings. I have attempted to write about each one of them with dignity, without romanticizing or judging their dalliances, and I occasionally obscure identifying details. The things men say to Gertrude, as a woman, in public—things like, "After nine years, I've grown tired of my wife. Run away with me!"—add both color and depth to our view of the local repartee. But Gertrude's private life is not on display here.

Population Chatter: Uncertainty in the Reproductive Realm

Departing from the focus on HIV, let me offer a second example of population chatter from Balaka. In the following fieldnote from April 2015, Gertrude is chatting with a shopkeeper she calls "Man, a bit old" at his store, a kiosk on the outskirts of the main market. She has been in Balaka for just a few weeks, and people tend to react to her as a "new face" when she moves about town.

> The owner greeted me and asked, "What are you buying today?"
> I said, "Baobab fruit."
> "Why? Are you pregnant?"
> "No, I am not."
> "Only pregnant women should eat that because it's sour. My name is Ahmed, and everybody knows me here."
> "Thanks. I am Gertrude, I'm new here, and I don't know a lot of people yet. Maybe we can chat."
> "Feel free. I don't have a lot of customers today."

Their conversation is long, almost an hour. They start chatting about business and livelihoods, then the difference between life in town and the villages. Ahmed raises the distinction that women in the villages give birth at home

while in town they deliver in hospitals. Gertrude asks whether people do better when they deliver at the hospital.

"I don't know if people receive anything if they deliver at the hospital, but
people are telling each other to stop giving birth at the hospital because they
are being mistreated by nurses, and apart from that, as of now, they just force
everybody to do an operation. They are doing the operation without a reason."

"Why are they forcing them?"

"They must be getting something from their bodies, and that's why they've
also brought this project of giving money to people who deliver at hospital.
Because when people are pregnant, it's not by mistake but by choice. So why
give money to those people?"

We laughed.

The man continued, "My daughter died after that operation. And people
are scared."

After telling Ahmed how sorry I was about his daughter, I realized that a
lot of time had passed and that I should get home, so I thanked him for the
chat and stood up to leave.

"No, don't go," he said. "There is one story that I want to tell you. A few
days ago a certain woman gave birth to triplets here at Balaka. The nurse told
her that two of the kids were born dead, and they should arrange for burial. So
the women came from her village to take the two dead bodies to the cemetery.
Now before going to the cemetery, the nurse told that mother, 'Although you
are going to bury the two, just know that the other one will also die.' That was
very sad. Already she had delivered through scissor, now the two kids died,
and further being told that the last one will die too? When they came back
from the cemetery, the nurse told the women that the other one had died. The
women went home with the dead body. Then the mother of the child said,
'Sorry, women. I know I have lost my triplets, but this child has been wrapped
with many clothes. Please can I take one *chitenje* [cloth wrapper] so that I can
use it? As of now I don't have money to buy chitenje.'

"The women took off the outermost chitenje, which the nurse had used
to wrap the dead child, and they gave it to the mother. But when they took it
off, the women were surprised. That child was breathing. They rushed to the
hospital to explain, then Zodiac Broadcasting Station [a radio station] went
there to investigate. And we don't know what will happen next. But that child
is, indeed, alive right now. And people are saying the other two were buried
alive. Now if this is a way to reduce our population, then that's a bad way. And
this is a true story. It happened at Mponda Hospital only a few days ago. So
just know that people will be afraid to give birth at the hospital."

I said, "Wow. That's sad. I had not heard."

Last, I said, "Thanks a lot for your time." And on my way home, I heard four men talking about the same story of the triplets. Around 3 p.m. the heavy rain started and no one came to chat.

Three weeks later, Gertrude passes Ahmed's kiosk, and he greets her by asking, "Do you recognize me?"

"Yes, we met a few weeks ago."

"Yes, and we chatted a lot. I told you the story about the triplets, and now I wanted to tell you that my daughter received money after giving birth at the hospital."

"How much?"

"5,000 kwacha [US$6.60]."

"Were you happy when you heard that she received money?"

"Yes, because when I asked her what the nurses did to her in order to receive the money, she told me nothing happened to her. Only that a lot of women complained that they didn't receive any money. She didn't understand why, because they had all started antenatal at the same time. I think some nurses are stealing the money from the patients they are supposed to be helping."

Then a week or so later:

On my way home, I bumped into the man who told me the story about the triplets. He recognized me again and greeted me and said, "Did you hear that the other child who was alive also died?" I said, "No. I didn't hear anything. What happened?"

"I don't know. I just heard the news from my friends, and I felt sorry for that woman because she can't be pregnant for nine months and lose all the children."

I said, "Yaaa. That's bad." Then he continued his journey while I also continued my journey.

This exchange doesn't mention AIDS at all. Instead, it offers an anguished example of everyday conversation about pregnancy and childbearing in Balaka. The conversation between an old man and a young woman covers a lot of ground, but the centrality of reproductive anxieties, the lack of trust in medical institutions, and the prevalence of maternal and child mortality merit exploration.

Again here the introduction of these two characters to one another is noteworthy. Gertrude enters a kiosk to buy some fruit, and the first question she is asked—even before names are exchanged—is, "Are you pregnant?" The topics of pregnancy and delivery belong to the ambit of everyday chitchat; they are not reserved for close friends or intimate exchanges. Ahmed, who has lived long enough to see the transition from a majority of women delivering at home to a majority delivering in the hospital, describes this as one of the major differences between town life and village life today. But something is not right. He cautions Gertrude that nurses are horrid and overly eager to perform cesarean sections, and he tells her that he has lost a daughter for these reasons. These are things a nice young woman, new to town, deserves to know.

In Ahmed's view, not only are nurses horrid and quick to operate; they're also malicious and may even murder poor women and their babies. Moreover, they're probably stealing the money they're supposed to be distributing to patients through the notorious RBF4MNH program. Who knows what they will do to you? The empirical literature provides no evidence that clinicians in Balaka are part of any plot to reduce the population and a lot of evidence that they are doing their level best to provide care in a grossly underresourced setting. But the optics are bad. Ahmed's personal experience of maternal mortality among his daughters is 50 percent.

Ahmed is correct when he says that people are scared. The uncertainty that characterizes the reproductive realm is acute. When this unnamed mother gave birth to triplets and buried all three, the story circulated for weeks, and Gertrude captured multiple iterations of the event in her daily writing. Everyone who heard or recounted the story ached for this mother. Nobody found the story unbelievable.

A Decade of Change

Thus far this chapter has provided a mini-history of the HIV epidemic in Malawi, a view of the political and policy changes that define the period, an overview of the TLT study design and objective, and snippets of population chatter in this community. From the perspective of academic demography, what exactly happens in Balaka during this ten-year period? I close this chapter with a thumbnail sketch of population change and an overview of the demographic trajectory of the TLT cohort as they move through the most eventful period of the life course. In the chapters that follow, I interrogate in detail the processes underpinning these trends and explain that these changes are experienced and understood as dilemmas of uncertainty.

Enumerating the entire population of the TLT catchment area twice—in 2009 and 2019—produced two full censuses, which I use here to establish the basic parameters of demographic change in Balaka. The patterns will come as no surprise to those familiar with population trends in sub-Saharan Africa. Against a backdrop of high population growth in Malawi as a whole

TABLE 2.2 Demographic overview of TLT catchment area, 2009 and 2019

	2009	2019
Population	57,591	78,433
Average household size	5.6	4.2
Thatched roof (%)	61	37
Owns animals (%)	53	40
No land (%)	16	28

Source: TLT Household Listings.

(from 14 million in 2009 to almost 18 million in 2019), table 2.2 documents a similar growth rate (almost 3 percent annually) in Balaka Boma, from 57,000 to almost 80,000. Within the study area, the growth occurs as a proliferation of households rather than an increase within households (household size declined during this period). Small houses are being built here, there, and everywhere. Balaka residents are constantly making and baking bricks and talking about their construction projects. Trucks, oxcarts, and bicycles haul bags of cement, iron sheets for roofing, panes of glass for windows, and the occasional porcelain toilet to sites of possibility. These in-progress structures are the crucibles of family formation, and like the other steps in building a family (solidifying a relationship, bearing and raising children, and maintaining a livelihood), these construction projects are filled with hope and uncertainty.

We also find evidence of urbanization within the study site. Not only are new structures going up everywhere, but they are being improved in key ways: fewer thatched roofs and more houses clad in iron sheets. Residents of Balaka live on subsistence agriculture and petty trade, but the agricultural conditions are increasingly strained as the pressure on land use becomes more severe. Over this decade, the proportion of households without land to farm increases, fewer households keep animals, and very few households in the boma subsist solely on agricultural activities. Infrastructure improvements like water access and toilets (as opposed to latrines) did not change much during this period. Electricity access, however, rose substantially— from 15 percent of households in 2009 to about 21 percent in 2019.

Although Balaka Boma is growing, its age structure is fairly stable (fig. 2.4). Balaka could be said to exemplify the classic pyramid shape of a developing context in that it exhibits high fertility and high mortality: a large base of many young people and a lean top as few people survive into old age. One interesting exception to the classic shape is the lower proportion of children ages 0 to 4 compared to children 5 to 9. This is a consequence of

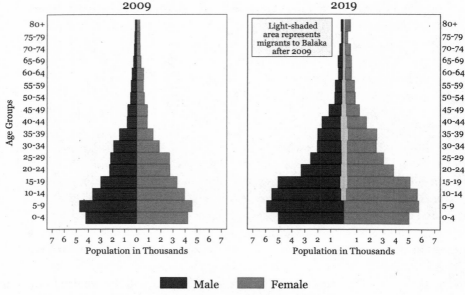

FIGURE 2.4 Population pyramids of the TLT catchment area, 2009 and 2019

Source: TLT Household Listings.

several factors: high infant and child mortality rates, recent fertility decline among women of childbearing age, and the fact that children between 5 and 9 may be migrating to Balaka to attend school, as the town is home to many schools and child fostering for the purpose of education is a widespread strategy across sub-Saharan Africa. Another important difference over this period is the visible thickening of the middle of the pyramid. Remember that life expectancy at birth rose a whopping ten years during this period (from 54 to 64) as ARVs became available and extended the lives of infected prime-age adults. Overall, Balaka is becoming more crowded, slightly older, more commercial, more built up—not just in terms of density of buildings, but also in the number of bicycles, motorcycles, and cars.[49]

Balaka's growth is a consequence of its fertility, mortality, and migration patterns. As stated earlier, mortality has been falling. Fertility is high but not high enough to sustain or explain a 3 percent annual growth rate. Taking 2009 as our baseline, all the 0- to 9-year-olds in Balaka in 2019 are "new" to the area—regardless of where they were born. But the growing number of 40- and 80-year-olds can only be explained by migration. The household listing we fielded in 2019 provides some answers to questions about the magnitude of migration. In constructing the population pyramid for 2019, I have used shading in the middle of the pyramid to distinguish, within each age group, those who were living here in 2009 from those who migrated to Balaka after 2009. This shows that Balaka is a major destination, especially for young people ages 10–14 and 15–19, many of whom move here for school. From ages 20 to 40 the main motivation for migration is marriage.

Turning to the sample itself, I sketch the basic sociodemographic contours of young adulthood in the domains of marriage, fertility, and HIV to show what the group collectively goes through over the study period, starting with the marriage trends. Starting at age 15—at which point about 2 percent of young women were married in 2019 (estimated from the household listing data, not from the TLT sample)—prevalence of marriage grows exponentially each year until it hits (indeed, exceeds) 90 percent, the common threshold for what demographers would consider a "universal" marriage pattern, at age 30. Nearly 40 percent of women are married by age 19, a clear majority (53 percent) are married by age 20. Men, in contrast, marry a little later, reaching the median threshold at around 25 and the universal threshold at 36.

When I call this period of the life course "eventful," I am referring not just to the number of women who transitioned from adolescence to adulthood through marriage—a linchpin of the social definition of adulthood in Malawi—but also to the overall density of vital events over these years.[50] Speaking just of the core sample of 1,505 women who started the study in 2009, we still had contact with 1,200 of them in 2015 and 1,022 in 2019. Completely suspending all the marriages and births that occurred before the TLT study began and examining only the vital events taking place between 2009 and 2019, this group of roughly 1,000 women participated in a total of 747 new marriages (both first marriages and remarriages, many of which are still ongoing) and 375 divorces, including separations. These women gave birth to 1,897 children; by 2019 about 35 percent said they already have all the children they want (around four), and the remaining 65 percent want one or two more children.

Of course, Balaka residents move away too. About 25 percent of our original respondents had moved away from Balaka by 2019—often to larger cities in Malawi (Zomba, Lilongwe, and Blantyre), sometimes to neighboring districts (especially Ntcheu, Mangochi, Salima), and only occasionally to international destinations.

Our respondents' proximity to death is also salient. Just 20 of our respondents died during the study period, and 30 of them lost spouses. But their *experiences* of mortality are prevalent and noteworthy; collectively, the TLT women reported 60 child deaths, 25 stillbirths, and 90 miscarriages.[51] Based on consistent reports of having attended between 1 and 1.2 funerals

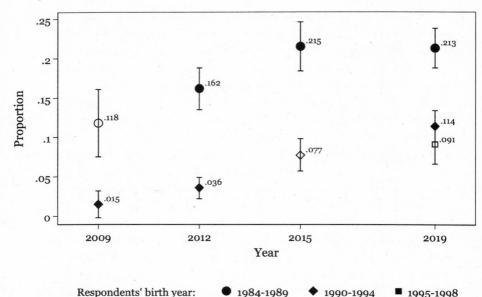

FIGURE 2.5 HIV prevalence by birth cohort at four points in time

Source: TLT, all waves.

Note: Birth cohorts are differentiated by shape. The hollow markers represent estimates for women ages 20–25 in the survey year and can be compared to assess period differences for this age group over time.

per month, I estimate that each TLT respondent attended nearly 150 funerals during the ten-year period. For most respondents, this included elderly relatives and community members, siblings, cousins, age-mate friends, and infants and young children.

The other vital event of interest for this population, of course, is HIV infections. Figure 2.5 shows exactly how HIV prevalence unfolds in the TLT sample, with an emphasis on the differences by birth cohort. When the study began in 2009, HIV prevalence among the sample was about 6 percent; upon closer examination, however, this "average" conceals quite a lot. Over 11 percent of women 20 to 25 were living with HIV, whereas among adolescents between 15 and 19 only about one percent was infected.[52] Three years later, HIV prevalence had increased in both groups but not equally. Among the younger cohort (born 1990–94) new infections doubled, from 1.5 to over 3 percent. Another doubling happened between 2012 and 2015, and the number of new infections continued to rise between 2015 and 2019, when it reached 12 percent.

For the older cohort the pattern is a little different. Already high in 2009,

we see large—5-percentage-point—jumps in HIV prevalence at both intervals, followed by a true flattening of the curve between 2015 and 2019. In other
words, after making it to age 25 or 30 without getting infected, very few TLT
women contract HIV after 2015. This stabilization of prevalence represents a
best-case scenario for people who care about global health. For an irreversible
condition such as HIV, a decline in prevalence can only come about through
high mortality rates, which would cause the numerator (i.e., adults living with
HIV) to decline more sharply than the denominator (i.e., all adults). The flat-
tened curve indicates that women with HIV are *living with* the virus and that
new infections beyond this point are rare.[53] We cannot know the future but
certainly hope that HIV prevalence among the 1990–94 birth cohort will likewise level out at its 2019 level—closer to 10 than 20 percent.

One additional data point adds a wrinkle to this generally hopeful portrait
of decline in new infections by cohort, even as prevalence increases over time
for each group. To assess HIV prevalence trends as a cohort phenomenon,
we strategically adjusted the age criteria for the refresher sample we enrolled
in 2019. Instead of refreshing the sample by adding women of exactly the
same age as the original women (who had reached ages 25–35), we expanded
the age eligibility criteria and enrolled a random sample of women between
the ages of 21 and 35. This allowed us to estimate HIV prevalence (and other
characteristics) for 21- to 25-year-old women and judge whether the emerging trend is cohort-specific or fully secular (i.e., driven by time, fairly uni-
formly). Following HIV prevalence among women ages 20–25 at three points
in time—the hollow markers in figure 2.5—shows tentative improvement at
best. Between 2009 and 2015, prevalence among this age group dropped from
11 to 8 percent, but it remained steady (even increased) between 2015 and
2019. Despite nationwide improvements on every HIV-related metric, with
prevalence levels of at least 10 percent among young adult women, Balaka's
HIV epidemic is far from over.

Having accumulated over more than forty years, the literature on HIV and
AIDS is both vast and deep, comprising more than 250,000 peer-reviewed
articles in medical journals and another 24,000 in the social sciences.[54] Scholars have written powerful accounts of HIV in sub-Saharan Africa, calling it
"a plague of paradoxes," "an exceptional disease," "a virus of vulnerability,"
and "a malady of misfortune."[55] However, the single most important thing I
have learned in two decades of research on HIV in Malawi—that emphasizing the unknown brings unique clarity to the grist of life amid a generalized
epidemic—has never circulated widely. In the face of ongoing endemic HIV
and the new epidemics before us, I suggest that HIV uncertainty and many

other unknowns of the social world can be studied, productively, using demographic tools and approaches. In the chapters that follow, I show what scholarship in this register might look like, by examining the phenomena of relationship formation and dissolution, fertility, HIV infection, and mortality in Balaka, with a focus on both the things themselves and the shadows of uncertainty, large and small, associated with each.

3

Uncertainty Demography

We all live with uncertainty; we experience it in varying degrees throughout our lifetimes and throughout the course of a day. Some uncertainty is situational—"Will my husband make it home tonight, or might he have gotten into an accident?"—and some is existential—"Will I live to see my granddaughter's wedding?" Some uncertainty is personal, while other varieties are shared. Compare "Do I have Alzheimer's, or am I just forgetful like I've always been?" to "Is she telling me the truth?" and "Am I ready for a baby?" to "Is our water safe to drink?" Despite its universality, some people live with more uncertainty than others, and some are more sensitive to it than others. In describing societies and time periods, we intuitively recognize some moments as being characterized by an acute awareness that the unknown carries a lot of weight in the world, the phrases "in these uncertain times" and "in an era of uncertainty" reverberating noisily throughout popular culture, scientific discourse, and even our personal correspondence. Making uncertainty central to demographic inquiry requires thinking about the concept in at least three distinct ways: how ordinary people experience uncertainty, how it defines particular historical contexts, and how researchers handle the concept.

Across the social sciences, scholars invoke the term "uncertainty" in their analyses of a wide variety of phenomena—from cohabitation to unemployment to anxiety to climate change to conditions of capitalism in an integrated, global economy.[1] Some fields operate with relatively settled understandings of what uncertainty means, especially with respect to profit and to measurement. Among quantitative scholars, the term is often used to represent the amount of error in an estimate of a quantity in a population, given the ideal of a true mean. Beginning with Jacob Bernoulli, this use of the term focuses on the mathematical quantification of uncertainty, typically with the goal of reducing it to facilitate better scientific inference.[2] Many economists and economic sociologists adopt Frank Knight's definition of uncertainty as applicable to situations in which it is impossible to specify numerical probabilities, in contrast to risk, which is susceptible to quantification. For Knight, profit is the reward for bearing uncertainty, and for economists following the simple Knightian tradition, risk is measurable, uncertainty is not, and that is the end of the discussion.[3] The narrow economic and statistical definitions are clear and precise but are not particularly well suited to the demographer's interest in the study of vital events: life, death, relationships, and health.

More useful for our purposes is to follow a branch of thought that begins with John Maynard Keynes and defines uncertainty by emphasizing the role of time given an unknowable future. One especially lucid intervention in this tradition distinguishes two concepts at the micro-level: *ambiguity*, missing information that could be known; and what the economist David Dequech calls *fundamental uncertainty*, wherein relevant information cannot be known, even in theory, because it depends on future conditions that do not yet exist and are not predetermined.[4] While ambiguity (the unknown) can be treated as a binary and may be resolved with new information or with the passage of time, fundamental uncertainty (the unknowable) is persistent, difficult to resolve, and may exist in degrees.[5] Focusing on macro-level processes, the historian Jonathan Levy likewise turns away from risk and identifies *radical uncertainty* as the inescapable category for historical analysis. To paraphrase Levy, radical uncertainty is a transhistorical quality of human existence that has particular relevance for understanding contemporary societies with a strong ("near gravitational") orientation to the future. Because the future is never predetermined by the past, it remains to some degree unknowable, despite being constantly subjected to the predictions and calculations, instinctive and deliberate, of ordinary people and experts.[6] Emphasizing the psychosocial weight of the unknown and the unknowable as a force in individuals' lives and a driver of societal change over the course of history, these approaches to uncertainty have clear relevance to the core concerns of demography: the patterning and predictability of vital events across space and over time.

Following these examples from the post-Keynesian tradition, this chapter reviews the kinds of research about uncertainty demographers have advanced already and articulates what *uncertainty demography* as an intellectual project might look like into the future. Advancing a demography of uncertainty rests on three contributions. First, I suggest that the substantive concerns of demography give our field an especially important role in understanding uncertainty in social life, especially our focus on the thresholds of life and death. Second, I synthesize some key insights from demographers who have already begun to move the field in this direction. Third, I offer a working definition of uncertainty and suggest some principles for studying it that reflect the intellectual habits of demography as an interdisciplinary field constituted by empirical insights from statistics, anthropology, economics, biology, and sociology. The phrase "uncertainty demography" (uncertainty, adj.—like economic demography or anthropological demography) captures two related but distinct intellectual moves as a pair: on one side, the proliferation of interest in uncertainty as a substantive topic for demography; and, on the other, the unique value of demographic approaches for rendering visible the role of uncertainty in social life, broadly.

Uncertainty for Demography

Centering uncertainty in questions about family formation, fertility, and the life course accomplishes three important things. First, while much of the foundational literature on risk and uncertainty begins with markets and profit, the true stakes of risk and uncertainty are nothing less than survival— our own and that of our loved ones. If mortality and survival are at the very core of the human experience of uncertainty and risk, the absence of mortality (and perceptions of it) becomes a conspicuous omission.[7] Locating the empirical study of uncertainty in an intellectual community focused on understanding vital events makes a great deal of sense and is consistent with the fact that mortality has always been a foundational topic in the history of probability and statistics. Second, spotlighting uncertainty clarifies the limitations of rational actor approaches to decision making and provides some workable alternatives for scholars working with empirical data.[8] The act of making uncertainty the object of empirical analysis directly refutes models that bracket imperfect information as part of a larger set of heroic assumptions to be made for the sake of a model. Third, centering uncertainty privileges people's lived experience over the researchers' habit of dismissing what people don't know by treating it as "missing data," "error," "ignorance," "bias," or "unobservable." This follows directly from anthropological demographers' habits of rethinking and redefining analytical categories in light of the locally relevant meanings and social practices. In this instance, treating the things that ordinary people describe as experiences of uncertainty as uncertainty brings emic integrity to our study of population processes.[9]

Several other defining characteristics make demography an ideal field from which to advance a robust, empirical engagement with the subject of uncertainty. The list of virtues includes but is not limited to careful definition of risk and the population at risk, a healthy obsession with measurement and data quality, and a supra-individual perspective that resists methodological individualism and can be bent to accommodate the cultural dimensions of uncertainty emphasized in anthropological and ethnographic perspectives. Seen in this way, the project of uncertainty demography is appropriate for addressing the resolvable and nonresolvable varieties of uncertainty people encounter in their daily lives while acknowledging that some uncertainties are deeply personal and that others are social, shared, and perhaps even structural.

A demographic approach to uncertainty follows the spirit of Bayesian statistics more closely than neoclassical economics. In the words of the statistician Dennis Lindley, "My view is that probability is the only mechanism for studying uncertainty. Almost every situation in this world has an uncertain element in it, partly because it involves the future, and the future is uncertain. Therefore probability must have a contribution to make toward almost any question you like to think about, no matter whether it is politics, economics, sociology."[10] A demographic approach to uncertainty easily sidesteps the Knightian focus on differentiating uncertainty from risk, because we work with our own, long-standing definition of risk—the robust definition of a trustworthy denominator for analyzing the occurrence of events.

> For demographers, the risk of a demographically significant event—such as birth, death, the onset of illness, marriage, migration, or labor force entry or exit—is the probability that the event will occur. . . . The demographic definition of risk ignores the desirability and impact of risked events. For example, sexually-active women of childbearing age are "at risk" of pregnancy, but the demographer's calculation of that risk does not consider if women regard pregnancy with delight or dread. Nor does the demographer's risk evaluation consider differences between pregnancy that is unwanted due to minor timing inconveniences and pregnancy that is unwanted because it would precipitate the mother's death. The demographic approach to risk emphasizes the explicit connection between the structure of risk experienced by a population and the structure of age—the time spent in a demographically significant condition— that the population develops over time.[11]

The demographic approach to risk is technical, and having a solid, technical, working definition of risk frees up space for scholars to focus on the substance of what uncertainty *is* rather than what it is not.

Uncertainty in Demography

This leads to my second point: What kind of contributions have demographers made already to the study of uncertainty in populations? From my reading

	Independent Variable (force in the social world)	**Dependent Variable** (outcome of social significance)
macro	How do *population-level uncertainties* influence demographic rates?	How *predictable and stable* are the *demographic rates and distributions* that define a population?
micro	How does *the psychosocial experience of uncertainty* influence vital events at the individual level?	How are *known unknowns* and *emergent plans* patterned and distributed in populations and dynamic over the life course?

FIGURE 3.1 Four general ways demographers analyze uncertainty

of the literature, demographers are contributing to the study of uncertainty through four distinct modes of inquiry. Figure 3.1 depicts the general taxonomy in a 2 × 2 table, which differentiates whether uncertainty is examined at the macro or micro level (i.e., is it conceptualized as a feature of the population or of the individual) and whether it is engaged as a driver of population change or as the outcome of interest (i.e., is it the independent or dependent variable in empirical analyses). Given that the essential core of demography focuses on rates, I begin in the upper-left quadrant, summarizing key insights about uncertainty as a macro-level force in the world, with consequences for demographic phenomena. The basic insight here is that population-level uncertainties produce demographic change through the sum of individual actions (voluntary and involuntary), which become manifest in aggregate rates. The relevant scholarship seeks to specify the kinds of societal uncertainties that produce demographic change and identify why these relationships exist.

UNCERTAINTY AS A POPULATION-LEVEL SOCIAL FORCE

At its most rudimentary level, the crucial theoretical link between fertility decline and mortality decline in demography's most important theory—demographic transition theory—hinges on uncertainty. In one leading account of this transition, high infant mortality rates generate uncertainty about child survival, women in historical populations bore many children in order to ensure that a sufficient number of them would survive to adult-

hood, and it was not until after infant mortality rates had fallen perceptibly
that fertility declines followed. Because fertility patterns tend not to follow
a logic of "child replacement" wherein women bear an additional child after
one has died, the consensus position is that child mortality levels are salient
to all women because they index an ambient sense of uncertainty about how
many of one's own children will survive to adulthood. This relationship has
been studied empirically in dozens of contemporary and historical contexts,
with the historical, ethnographic, and quantitative evidence all pointing to
the uncertainty surrounding child survival rather than the infant mortality
rate itself as the crucial link.[12] Consider, in contrast, Becker and Barro's reformulation of the economic theory of fertility, which imposes the following
assumption: "parents ignore uncertainty about child deaths and respond only
to changes in the fraction p of offspring that survive childhood."[13] Compared
to standard economic approaches, demographers are more resistant to brack-
eting uncertainty as a necessary assumption and, indeed, tend to emphasize
uncertainty in their explanations of demographic change.

Looking beyond mortality, perhaps the most comprehensive example of
macro-level uncertainty as a driver of population change comes from one
of John Caldwell's lesser-known papers. Theorizing broadly about fertility
transitions, Caldwell argues that social upheaval manifests demographic
change through a two-step process: first, temporary adjustments to a period
of uncertainty about the future; and second, a continuing adjustment to the
new social, political, and economic conditions that become firmly established.[14] Analyzing thirteen social crises from around the world for which
adequate demographic data could be found, Caldwell's cases include the
seventeenth-century English Civil War; the French Revolution; the American Civil War; postdictatorship transitions in Spain, Portugal, and Chile;
and the fall of communism in Eastern Europe in the late twentieth century.
In Caldwell's view, fertility decline almost never unfolds in linear fashion
under conditions of incremental social change; it occurs in fits and starts, as
marriage and fertility rates plummet in the short term when marriage and
childbearing are deferred in response to uncertainty and then only partially
recover once a new normal emerges. Through historical analysis of demographic and economic data, Caldwell persuasively spotlights uncertainty as
a unique and consequential force, differentiating it from both the unfavor-
able economic conditions that characterize upheavals and from mind-set
change—salient ideological transformations that often emerge in revolu-
tionary periods.

Theorizing across these cases, Caldwell elevates uncertainty over economic hardship in the following way.

What is common in all cases of upheaval is not the growth of material adversity but an increase in feelings of insecurity. In every case, most of the people involved believed that what lay ahead was unknown and might be better known as time passed. There were excellent reasons for delaying marriage and family formation until it could be seen what the future was going to be like.[15]

Anticipating the objection that social upheavals may bring about—deliberately or unintentionally—entirely new ideologies that are relevant for demographic processes, he likewise prioritizes uncertainty over "mind-set changes" in terms of its explanatory power.

It is very clear that change in the individual outlook, philosophy, or worldview does not on its own depress fertility. What is effective is change in legislation or the economic and social systems that provide a different context for individual behavior. Those changes are, in a sense, the result of the sum total of individual actions, but only a minority of the population provides the ideological leadership; perhaps only a minority supports the new social directions. What dominates most situations is a feeling of personal and family insecurity and a fear of being committed to new demographic acts before it is clear what the world will be like when those acts are consummated.[16]

In sum, from a sweeping analysis of social upheaval in the historical record, Caldwell attributes pivotal periods of accelerated demographic change to widespread uncertainty rather than to material adversity or to ideological transformations.

The ideas that flow from Caldwell's analysis of upheavals are compatible with the insights of the sociologist Ann Swidler, who, theorizing about culture rather than demography, distinguishes between settled and unsettled lives (aggregated into settled vs. unsettled times) as historical moments in which cultural norms are highly visible, as tradition gives way to a particularly powerful combination of ideology and innovation.[17] A limitation of Swidler's approach is the puzzle of how to identify an unsettled time, except for retrospectively, according to the amount of change that resulted. However, if unsettled times can be empirically distinguished from settled times— for example, indicators to gauge larger than usual amounts of uncertainty in a population, general or specific—scholars' capacity to predict and understand uncertainty as a driver of population change could be greatly enhanced. Excellent research on demographic responses to global climate change is moving precisely in this direction, emphasizing the disruptive force of climate variability, in addition to rising levels of global temperature and atmospheric carbon dioxide, and demonstrating clearly that in the case of the climate crisis, uncertainty carries force of its own.[18]

More recent research clarifies that the macro forces of uncertainty are not only relevant for iconic historical events and seismic sociopolitical shifts but also central to analyzing contemporary economic, epidemiological, and social change—big and small. Explaining the emergence of "lowest low" fertility in Europe during the early 2000s, Melinda Mills, Hans-Peter Blossfeld, and others point to youth unemployment and job instability as indicators of palpable economic uncertainty for young adults that leads to the postponement of marriage and childbearing.[19] In the wake of labor market transformations and changes to returns on education, they observe longer periods of coresidence with parents, marriage postponement, delayed fertility, and an accompanying reduction in birth rates across much of Europe. Advancing a multiple-equilibriums model of demographic change, Kohler, Billari, and Ortega assert that fertility starts being delayed when structural aspects of uncertainty in young adulthood begin to rise, according to macro-level metrics, after which time the mean age at first birth adjusts itself to the new, stable situation.[20] Because marriage and childbearing are social phenomena,[21] these shifts are subject to a social multiplier effect, so even relatively small increases in uncertainty that might make little difference to any one individual's fertility can produce large delays in fertility at the population level.

In contrast to Caldwell, who advanced causal connections without directly measuring uncertainty, a more recent generation of insights about uncertainty uses macro-level indicators to proxy uncertainty in defined populations: nation-state, community, or census tract. In this sense, uncertainty is measurable and gets operationalized at the macro-level through strong proxies like the unemployment rate, the inflation rate, housing availability, or the infant mortality rate. Here uncertainty exists in degrees, and some populations have more of it than others—with high levels of youth unemployment, for example, indexing greater uncertainty about the future than a regime of nearly full employment, regardless of one's own employment status or ideal family size.

Seeking to explain delayed marriage and falling fertility across the United States and Europe, Chiara Comolli argues that economic uncertainty has an effect above and beyond structural market conditions.[22] Acknowledging that "it is more complicated to design accurate indicators of economic insecurity, and to identify their impact on fertility, than it is to design accurate indicators of the material conditions of the economy," Comolli nonetheless creatively identifies independent indicators of uncertainty, such as economic policy uncertainty, sovereign risk, and consumer confidence and finds a negative fertility response in twenty-two of thirty-two countries.[23] Like Caldwell, Comolli concludes that fertility rates are responsive to the perceived uncertainty generated by the recession in ways that extend beyond the tangible material conditions of the economy itself.

Exploiting state-based variation in the United States in the wake of the Great Recession, Daniel Schneider advances a similar argument about uncertainty's role in reducing fertility. Pointing to greater fertility declines in states with high foreclosure and unemployment rates, Schneider argues that uncertainty lowers fertility intentions (i.e., volitional change) and points to two other important pathways through which uncertainty may reduce fertility: delayed marriage patterns and stress-induced miscarriage. Because other studies clarify that stress has negative health consequences (including miscarriage), the nonvolitional physiological pathways between uncertainty and fertility are entirely plausible. Not only does Schneider see uncertainty as relevant for the demographic consequences of the great recession; he argues for a greater focus on uncertainty for demography generally: "The focus on uncertainty is especially important given that the increasing insecurity of work may make economic uncertainty a more certain feature of the future U.S. economy and thus a potentially important driver of demographic behavior over the coming decades."[24] Writing about macro-level uncertainty in Russia and Ukraine, Brienna Perelli-Harris, however, expresses concern that the evidence for economic uncertainty as a driver of fertility decline is insufficiently strong empirically and may be overstated. In a series of excellent articles, Perelli-Harris urges researchers to move beyond conventional measures of economic uncertainty and think more carefully in two directions: concrete adjacent factors like available housing and functional government and fuzzier psychosocial dimensions of uncertainty, including belief in progress, anomie, and hope for the future.[25]

If uncertainty is conceptualized as a macro-level force in the social world, epidemics differ substantially from the economic sphere. However, they may function similarly because they too represent a supra-individual force that can influence population change. One important dimension of epidemic influence is involuntary: epidemics have compositional and physiological consequences. Changing mortality patterns brought about by new diseases alter the size of a population, its age structure, and the health and fecundity of the surviving population, thereby affecting the number of births in purely mechanical terms. Another route of influence is voluntary, as decisions about family formation often shift in response to new diseases, and it is with respect to the voluntary consequences that substantial explanatory power has been given to uncertainty rather than to the disease itself. The AIDS crisis in sub-Saharan Africa is thought to have altered the fertility patterns in most affected countries through a combination of volitional and psychological pathways. Early in the epidemic, the demographers Basia Zaba and Simon Gregson observed a population-attributable decline in total fertility of about half a percentage point for each percentage point of HIV prevalence in the general population.[26] To the extent that fertility rates declined in light of Zika outbreaks in Brazilian states, this was the result of uncertainty about the possibility of healthy childbearing.[27] In the recent example of the COVID-19 pandemic, mortality is overwhelmingly affecting older adults who have already completed their childbearing, but uncertainty has been influencing birth rates among the young by eroding fertility desires as, for many, planning for the future seems impossible under the perpetually shifting conditions of a global pandemic.[28]

PERSONAL UNCERTAINTY AND DEMOGRAPHIC EVENTS

Population-level uncertainties like drought, revolution, shifting unemployment rates, or hyperinflation do not have to affect everyone in order to shape demographic rates. Uncertainties are distributed unevenly in populations, with some individuals experiencing acute uncertainty and others relatively insulated from it. This insight shifts us to the next mode of inquiry, wherein demographers writing about uncertainty as a driver of demographic change emphasize the personal nature of uncertainty as a lived experience. Moving counterclockwise to the bottom-left quadrant of figure 3.1, a growing body of literature argues that the lived experience of uncertainty has consequences for demographic behaviors and attempts to measure it at the micro-level to harness variability in the experience of uncertainty and its effects. This body of research is methodologically diverse, drawing heavily on survey research (especially longitudinal studies that can measure change over time), and is also well represented by ethnographic, in-depth interview, and focus-group studies on demographic topics.

Illustrating the crucial bridge between anthropological and demographic perspectives, scholarship by Jennifer Johnson-Hanks has established the salience of uncertainty for intentional action in both general and specific ways, asking: What kinds of reproductive futures do young, educated Cameroonian women hope for? How do they try to bring about those potential futures? How are these intentions and actions influenced by the uncertainty of everyday life in contemporary Cameroon?[29] Beyond the specific case of young Beti women's reproductive lives, this work has inspired dozens of empirical contributions attempting to manifest uncertainty in a serious way in demographic research.[30] The insights open doors to important comparative and global questions, including: How do young people make a living and make life meaningful under conditions of crushing economic uncertainty? And how do they relate to time as an object when acting in the present with respect to the future?[31]

Some researchers working in a quantitative register measure personal uncertainty directly, while others infer uncertainty from strong proxies. One example of the kind of reasoning I find particularly valuable points to the role of variance, rather than levels, for capturing personal experiences of uncertainty. Circling back to the foundational relationship between fertility and mortality as one of uncertainty, John Sandberg's research on fertility patterns in rural Nepal demonstrates that uncertainty about child survival is associated with accelerated childbearing.[32] Comparing women who observed high levels of infant mortality among their friends to those ensconced in low-mortality networks, Sandberg found earlier first births and shorter birth intervals among the former. Moreover, where infant mortality was low but highly variable (i.e., difficult to predict), childbearing patterns more closely resembled those observed among high-mortality-network women, the mechanism being uncertainty about children's survival rather than "pure replacement." Even within a high-mortality context, Sandberg shows that the experience of uncertainty varies, that that variability could be measured empirically, and that measured uncertainty has observable consequences for the fertility trajectories of individuals.

Without necessarily referring to it as such, recent studies from the United States and Malawi have harnessed this logic of existential uncertainty as a driver of fertility, relying not on aggregate-level mortality measures but on adult mortality in one's personal network. Michigan-based studies demonstrate that exposure to violence, measured by geocoded homicides, increases young women's desires to become pregnant,[33] while a study from Malawi suggests that nonvolitional forces are also at play: young women who attended funerals in the previous month had a higher net risk of conceiving than those who attended none, and the relationship seems to be driven by unintended, rather than desired, pregnancies.[34]

Far more abundant than these studies of existential uncertainty is the literature on the demographic consequence of economic uncertainty for individuals. This area of research has been especially fruitful in Europe, where scholars have been combining high-quality survey data with rich administrative sources to consider the demographic consequences of economic uncertainty through events like German unification in the 1990s, Russia's transition to a market economy, the effect of the 2008 recession across Italy, and shifting employment regimes in Japan.[35] Among the key distinctions between this literature and macro-level studies that demonstrate a negative consequence of economic uncertainty on marriage and fertility rates are the emphasis on personal experience, an individual-level approach to measuring uncertainty, and a focus on the timing of key life course events: marriage, moves, births, and deaths. A shared challenge is the task of adequately differentiating the subjective uncertainty an individual experiences from that individual's objective conditions. For example, are outcomes different for a woman in an objectively precarious occupation who perceives her employment as stable into the future (perhaps even mistakenly) in comparison to one who experiences both objective and subjective uncertainty?

One of the strongest recent studies to emphasize personal uncertainty was conducted by Danilo Bolano and Daniele Vignoli, who carefully link the experience of employment uncertainty to union formation (i.e., legal marriages and de facto cohabitations) in a sample of Australian adults.[36] Differentiating between objective and subjective uncertainties, they observe no differences in union formation between permanent workers and those on fixed-term contracts. However, the lens of subjective uncertainty adds crucial insight to the patterns; women in permanent positions with low levels of job security postpone union formation, and subjective appraisals of job security are even more important for nonpermanent workers. Beyond the specifics of the Australian case, this work helps underscore the importance of considering uncertainty as a puzzle of temporal scale. Contemporaneously measured, objective indicators of job security tell us little about how union formation in Australia is patterned, but forward-looking measures built to acknowledge the prospective nature of uncertainty indicate that relationship formation is strongly influenced by individual-level economic uncertainty. Consistent with insights from cultural and economic sociologists, the uncertainty that matters is about the future, not the present.[37] And while historically grounded life course research tends to emphasize the impact of past events on a phenomenon of interest, this approach to the study of uncertainty emphasizes the "shadow of the future" as an independent force in decision making and demographic outcomes.[38]

Beyond existential and economic uncertainty, personal biographies can be marked by uncertainty through an experience of family instability, poverty, or a combination of the two. Considered in the US context, uncertainty tends to beget more uncertainty. In a new book on young adulthood in the United States, the sociologists Rob Crosnoe and Shannon Cavanaugh operationalize uncertainty as early childhood poverty and family instability, noting that there is a great deal of variation in how young people form families and pursue socioeconomic attainment between their late teens and early twenties.[39] Using sequence analysis to identify common trajectories, they find that early-childhood experiences of family instability and family uncertainty are the most powerful determinants of how family and economic lives unfold. Even the economic conditions so many demographers have focused on (e.g., community-level labor market conditions, whether the transition unfolds during an economic recession or boom) are less influential than the uncertainty manifested through family instability for young adults in the United States.

Some young adults go through a lot of changes in their late teens and midtwenties, but these changes fail to produce anything resembling forward movement; they are "churning" (i.e., stuck in place without a clear path forward). The more instability and uncertainty individuals experience as a child, the more time they spend in a churning state as young adults, while those with stable childhoods are far more likely to make a clean transition from college to the labor force (full-time) while delaying (voluntarily) childbearing and marriage. But there is a puzzle here. Cavanaugh and Crosnoe observe substantial levels of instability and uncertainty in family formation, socioeconomic attainment, and mental health in their quantitative data; however, when given the chance to talk about their feelings of uncertainty and stress or to ruminate on how their lives might have turned out differently, young adults focus almost exclusively on the uncertainty of socioeconomic attainment and have little to say about the family dimension. As we saw earlier with Alice's respondent (see chap. 2), the emphasis in the demographers' explanatory models sometimes diverges from the processes ordinary people emphasize when narrating their own experiences of demographic phenomena. Such paradoxes present opportunities to examine which population-level processes are visible as opposed to invisible to ordinary people navigating their own worlds. Perhaps young adults in the United States do not dwell on patterns of family formation, or perhaps they are so consumed with socioeconomic anxiety about the future that this concern dwarfs everything else.

UNCERTAINTY AS AN OBJECT OF DEMOGRAPHIC INQUIRY

In addition to being a force in the social world, uncertainty is a phenomenon of inquiry in its own right, the dependent variable in analyses of micro-level phenomena. Demographers working in this third quadrant, the bottom right of figure 3.1, seldom invoke "uncertainty" as the key word to describe what they are studying. Nonetheless, several pertinent examples illustrate the salience of what people don't know—at the personal and population levels—as an important and independent demographic indicator. Since the emergence of widespread, comparative microdata in the World Fertility Studies, the

study of fertility has become strongly informed by the role of fertility preferences and desires for understanding childbearing norms and likely trends.
Non-numeric responses to questions about ideal family size have been widely
studied, both as a problem for researchers who would like everyone to give
a numeric answer and as a valuable indicator of a "pre-transition mindset,"
the belief that fertility lies outside of the ambit of one's own control or, in the
famous words of Ansley Coale, outside the calculus of conscious choice.[40]
Writing about presumptions of numeracy in historical and contemporary
populations in a Population Association of America presidential address
given in 1992, Etienne van de Walle mentions a survey collected in Nigeria in
the early 1980s, in which more than 50 percent of women gave a non-numeric
response (answers like, "I don't know" or "Up to God") to questions about
how many children they wanted to have.[41]

Van de Walle's now-famous exchange with Maimouna from Bamako (age
28, seven children) illustrates that "don't know" responses are not a missing
data problem but a distinctive attitude about fertility that is itself a worthy
subject of inquiry.

Q. Maimouna, how many children would you like to have in your life?
A. Ah, what God gives me, that is it . . . I cannot tell the number I will have
   in my life . . . [laughs]
Q. It is true that God is the one who gives the child, but if God asked the
   number of children you wanted, how many would you say?
A. Oh, me, I cannot tell the number of children to God. What he gives me is
   good, that's enough. To say that I can stop and say the number to tell God
   what to give me, I could not do so.
Q. Even if God asks you?
A. Even if he asks me, I cannot say it.
Q. Would you like to have many children or not many?
A. Only what God gives me, that's what I want.
Q. Do you want more than those you have now?
A. What I say is that what God gives me, that's what I want.
Q. And if God gives you 12 children now?
A. Ah, if God gives me 12 children, then God created them.
Q. So you like that?
A. Ah, what God makes, that is that.[42]

Writing thirty years after van de Walle to elaborate non-numeracy as a
trend, Margaret Frye and Lauren Bachan identified a trend of global decline
in non-numeracy over a period of twenty years, from the early 1990s to the

early 2010s.[43] Rather than treat non-numeric responses as a missing data problem or a selectivity issue, Frye and Bachan treat non-numeric responses to questions about fertility preferences as a statement of uncertainty about ideal family size (IFS), and this becomes their subject of demographic inquiry. The observed decline over this period is both steep (with non-numeracy in Burkina Faso falling from over 20 percent in 1994 to less than 4 percent in 2010) and global (with 22 of 32 countries exhibiting measurable decline during the observation period). Non-numeric responses are also strongly patterned; educated women and those knowledgeable about modern contraception are unlikely to provide non-numeric IFS responses, whereas women who have suffered the death of a child often give non-numeric responses. In other words, fertility-specific uncertainty about ideal family size is patterned and linked to another demographic uncertainty: mortality. Overall, women who give uncertain answers about the families they would like to have are distinct from those who answer with numbers, regardless of whether those numbers are large or small.

Even in contexts where numeric reasoning about fertility is ubiquitous, evidence points to fertility preferences as uncertain, unstable, and subject to change with changing circumstances. In fact, some of the field's most compelling scholars have been placing uncertainty at the center of the puzzle. Phil Morgan began writing about the crucial role of uncertainty for understanding fertility in the United States nearly forty years ago.[44] In a well-known critique of standard survey practices for research on fertility intentions, Nora Cate Schaeffer and Elizabeth Thomson advanced a theory of grounded uncertainty, focusing on the methodological and substantive implications of "I don't know," "that doesn't apply to me," and "it depends" answers in survey research about fertility.[45] More recently, Máire Ní Bhrolcháin and Éva Beaujouan have advanced an ambitious research agenda that emphasizes the uncertainty surrounding childbearing in Europe, demonstrating, for example, that about 30 percent of British women were uncertain about the number of children they want to have.[46] Depending on the measurement, between 10 and 40 percent of women are uncertain about their fertility intentions in cross-sectional data from Europe and the United States. A key insight from Ní Bhrolcháin and Beaujouan is that uncertainty in fertility intentions should not be thought of as a residual category, attributable to measurement errors or a lack of knowledge on the part of the respondents, but a demographic concept worth studying in its own right.

A final example of fertility research that spotlights uncertainty as an object of inquiry is evident in comparative historical research by Suzanne O. Bell and Mary E. Fissell, who trouble the presumed pregnant/nonpregnant binary that dominates the field, arguing that the simple binary blinds scholars to precisely the family planning and reproductive health strategies we should be investigating.[47] While many of us have grown accustomed to the now-forty-year-old notion that pregnancy can be identified early and comfortably at home, in private, with a rapid test, this technology is relatively new and is still, today, unavailable to women across most of the globe.[48] For millennia, women have navigated the world with imperfect information about their pregnancy status, often for fairly long periods of time. Throughout most of human history, missed menses could be just as easily attributed to illness or poor nutrition as to pregnancy.[49] Rooted in the long-standing tradition of the history of medicine and new insights from critical demography, Bell and Fissell note that early pregnancy is characterized by months of hope, suspicion, uncertainty, and denial—a crucial, recurring, and overlooked stage of the reproductive life course.

Of course, uncertainty reduction can be a driving force in human behavior, and this applies to pregnancy too. Women have always taken steps to discern uncertain pregnancies at early stages. Ancient Egyptians assessed sterility, diagnosed pregnancy, and predicted fetal sex by "watering" different cereals with women's urine and tracking the germination patterns.[50] But even after confirmation of a pregnancy, reproductive uncertainty continues. Pregnancies themselves are fragile and uncertain—especially but not only in low-resource settings and among "at-risk" populations.[51] Today, questions about reproductive uncertainty have renewed salience, especially among scholars anticipating the future of fertility research—one in which aggregate patterns will be non-negligibly informed by assisted reproductive therapies. These therapies are relevant on two levels: as a set of technologies that influence fertility patterns and as a bundle of personal strategies for managing uncertainty and manipulating the time horizons on which a future family can unfold.[52] Consistent with insights from the theory of conjunctural action, this research emphasizing the inherent uncertainty of pregnancy underscores the importance of analytically prioritizing the contexts in which events occur over the traits of the individuals experiencing them.

Although fertility uncertainty is by far the most well-researched variety of uncertainty to be engaged by the demographic literature as an outcome, a handful of insightful studies focus on personal uncertainty with respect to relationships and life expectancy as noteworthy objects of inquiry. Together, these studies suggest that micro-level uncertainty is emerging from within the field as a priority topic. As discussed in the introduction, Patuma's uncertain marital status may not be an objectively prevalent relationship status in the population as a whole; however, in populations where divorce and re-marriage rates are high, uncertainty about a relationship can be salient even if it isn't widespread at any single point in time. Writing about Black women in the US context, Linda Burton and Belinda Tucker made uncertainty the focus of their analysis. Instead of following the Moynihan Report's analysis of family pathology, Burton and Tucker used in-depth interview data to "interrogate the role of uncertainty as context, engine, and barrier for relationship maintenance."[53] Following an argument made by the development economist Geof Wood,[54] they characterize uncertainty as *the* determining phenomenon for impoverished persons, pointing to the pervasive absence of predictability about the future. For Burton and Tucker, this lack of predictability has roots in a general insight about poverty poignantly summarized by their respondent Clara—"It's like flying blind every day, never knowing what to expect"—and in existential uncertainty, that is, premonitions of length of life for their partners and themselves.[55]

A small and focused literature on subjective survival beliefs cuts straight to the heart of uncertainty in demography: mortality. Given that no one knows the hour of their death, how long do we think we have on earth? And are people who understand something about population-level statistics more accurate than those without any kind of statistical foundation to guess from?[56] Some demographers have engaged subjective survival beliefs as an independent variable and assessed their predictive power relative to clinical assessments.[57] Increasingly, however, subjective survival beliefs have become their own object of inquiry: patterned in populations according to well-established lines of social inequality and indicative of particular mind-sets or dispositions with respect to the material world. Research by Charles Manski, Baruch Fischhoff, and colleagues shows that US teenagers wildly overestimate the likelihood of their own mortality, while the consensus about older adults is that they underestimate how long they will live.[58] If there are general takeaways from this literature, aside from its value to actuaries and designers of life insurance policies, they would be that rational-choice theories provide a poor fit to data on subjective survival probabilities from around the world, that ordinary people regularly update their survival beliefs in light of new information (especially about health), and that people do not reason about mortality with population averages as their reference point but are instead guided by heuristics and heavily influenced by salient events within their personal networks.[59] Ordinary people are constantly reasoning with uncertainty about how long they will live, and they do it in ways that deviate substantially from demographic models.

INFERRING UNCERTAINTY FROM AGGREGATE
VIEWS OF POPULATION STRUCTURE

If individual-level mortality perceptions represent the pulse of demographic research on uncertainty, the process known as mortality rectangularization is the heart. I locate this process (along with others) in the fourth quadrant of figure 3.1, where demographic research about uncertainty is perhaps the most "classically" demographic, depicting the structure of the whole population and rates of change over time. Again here scholars working in this register rarely use the term "uncertainty" to describe the focus of their research, and none of the examples I draw on are key worded as studies of uncertainty. Nonetheless, the essence of mortality rectangularization, the population turnover rate (PTR), and life course destandardization represent clear and measurable forms of macro-level change that when in flux necessarily stretch social institutions, traditions, and settled ways of living life. Regardless of whether the shifts are perceived accurately in a population (or at all), I argue that the dispersion and predictability of these events constitutes a set of clear and crucial measures for distinguishing "normal" times from uncertain times. And because empirical work making claims about levels of uncertainty needs to be able to differentiate time periods saturated by uncertainty from periods characterized by less uncertainty, I argue that vague, decorative statements about "uncertain times" cannot provide the foundation for serious scholarship about uncertainty. The future is always uncertain, so who is to say whether Malawi's HIV epidemic of 2000–2010 is more or less uncertain than Italy's experience of the COVID pandemic of 2019–present without some kind of empirical barometer for doing so?

In addition to their utility to demography for its own sake, studies of population-level change that identify and elaborate population composition and processes "under the surface" are valuable levers for gauging uncertainty in populations and making fair comparisons about levels over time.[60] In terms of operationalization, these measures tend to harness variance and rates of change to index uncertainty. Importantly, many of these processes are invisible to the eye from within a population—or perhaps perceived only as incremental changes, narrated in personal biographies or intergenerational comparisons. While population growth and mortality levels, for example, are readily visible to anybody who is paying attention (narrated in real-time through population chatter with comments about crowding, housing availability, funeral frequency), crucial dimensions of population composition often go unnoticed, while others are noted without being considered noteworthy. An observation such as, "My grandmother had her first birth at age 22, my mother hers at age 25, and I had mine at 29," is unlikely to be cited as an example of massive social change; however, as evidenced by the best examples of research from quadrant 1, relatively small individual-level actions of postponement often aggregate into noteworthy fertility declines, and the destabilizing effects of subtle changes in population-level characteristics can be substantial in terms of the effects on social institutions and on morale.

Writing about aging, natural death, and the compression of morbidity, the physician James Fries was the first to describe the aggregate-level process with the emphasis on its geometry.[61] As mortality declines in societies with abundant food and access to medical care, not only does life expectancy get longer, but mortality becomes compressed (concentrated at older ages), and so does morbidity, as chronic illnesses can be postponed and (to a point) separated from the aging process. Writing in 1980 based on observations from US health and mortality data, Fries shifted the focus from the average length of life to the distribution of deaths. Presuming 100 years as the natural limit on the human life span, Fries observed that with the decline of premature death and the analytical suspension of deaths by violence, nearly 95 percent of natural deaths take place between the ages of 77 and 93. This key feature of the demographic transition is too often overlooked: more important than the fact of lives becoming longer in the United States between 1900 and 1980 is the fact that death became predictable, with tangible consequences for population structure (i.e., an aging population) and a crucial psychosocial insight: "Paradoxically, the predictability of death may prove soothing."[62]

The conditions of rectangularized mortality and morbidity represent a milieu in which, consciously or unconsciously, the population as a whole makes decisions, big and small, with a shared assumption of a vigorous, long life. Conversely, in contexts in which mortality is more evenly distributed across the age spectrum, that assumption does not hold. Reflecting on mortality in comparative perspective, using data from Sweden, Japan, and the United States, the formal demographers John Wilmoth and Shiro Horiuchi identify ten distinct points in the rectangularization process, including the fastest decline, the quickest plateau, and the sharpest corner.[63] These precise measures are most useful to demographers seeking to understand the formal relationships between mortality decline, population growth, and aging. However their key measure (the lifetable interquartile range) has relevance far beyond demography, because it summarizes a set of conditions that is relevant to every other social structure and indexes a (perhaps even *the*) fundamental uncertainty for populations.

A second example of a truly macro-level indicator of uncertainty can be found in the notion of the population turnover rate. Population growth has long been the singular focus of demographic change—with periods of rapid growth being identified as fodder for political and social instability and the slowing of population growth indicating a crucial juncture in the phases of the demographic transition. The PTR captures something different: the speed at which demographic replacement occurs in a population, given the total quantity of births, deaths, immigration, and emigration. Elaborating the relevance of the PTR for understanding the overlapping COVID-19 and migration crises in Europe, the demographer Francesco Billari notes some key patterns: peaks in pretransitional turnover rates are likely to have been reached during years of mortality crises in the preindustrial world and, under assumptions of zero migration, PTR is lowest when population growth is negative.[64] The observed heterogeneity in PTRs is vast, and periods of crisis tend to be characterized by high turnover rates.[65] Examining the empirical trends for Italy over the past hundred years, Billari finds that the general trend has been a downward one, with two exceptions: peaks during the world wars and the reemergence of "fast" demographic change beginning around 1990. To interpret the PTR as an indicator of uncertainty, both quantities and variability matter. If all we knew about a country was that its PTR was 52.7 per 1,000 for 1990–95 and 42.8 for 2015–20, we might reasonably conclude that the later period was more certain than the former—characterized by greater level of stability (i.e., persistence of the same human beings) in the population overall. Or we may emphasize the fact that a context characterized by a declining PTR is experiencing change in a way that a society experiencing stable rates (say, 60.2 in both 1990–95 and 2015–20) is not. Thought of as the background noise against which daily life is lived, both the levels and changes in PTR are salient to how large and small decisions are made, norms constructed, and values transmitted. Researchers might harness the PTR (both levels and changes) as an indicator of uncertainty, as it captures something about the demographic foundation on which the rest of social life rests, regardless of whether these are perceived by those living within the population.

A third and final example of how population-level uncertainties can be made visible through demographic tools emerges from life course theory, specifically the trend of life course destandardization in contemporary societies, measured using sequence analysis techniques. Life course approaches to studying the transition to adulthood, in particular, emphasize that socially defined events are enacted in individual lives and unfold as a trajectory, in which the timing and ordering of events intersect in a larger context. In societies where the pathway to adulthood is strongly scripted, the biographical steps are synchronized within cohorts and guided by fairly rigid age norms. Deviations from the dominant trajectory may be judged as "unacceptable"

and socially sanctioned, sometimes severely. The process of destandardization refers to greater heterogeneity of sequences in a population and a less
predictable ordering of events through the transition to adulthood, as biographies are increasingly individualized and less constrained by cultural norms.
Just as mortality and morbidity rectangularization represent greater certainty
about longevity and healthy life expectancy as variance around mortality declines, life course sequence measures harness variance to communicate how
predictable or unpredictable the pathway to adulthood is within the population as a whole. The relevance for uncertainty demography is not to judge
whether it is good or bad to have a strongly standardized life course or to determine what level is optimal but to infer that populations with more strongly
scripted life course trajectories could be deemed more certain *on the specific
dimension of family formation* than societies characterized by highly variable
trajectories and no clear dominant script. Research by Luca Pesando, Maria
Sironi, and colleagues demonstrates that the destandardization process documented in Europe is also under way in most low- and middle-income countries, and they provide an elegant example of how researchers can capture
and classify contexts according to the pace of change.[66] Periods of discernible destandardization could reasonably be read as uncertain times, indexing
a supra-individual process of social change in which a relatively clear view
about how to move from one stage of life to another becomes cloudy.

Do these demographic measures of population structure capture economic uncertainty? Absolutely not. Might they be valuable for proxying the
predictability (real and perceived) of the landscape in which the drama of
daily life plays out? I believe so. Given the seemingly unbounded desire to
make claims about uncertainty and the shortage of concrete strategies for
assessing it empirically, I suggest these indicators are strong candidates for
consideration as scholars writing about uncertainty attempt to assess its relative level in the populations they study.

The Contours of Uncertainty Demography

As seen from the examples in this chapter, demographers already have a
strong start in advancing empirical work on uncertainty from a variety of
methodological perspectives and a wide range of geographic contexts. However, demographic scholarship has innovated very little in terms of offering
new definitions of uncertainty; our working definitions tend to be presumed
rather than articulated and borrowed from across the social sciences rather
than constructed in-house. Whether measured with survey items, proxied
from found data sources, or drawn out of ethnographic observations, uncer-

tainty tends to be measured and operationalized clearly (if inconsistently) in our research. Yet the lack of a clear and shared definition strikes me as uncharacteristically sloppy and incoherent for a field that takes operationalization and measurement so seriously in most other ways. I close this chapter by offering a definition that works for demography and setting out some parameters to guide what a more coordinated and robust approach to uncertainty demography could look like into the future.

Definition: "Uncertainty refers to epistemic situations in which the salience of the unknown and the unknowable eclipses the relevance of known factors."

1. Uncertainty is a specific category, rather than a residual category. Scholars can define it as the presence of a particular thing rather than the absence of another thing.

2. Uncertainty relates both to present circumstances and to the anticipation of future events.

3. Uncertainty is measurable—perhaps not directly, but it can be inferred by good proxies and observed by skilled ethnographers—and worth measuring.

4. Personal uncertainty is experienced by individuals and is experienced in degrees. Despite being a transhistorical universal quality, one can have more or less of it.

5. Personal uncertainty is unevenly distributed in most populations and often follows known fault lines of social stratification.

6. Personal uncertainty may be measured by probability degrees, using the kind of intuitive language of prediction that permeates everyday conversation.

7. Uncertainty is a supra-individual force as well. At the population level and in human history, uncertainty is irreducible to the feelings of uncertainty individuals experience.

8. Some historical moments (defined by geography and time) are characterized by more uncertainty than others, but it would be a mistake to assess collective varieties of uncertainty based on intuition alone or tautologically by the amount of change that gets produced.

9. Collective uncertainty can be indexed by aggregated levels of personal uncertainty or proxied by measures of distribution and variance that capture the predictability of events in a population.[67]

10. Uncertainty has measurable consequences. It can cause or exacerbate suffering (e.g., stress, poor health, poverty). Alternatively, it can be fruitful—a productive condition that drives innovation and creativity.[68] The force of the uncertainty surrounding a phenomenon can be more (or less) powerful than the force of the thing itself.

As I drafted and revised the chapters that follow, I took much inspiration from scholars who have thought carefully about how to identify and understand the role of uncertainty in population processes. And it genuinely surprises me that these distinct modes of engaging uncertainty have not, to my knowledge, already been assembled into a framework that allows us to coordinate insights, measures, and strategies for building collective knowledge about the role of the unknown and the unknowable in the world. Perhaps, contra Vance, uncertainty is one of the conceptual binders that organizes a wildly diverse set of topical findings in a cumulative and coherent way. In the remaining chapters, I empirically analyze a variety of uncertainties among young adults living in Balaka, Malawi, between 2009 and 2019. My analyses begin with HIV-related uncertainty and link to other kinds of uncertainty, including relationship uncertainty, livelihood uncertainty, reproductive uncertainty, and existential uncertainty. At each stage, I spotlight uncertainty and the phenomenon it, like a shadow, is projected from. I offer empirical examples from each of the four quadrants depicted here, with uncertainty examined as both outcome of interest and force in the world, as a personal experience and as a population-level phenomenon.

4

The Scope of HIV Uncertainty

UNAIDS defines a generalized HIV epidemic by two criteria: more than one percent of the population is infected with HIV, and the virus is not concentrated in any specific subpopulation or risk group.[1] Prevalence is measured by serostatus, the presence of antibodies in a blood sample, and is typically stated as a percentage. We often assess the severity of an epidemic by comparing prevalence in one society to another: with 9.5 percent of all adults infected with HIV, Malawi's epidemic is more severe than Kenya's (4.5 percent prevalence); within Malawi, Balaka's epidemic (14 percent) is more severe than Rumphi's (6.7 percent). Serostatus is the focal point of the HIV literature, and rightly so; serostatus is what matters for securing life-prolonging treatment, for providing appropriate maternal care, and for anticipating mortality shifts.

In this chapter I outline the scope of uncertainty in Balaka, arguing that the most socially salient feature of an epidemic is not the proportion of those who *have* the condition but the proportion of those who *do not know* their status, that is, the proportion uncertain. Through ethnographic vignettes from Gertrude's fieldnotes, I show what HIV certainty and uncertainty sound like in everyday conversation. I then present analyses of the TLT survey data that focus on what people don't know about their status when asked about the likelihood of HIV infection, present and future. I show that HIV-related uncertainty weighs heavily in this population, even though HIV prevalence itself remains quite low among adolescents, in particular. Uncertainty about HIV is an entirely different statistic from the proportion infected and the rate of spread; this large, uncertain population is a group scholars need to know much more about. If human behavior is responsive to uncertainty, and theory suggests this is the case, reliance on serostatus for understanding the force of HIV in a population will mislead researchers, clinicians, and policy makers who seek to understand how HIV shapes behaviors and outcomes for individuals and within populations.

Tapwater Conflict

Balaka Boma is characterized by persistent water shortages. This is the result of poor infrastructure, including the malfunctioning dam that supplies the southern region, which is exacerbated during times of drought. The water shortages are consequential, by which I mean they rearrange everything, starting with the creation of very long lines at the boreholes where you would need to arrive before 5 a.m. to avoid a wait of many hours for your turn. Not surprisingly, water shortages lead to conflict between neighbors. A water problem early in the morning provides the backdrop for the vignette that follows. It involves Blessings, a neighbor Gertrude sees regularly but doesn't yet know well, and "Father of Stella,"[2] Gertrude's neighbor and landlord, a notoriously difficult man. Their houses are located within the same compound, which shares a community tap.

> Later in the morning Blessings came to fetch water at our tap; she said she didn't have drinking water at her home. Father of Stella asked her, "Who gave you permission to come and draw water here?" She said, "No one did." And he sent her away.
>
> She asked me to escort her to the borehole; as I was escorting her she complained that Father of Stella is always harsh to the people around him. "Maybe the ARVs are making him be very harsh to everyone."
>
> The remark surprised me, so I asked, "But is it true that all the harsh people are on ARVs?" And she said, "No, some when they are on ARVs they act abnormally, as he is doing; others, they behave normal."
>
> "But how can you differentiate a man who is on ARVs and a woman who is on ARVs?"
>
> "With these ARVs you can't differentiate them; two of my kids are HIV positive, but you can't tell by looking at them."
>
> "Really?"
>
> "Yes, really. My husband died of that because he was not taking ARVs. He said he couldn't take ARVs because of the belief of our church. At the Jehovah's Witness church, we don't believe in any kind of medicine. And that made my husband die. For me? I don't follow those rules; if I followed them, I would also be dead, and my kids would be left alone so young."
>
> I asked how old those kids are, and she said, "One is 8 and the other one is 10." She continued, "Had it been that they were born today, my kids wouldn't be affected, because the nevirapine that the mothers get when giving birth, it helps a lot. My oldest daughter got infected by her husband, and she realized

it when she was pregnant because now they do compulsory testing at the hospital, and when her child was born she was born negative."

"When did your daughter start taking ARVs?"

"At the hospital, at the very same time they realized she is positive." She continued, explaining that even nowadays all the people who are found HIV positive are told to start ARVs right away, regardless of their CD4 count.

"How come?"

"That's what people are saying. They are saying that if we wait for the CD4 count to get low, then a lot of people will keep dying because they will be thinking of their status. Better to have the ARVs working on their body. Also, sometimes when they tell people, 'Go to the hospital for a CD4 count checkup,' they never go. So they decided that if you are HIV positive you should start taking ARVs right away. I learned a lot about HIV while going to collect ARVs for myself and my two girls."

She said that she feels bad[3] because her husband didn't think of how the kids would be affected or about who would take care of them when he dies. "I am managing through the business that I am doing, and that's why I don't sit around at home. I go to the market to sell different things." Things have gotten better since the government abolished primary school fees. But recently the kids were told to pay 950 kwacha per month for projects at school, and that caused an uproar because people thought the government was asking the primary school students to pay fees. She said she has another child in secondary school and is starting to worry about how is she going to manage to pay for all the kids once they move from primary to secondary school.

After escorting her home, I turned back, and she said, "Thanks for a good chat, let me cook for my kids before they come back from school."

When I reached home, Father of Stella got angry with me and asked why I escorted that neighbor, and I told him, "She's my friend, that's why."

"So, are you the one who told her that she can fetch water here at my compound?"

I said, "No. I didn't." And I went inside.

This is what certainty about HIV looks like in Balaka: a known infection, unambiguous, acknowledged, well managed, and unfettered by stigma or shame.

After being shouted at rudely while trying to meet a basic need for water, Blessings vents her frustration to a friendlier face she has seen a few times before: "What a jerk; must be his meds." At first, the jab seems discriminatory. But she goes on to share more, that she is infected, affected, and how. Her husband is dead. Her small children were born HIV positive just months before single-dose nevirapine became widely available in this district. Her older daughter is living with HIV—contracted through a different route of transmission—and just gave birth to a healthy baby thanks to the recent policy shifts that prioritize HIV-positive mothers. Blessings's openness about her HIV status is striking, and her description of the policy changes is astoundingly accurate. By navigating the treatment possibilities for herself and her children over the course of a decade, this woman has become a bona fide expert.

This narration of policy changes with respect to HIV treatment led Blessings straight into a discussion of her other worries, specifically, the burden of surprise school fees. We see that even for an HIV-positive woman caring for two HIV-positive kids, HIV is just one layer of the difficulties she is facing. Talk about HIV is readily woven into everyday interactions, but in this conversation the water shortage and the school fees are Blessings's pressing complaints. Heard and interpreted as population chatter, the personal and policy-level information about HIV flows easily between newly acquainted women as they go about the mundane work of fetching water and share an eye roll at an irascible man.

Bitten While Breastfeeding

A similarly casual discussion of life's trials and tribulations occurs when a woman is unsure of her HIV status. Gertrude's conversations with other women usually take place while they are engaged in some kind of domestic pursuit, such as fetching water, frying donuts, shelling peas, and sorting hair. In this vignette, Gertrude sets out to meet Tiyamike, a gifted hair stylist who is getting started as an entrepreneur. Gertrude goes to a nearby compound to assist Tiyamike with her first paying client, Linda. Like Gertrude, Linda is new to Balaka, having relocated from Blantyre.

> When I got to the compound, I found Tiyamike, who had already started braiding Linda's hair. As we were braiding her hair, a child started crying, and Linda asked me to go and get the child from inside the house. I asked, "Is this your child?" She said, "Yes, but my husband stays in Blantyre. We divorced." Linda said that she finished secondary school and got married right after that, but the relationship started when she was in form two [second year of secondary school]. "My marriage ended while I was pregnant with this child because my husband had a lot of girlfriends. He's handsome, so women were just accepting him whenever he asked, and when we quarreled, he would even brag that no woman can ignore him because he is so handsome. After I left the house, he got married immediately, but that marriage also ended. The only good thing from that relationship was that when he had money, he was generous. He is still there working in Blantyre, but he doesn't come to see the child."

Then Linda continued, "My child looks abnormal because I stayed in labor pain for 3 days before the child was born, and the nurses forced me to deliver, and when the baby came out she didn't even cry. The nurses tried their best to make the child cry."

I said, "Where was she born?"

"Queen Elizabeth, Blantyre.[4] The child is 18 months, but she is unable to walk. She doesn't even speak. And the child has been getting ill often. But my husband doesn't care; he left all the responsibility with me, and I am now staying with my sister who works here in Balaka. She encourages me not to go back to him. After he and I split, he got remarried but divorced again. Now he wants me back. He's been calling me and asking me to return, but as of now I am applying for different jobs so that I can work and take care of the child. Before we got married my husband had impregnated another girl. His parents didn't like her because she was very, very rude. My in-laws were happy when he got married to me. I was the one taking care of her child. That one started prostitution and just left the child with my mother-in-law. When we were first together I was not getting pregnant quickly because I wanted to see if he would indeed marry me, and only after we got married is when I became pregnant. The other mother, the one who was prostituting, she died recently in a horrible car accident."[5]

"When did you get married?"

Linda said "2012." She said she was using injections[6] to prevent the pregnancy at first.

I asked, "Did you agree with your boyfriend to use injections?"

She said, "No, I was just doing it on my own."

Then Linda's child cried again, and Linda started breastfeeding her. As she was breastfeeding, the child bit her. Linda winced and corrected the child, saying, "Don't you bite me because I might be HIV positive."

"Why do you think that?" I asked.

"I have slept with different men without a condom, and I went for HIV testing when I was pregnant for this child, but that was in 2013, and since then I haven't gone for testing again."

"Why not just stop breastfeeding if you have doubts about yourself?"

"I will stop breastfeeding her when she's 2 years old, but now she is too young."

After braiding, Linda paid 1,000 MK to Tiyamike. To me, she said, "Thanks a lot for chatting and being friendly."

I said, "Thanks a lot for knowing each other." Then her sister came back from work. She came with her husband, and we just greeted each other and said goodbye.

In contrast to the previous exchange, this vignette provides a clear example of what HIV-related uncertainty looks and sounds like. "Don't you bite me because I might be HIV positive" communicates a genuine and accurate concern about mother-to-child transmission (through blood and/or breast-milk) on the part of a woman who does not know her current status. Linda articulates her uncertainty as an aside and expresses it as a light annoyance. Given the testing protocols of 2015 and the fact that she gave birth at the best hospital in the country, we can deduce that Linda's last HIV test is about 18 months old. She is forthcoming about having had unprotected sex with a few partners and, if she were disclosing this information to a health practitioner, she would be recommended for a retest that same day.

But Linda is not panicked about her HIV status. Her uncertainty is ex-pressed matter-of-factly, to her baby and (audibly) in the company of strang-ers. It may be something she has grown used to. Linda may not presume that this uncertainty is shared by Gertrude, but she definitely presumes that that "might be" will be understood, rather than judged, by her interlocutor. An implicit, declarative, woman-to-woman, "You know what I mean . . . ," colors the whole exchange. The pressing issues truly bothering Linda are the other uncertainties she complains about: the developmental delays she's observing as her child grows, the tempestuous relationship with her former husband, her responsibilities to his kin, her livelihood concerns, her desire for indepen-dence, and her self-consciousness about relying on her sister and brother-in-law. In this way, Linda's overall disposition closely resembles that of Blessings, whose HIV status entered the exchange as a noteworthy, not a crucial, detail. In sum, Linda is unambiguous in her articulation of AIDS-related uncer-tainty, which I argue has consequences for her health, her relationships, and her decision making writ large. But this uncertainty ranks lower than other matters, because everything else is more urgent. Linda reminds us about the paradox of HIV: while looming, threatening, and still deadly, it is no big deal in comparison to all the rest of life's concerns.

Beans: A Flexible Tool for Gauging Subjective Probability

Scholars working across disciplines and literatures invoke the concept of un-certainty regularly, but it to be leveraged without much clarity and almost no empirical ambition. I argue here that uncertainty about HIV is a distinct and important feature of the epidemic that has not yet been treated seriously by previous research. In contrast to those who consider uncertainty immeasur-able, I insist that uncertainty can be examined empirically and that doing so is essential for understanding HIV in Balaka and in other contexts character-ized by generalized epidemics today. How, then, do we go about measuring it?

My key measures for studying uncertainty are derived from a section of the TLT questionnaire that was designed to gauge each individual's perceived likelihood of risk using an interactive solicitation method in which respondents were given a cup containing ten white beans and an empty plate and asked to move onto the plate the number of beans that best represents the likelihood of a certain thing happening. Naturally, we did not begin the interview by asking respondents about sensitive issues using terms like "probability" and "likelihood." In fact, the Chichewa language contains a variety of terms for risk, hazards, and possibility, but the notion of chance in probabilistic terms has no direct equivalent.

A little more than halfway through the first TLT survey, we introduced a section that moved away from the standard question-and-answer format that characterizes most survey research and engaged our respondents by having them answer these questions interactively—more like a game than a conversation or a quiz. Each interviewer started the section by giving a long instruction explaining the gist:

> I would like to ask you questions about the [probability/chance/likelihood] that certain things will happen. There are ten beans in this cup. I will ask you to pick some of the beans and put them in the plate. The number of beans that you are going to put in the plate will reflect the probability that something will happen. One bean means there is very little chance that something will happen. If you do not put any bean in the plate it means you are certain that there is no likelihood that something will happen. If you put additional beans in the plate it means the chance that something will happen will also increase. For example, if you put one or two beans in the plate, it means there is little chance that something will happen. Even though there is little chance, that something could happen. If you put five beans it means there is equal chance that something happening or not. If you put six beans it means the chance that something will happen is slightly greater than not happening. If you put all ten beans, it means you are certain that whatever the case something will really happen. There is no wrong or right answer. I just want to know what you think.[7]

We then asked about simple things like going to the market: "Pick the number of beans that reflects how likely you think it is that you will go to the market at least once within the next two days. Within the next two weeks?" Zero beans means there is no chance of a stop at the market; ten beans, certainty of a visit to the market; and five beans, a scenario everybody recognizes as fifty-fifty. For our research, we did not actually care about the likelihood of anybody going shopping within two days or within two weeks, but these warm-up questions helped us ensure some of the quality standards survey researchers hold dear: comparability, reliability, and validity. In each interview, the interviewer took some time to confirm that the respondent truly understood the exercise and the notion of probability. The likelihood of going to the market within two weeks has to be greater than it is for a two-day window. Just a few respondents had a difficult time understanding it at first. In these cases, our interviewers also ticked boxes to flag for data analysts that this was the case. These indicators can be extremely useful for analyses. Respondents who give probabilistic answers that make little sense or contradict the answers they gave in other portions of the survey can be examined more closely by education level or by the interviewer's assessment of whether this section was challenging to administer.

From the shopping scenarios, we moved on to games: "Pick the number of beans that reflects how likely you think it is that you will win if we play a game of Bawo after this interview." Bawo is a mancala-style count-and-capture game often referred to as "African chess."[8] Like chess, bawo is a game of strategy and skill; almost everyone knows how to play it, and it is taken seriously. Both male and female respondents thought they could eke out narrow victories over the TLT interviewers, placing (on average) 5.5 and 5.3 beans, respectively. These interactions tended to generate lots of laughter between interviewers and respondents and helped build rapport and provide a break in the very long conversation underpinning the TLT survey (each visit lasted between one and a half and two hours).

After making sure the respondent understood the exercise and asking about simple and straightforward events that may or may not occur along specified time horizons, the interviewer moved to questions about more sensitive issues. Interested in economic transfers within the family network, we asked about the likelihood that the respondent would have to provide financial assistance to kin in the coming year or, conversely, receive it from others. Beans questions designed to gauge relationship stability asked whether one would still be with the current partner a year from now and sometimes revealed surprising levels of pessimism or ambivalence about ongoing relationships.

To estimate uncertainty related to HIV, I leverage a series of three questions designed to measure precisely this: "Pick the number of beans that reflects how likely it is that (a) you are infected with HIV right now, (b) you will become infected with HIV during the next 12 months, and (c) you will become infected with HIV during your lifetime." If a respondent put ten beans on the plate, indicating she was certain of infection at any one of these points in time, there was no need to ask the question along expanded time horizons. The interviewer stopped the HIV questions there and moved on to the next topic, also using beans.

The beans measures are useful for a few reasons. Most important, our interviewers loved it. Asking randomly selected people pages and pages of invasive questions about sensitive issues with respect to nearly every aspect of their life is a difficult job. In addition to asking about HIV, we collected full pregnancy histories from women, which in a context of high mortality involves documenting the deaths of children, recounting miscarriages and stillbirths, and explaining the suffering that accompanies infertility. We collected marital histories and, through these, listened to countless stories of love, betrayal, and loss. Our interviewers told us that respondents were able to relax during the beans section. And when we held our debriefing meetings at the end of each day, our interviewers often emphasized the extent to which the beans method was a kindness; it allowed respondents to stay quiet and share sensitivities, fears, and realities without having to say difficult things aloud. Some respondents dealt with the beans solemnly, putting their heads down and "playing" through the entire section without ever engaging the interviewer with words and without making eye contact. Others chatted throughout the series of fifty-nine questions, narrating their answers with stories, some dark and some hilarious.

Shifting from the interviewer's experience to data quality, from my first, cursory examination of these data, it was immediately clear that they are more complete than the alternatives. A high-quality survey fielded in 2009 in Mozambique asked women (ages 15–44) about their perceived likelihood of infection: "Many things can happen in the future, but in your opinion, do you think that in two years from now, is it very likely, little likely, or almost impossible that you will be infected with AIDS virus?" Five percent of women responded "very likely"; 25 percent, "not likely"; 11 percent, "almost impossible"; and 58 percent did not know or could not answer the question.[9] Likert-style questions about the likelihood of HIV risk fielded in three districts of rural Malawi between 2001 and 2010 reliably produced 15 percent nonresponse in large samples (i.e., the respondent refused to answer or said "don't know").[10] In contrast, at our baseline interview only three (of more than 2,500) respondents, using beans, failed to answer our question about their current likelihood of infection. While no measure is perfect, these measures are strong in that they are valid, reliable, and flexible.[11]

Sara and I validated the beans approach to measuring current infection in the first paper we published using the TLT data. We examined its predictive power vis-à-vis HIV biomarker data collected from a subset of TLT respondents immediately following their first survey.[12] We also compared the performance of the beans measure to another commonly used subjective measure: "How worried are you about HIV?" Indeed, HIV prevalence in the tested subsample tracked closely across the spectrum of beans, and while the same, positive relationship was observed for the more general "worry question," the relationship is much weaker and the correspondence less precise.

The beans measures are reliable in that, to the best of our knowledge, respondents answer consistently regardless of who is asking, and the answers tend to be internally consistent—both within the questionnaire and when compared to other aspects of the survey. To paraphrase Charles Manski's conclusion about subjective probability measurement in US-based survey research, the measures work.[13] Women who report high likelihoods of current infection (unconfirmed) also report having recently experienced some significant weight loss or some of the other symptoms of poor health we often associated with advanced HIV infections. In contrast, women who report no and very low levels of risk tend to have had few sexual partners in their lifetimes and when we asked them about the quality of their romantic relationships, articulate high levels of trust in their primary partner. On several occasions, respondents who initially reported few sexual partners (just one or two) and then disclosed a high likelihood sometimes went back and revised their answers to the sexual behavior section, offering interviewers a "truer" version of their sexual history than the one they had led with.

Finally, the beans measures are flexible in that researchers can analyze them in a wide variety of ways. One can use the beans distribution to categorize respondents along a gradient of perceived risk that maps onto the standard Likert scale response categories (i.e., no-risk, low-risk, medium-risk, or high-risk), unfettered by the missing data problem generated by other approaches. One can impose a simple, stark distinction between those who think of themselves as insulated from the epidemic (zero beans) and everyone else. Or one can use them to differentiate those who know they have HIV (ten beans) from those who are anything other than certain. Or one can choose not to commit to any one of these approaches but rather approach the data with the objective of examining it from multiple angles, rotating it regularly to see what unique insight becomes visible from each new view.

To demonstrate the scope of HIV uncertainty, I analyze the longitudinal data using models designed to estimate how long, on average, it takes for things that sometimes happen to happen.[14] Hazard models were originally developed in the 1970s to measure mortality, estimating time to death as an interpretable rate. Since then, hazard models have been adapted to examine phenomena that are neither universal nor inevitable: time to first birth or first marriage, time to an HIV infection or to a cancer recurrence. Here I use hazard models to estimate HIV incidence (i.e., new infections) in the TLT cohort before leveraging the tool for a less traditional purpose, namely, to show how

long young men and women in Balaka "survive" until experiencing either
acute uncertainty or any uncertainty about HIV.

HIV Uncertainty: The Initial Snapshot from 2009

Grounded in the basic facts about the arc of Malawi's AIDS epidemic outlined
in chapter 2 and, specifically, the age- and sex-specific prevalence estimates
described in chapter 1, I begin an exploration of the epidemic in subjective
terms. How do people living in the middle of an ongoing epidemic assess
their status? How do they perceive the landscape of risk that surrounds them?
How accurate are their assessments? What can we learn about uncertainty by
taking and treating subjective views seriously?

The cross-sectional view, taken at a single point in time in summer 2009,
provides the starting point. Figure 4.1 shows the distribution of responses to
the beans questions about HIV infection, asked along three time horizons, for
men and women combined. On the first day of their first interview, a majority
of young adults were confident that they did not have HIV. When asked about
the present moment, over 60 percent put zero beans on their plates. Very
few indicated a known infection by putting ten beans (19 women—about one
percent of the sample—and just one male respondent). Conversely, nearly
40 percent of young adults indicated to us, with beans, some level of uncertainty about their HIV status. Calibrating that figure of 40 percent uncertainty to the amount of HIV in this population (6 percent at the baseline
survey), this cross-sectional view provides our first glimpse of what I refer to
as the epidemic of uncertainty.

Importantly, the perceived risk of HIV is a dynamic thing that individuals
assess along distinct time horizons. The picture of perceived risk shifts dramatically when we asked respondents to use one year from now as their frame
of reference. As is clear from the second panel of figure 4.1, the proportion of
people putting zero beans on the plate dropped by 20 percentage points. The
proportion of respondents who anticipated infection (with certainty) rose to
just under 4 percent, and, as a consequence, our estimate of prospective uncertainty rises to about 60 percent. In response to questions about the lifetime
probability of infection, five beans—a fifty-fifty proposition—is the modal
answer, and a state of uncertainty (between one and nine beans) characterizes 80 percent of the sample.[15] Again, calibrating 60 percent uncertainty on a
one-year time horizon to prevalence among women 25 to 29, which stands at
about 8 percent, the epidemic of uncertainty looms large, both in magnitude
and as a proportion.

There is, of course, no conversion formula for translating the prevalence

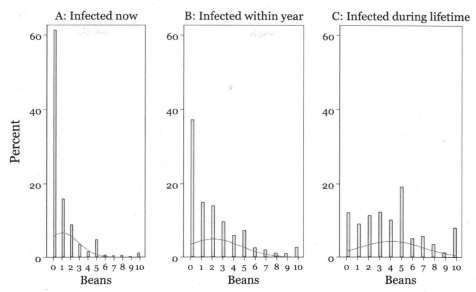

FIGURE 4.1 Perceived likelihood of HIV infection among young adults (ages 15–25) in Balaka, 2009

Source: TLT-1, wave 1.

Note: This figure is substantively identical to figure 1 in Trinitapoli and Yeatman 2011.

of a condition into a measure of the uncertainty that surrounds it. But this simple, descriptive, snapshot view shows us that at 6 percent HIV prevalence, almost 40 percent of the population believes, at the moment the question is posed to them, that they could be infected. Despite the fact that prevalence in this population has never exceeded 15 percent of the adult population in Malawi, nearly half of respondents think that they are more likely than not to become infected during their lifetime (see fig. 4.1). This snapshot of risk perceptions, capturing a single point in time, helps situate Linda's experience within the larger population and approximate uncertainty to capture the *reach* of the epidemic in ways that extend beyond prevalence, incidence, mortality, and even the caregiving burden. Some state of not-knowing defined a sizable minority of the population at the moment we first met them and nearly saturates the population when young adults were asked to reflect on what the future holds. HIV uncertainty is a condition that affects far more of the population than will ever be directly affected by the virus itself.

Uncertainty Prospectively (2009–2011)

Asking young people to think and speculate about their HIV status, present and future, provides a new perspective on the epidemic. At any given point in time we can compare the reach of uncertainty to the traditional epidemiological measures, like prevalence and incidence. Even more powerful is the dynamic, prospective view. Repeated measures of these same questions—asked in exactly the same way during each subsequent visit to the TLT research center—allow us to track risk and uncertainty in this population as these unfold over the three-year period. I analyze the data on two levels: the macro-societal level, with an eye to metrics of prevalence and population-based concerns, and the micro-individual level, with an eye to the factors and events that instigate, exacerbate, and abate uncertainty and risk for individuals as they move through the challenges of young adulthood.

Figure 4.2 depicts five analytically crucial groups for situating uncertainty and understanding how I operationalize the concept using the beans measures. The key insight is locating uncertainty (i.e., not knowing) along a linear spectrum of "risk." Imagine grabbing the likelihood scale by its middle and yanking it up to isolate the experience of *acute uncertainty*. Acute uncertainty includes respondents who placed four, five, or six beans when asked the question, "How likely is it that you are infected with HIV right now?" A broader definition of uncertainty includes those who indicate *any uncertainty* about their current status—any answer between one and nine beans. The phenomenon of *vulnerability* relates to risk and overlaps with uncertainty (its similar and distinctive features are discussed in greater length in chapter 8).

Two varieties of certainty characterize the poles of figure 4.2. The *insulated* population is defined as those who place zero beans, confident of their seronegative status and unaffected by HIV uncertainty. At the other end of the spectrum are those who report a *known infection* using ten beans. Both

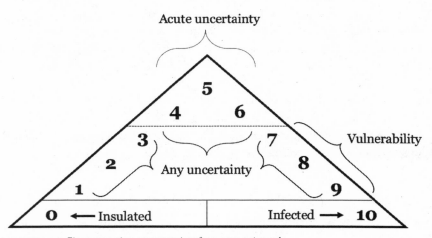

FIGURE 4.2 Five perspectives on uncertainty from a ten-point scale

certainties are defined by individually measured perceptions, which may or may not be clinically accurate. As stated in chapter 1, the Thomas theorem would prioritize perceptions of HIV status over any clinical measure, treating perceived infections as fully "real." The empirical contributions of the analyses presented in this book rest on two subtle analytic moves for estimating the HIV epidemic and its consequences: (1) privileging perceived status over serostatus without denying the existence of a biological reality and (2) disturbing long-standing assumptions about HIV status as a clinical binary by spotlighting the state of being uncertain. Centering uncertainty adds a whole new dimension to the portrait typically composed of the standard metrics: prevalence, incidence, and mortality (as in fig. 2.2).

To illustrate, let us look at three respondents—Miriam, Promise, and Sophie—each of whom occupies different areas of the uncertainty pyramid over the course of the TLT study (see table 4.1). Miriam placed five beans on the plate when asked about her current HIV status at wave 1, and she received a negative result from the HIV test at wave 1. During wave 2, Miriam gave the same answer about her current HIV status (still uncertain) and got the same test result: negative. Not shown in the table is the fact that during wave 2 Miriam suspected she might be pregnant and that pregnancy was confirmed at the research center with an HgC urine test. Following the recommendations, Miriam attended antenatal care later that month. When she was tested for HIV at ANC (a standard procedure), Miriam learned that she had contracted HIV and began to receive ART through the Option B+ program to

TABLE 4.1 Data structure for three cases

	Miriam		Promise		Sophie	
Wave	Perceived	Biomarker	Perceived	Biomarker	Perceived	Biomarker
1	5	–	2	–	0	–
2	5	–	3	–	0	–
3	10	+	.m	.m	0	–
4	10	.c	.m	.m	0	–
5	10	.c	.m	.m	0	–
6	10	.c	.m	.m	0	–
7	10	.c	9	–	0	–
8	10	.c	8	–	0	–

Note: The biomarker notation is as follows: – indicates seronegative; + indicates seropositive; .c is censored such that the test result can be inferred from the previous biomarker data point but was not gathered directly; .m is missing such that it cannot be inferred in real time but can be backfilled by analysts if a later result is negative.

avoid transmitting the virus to her baby. In wave 3 Miriam contributes both a perceived infection and a confirmed infection to our estimates—"perceived" because she placed ten beans on the plate when asked about her status and "confirmed" because she agreed to be tested again at TLT so that we could document her status. Miriam is affected by HIV in multiple ways: she experiences acute uncertainty, she becomes infected, and she perceives that infection as a certainty, moving between the peak and the right-hand corners of the pyramid.

Like Miriam, Promise communicated uncertainty when she first began the study, placing two and three beans during waves 1 and 2, respectively. During waves 3–6 she had migrated to South Africa for work and missed several interviews. When Promise returned to Balaka to visit her family in mid-2011, her perceived risk had increased markedly: she placed nine, then eight beans on the plate. Despite the elevated risk she expressed as a return migrant, Promise tested negative at wave 8, contributing four waves of "any uncertainty" and no HIV infection (clinical or perceived) to the analyses that follow.

Of the three, only Sophie contributes a full eight waves of certainty to the TLT data set, consistently locating herself in the left-hand corner of our uncertainty pyramid. Sophie is unusual in feeling insulated from the epidemic throughout three years of young adulthood. Although Sophie knows many people who have died of HIV and lives with a man in an ongoing sexual relationship, she *knows* that she is negative.

LEVELS OVER TIME: REPEATED CROSS SECTIONS

The TLT data enable us to study HIV simultaneously in epidemiological and experiential terms and to do so over time for this cohort of young adults as they move through an especially vulnerable period of the life course. A first step in expanding this view is plotting the data at each wave to identify salient patterns and emerging trends. Figure 4.3 depicts the results, cross-sectionally, for all eight waves of data, using the randomly selected subsample from whom we collected HIV biomarker data at every wave.

Population prevalence is a standard measure for any epidemic. The rising line for the HIV biomarker data represents the prevalence of confirmed HIV infections in the population and underscores just how perilous this period of the life course truly is in this part of the world. While HIV prevalence among young men stayed stable over the study period, at about 2 percent, in just thirty-two months, prevalence among young women doubled—from 6 to 12 percent.

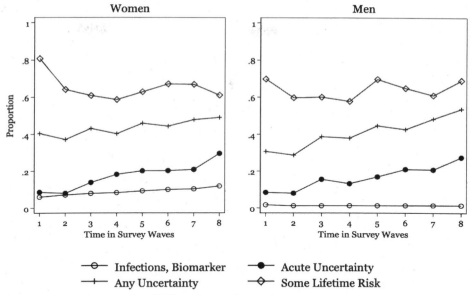

FIGURE 4.3 Aggregate view of HIV prevalence and uncertainty, 2009–2011

Source: TLT-1, waves 1–8.

The doubling of HIV prevalence in a population over a three-year period is arresting. But figure 4.3 shifts the lens by indexing the prevalence trend (focus on the virus) to the epidemic of uncertainty. I focus again on the subset of respondents who received HIV testing and counseling once every four months from 2009 to 2011, and I present the results separately for men and women. We already saw the ratio of actual HIV to any uncertainty about it in the first cross section: 6 to 40 percent for women in 2009. This ratio is remarkably stable over the study period. Acute uncertainty (measured contemporaneously, four to six beans, and depicted with solid black circles) rises moderately over time, while the prevalence of any uncertainty (between one and nine beans) hovers at around 40 percent throughout the study period. The proportion of young adults who perceive any vulnerability—at least one bean on any of the three time horizons—declines after the first interview and then stabilizes at around 60 percent. These levels of uncertainty persist in this population in the face of the highest-frequency testing regime that has, to my knowledge, ever been imposed on a nonclinical, population-based sample. Among men of the same age, the overall pattern is similar: although HIV prevalence is low (less than 2 percent), both acute and any uncertainty exhibit a clear climbing pattern over time.

Although young men and women in Balaka may not know the exact facts about the age-specific infection rates in the same way demographers do, they *perceive* this period of the life course as dangerous, and this sense of danger swells as they move through young adulthood. The repeated cross-section view shows both change and stability in Balaka's epidemic over the three-year period. We see simultaneously the severity of the epidemic through the magnitude of rising HIV prevalence among women, the extent to which prevalence pales in comparison to the uncertainty that characterizes this population, and the relative symmetry in the subjective estimates over the three-year period for both men and women. We begin to see Balaka's HIV epidemic as an epidemic of uncertainty.

SHIFT TO A SURVIVAL FRAMEWORK

HIV is spreading in Balaka, especially among women. Mortality rates for young PLWHA are mercifully low, so the proportion of women living with HIV accrues over time. But what about the uncertain population? Are the same 40 percent of women hovering in a state of uncertainty over this entire period? The same 60-some percent in a state of vulnerability? Or are these groups churning, indicating that the uncertain state is temporary and resolvable? These answers cannot be discerned from the repeated cross sections (prevalence) but can be addressed using individual-level longitudinal data over time to count new cases (incidence). Because the differences between men and women are pronounced, I explore the gendered nature of HIV infections and uncertainty in some detail here.

The lines in figure 4.4 are based on hazard models and represent the rate at which women and men in the TLT study become infected with HIV (measured with a biomarker) and the rate at which they perceive new infections (measured with beans). The lines begin at time 0 (prior to the start of the study) with the entire population of respondents (100 percent) and decline at each wave as individuals become infected. In contrast to ratio measures like prevalence, hazard models calculate rates by introducing an additional important analytic shift to the denominator. Rather than represent HIV-positive individuals as a proportion of the population, using a consistent denominator of individual persons, we represent new HIV infections (events) as a function of time, where each individual's time at risk is pooled across the sample, adjusting for the facts that once infected individuals are no longer at risk of infection and, similarly, that respondents who die or drop out of the study are no longer observed and therefore stop contributing their time to the pool of risk against which the event is calculated.

The left-hand panel of figure 4.4 repeats the knowledge gleaned from the

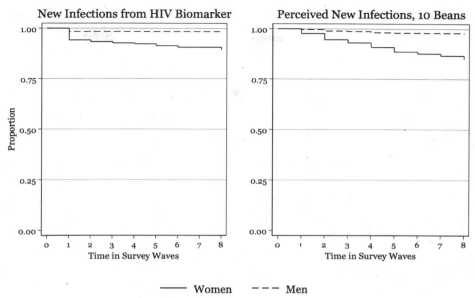

FIGURE 4.4 Incident HIV infection (confirmed and perceived) in the TLT sample, 2009–2011
Source: TLT-1, waves 1–8.

crude, aggregate prevalence measures presented in figure 4.3 but measures it more carefully—as a true rate, a function of time. Though based on a relatively small sample (400–450), our incident rate of 6 per 1,000 is consistent with estimates based on much larger samples and with estimates derived from simulations.[16] The right-hand panel shifts the focus, treating perceived infections (ten beans) as the outcome of interest. In the absence of biomarker data on serostatus, one could use perceived infections to approximate real infections and come away with a pretty accurate view of the landscape. Using perceived infections alone would overestimate the force of HIV in the population (both prevalence and incidence, among both men and women); slightly more people think they have HIV than the proportion who actually test positive, and this is consistent with other research from Malawi showing that in endemic contexts most people overestimate their risk of contracting HIV.[17]

But what about uncertainty? Using data from all eight waves (again, these are four-month intervals), I model the epidemic of uncertainty using the same methods used to calculate an infection rate. I begin with the entire cohort (at time 0) and then, beginning with the first interview (time 1), eliminate each individual who experiences the uncertain state as if it were an "infection" or a "death." What could not be read from the single wave of data presented in figure 4.1 or from the repeated cross-sectional view (fig. 4.3) is now legible

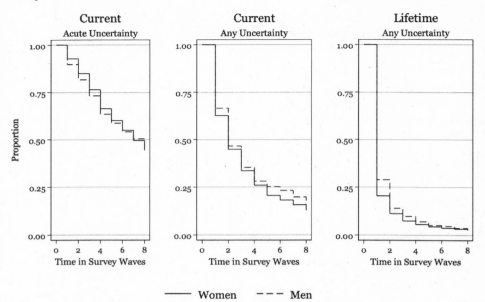

FIGURE 4.5 Incident uncertainty, defined as acute uncertainty or any uncertainty (current and lifetime)

Source: TLT-1, waves 1–8.

in figure 4.5. Balaka is not populated by a small group of worried individuals who are avoiding the clinics and hovering in a state of uncertainty over the three-year period. At baseline, the percentage of women placing between four and six beans is 7 (10 percent of men) and increases steadily throughout the study, characterizing over 20 percent of respondents during the final two waves. The hazard models clarify that a great many people cycle through these states of uncertainty. By the end of the observation period, 50 percent of respondents have spent time in the state of acute uncertainty. And while gender differences in actual infections are pronounced at this stage of the life course, uncertainty is distinct in that it features no difference by gender.

Expanding the definition of uncertainty from acute to any necessarily produces a steeper hazard function. Even so, when I define uncertainty as between one and nine beans, the magnitude is dramatic. Less than 20 percent of the sample "survives" the three-year period knowing their HIV status confidently throughout this portion of the study. Importantly, these hazard models are concerned only with respondents' assessments of their current likelihood of infection. Expanding the time horizon further to incorporate respondents' prospective views of infection in the coming year during their lifetime, exactly 34 respondents—21 women (of 1,500, including Sophie) and 13 men (of 600)—survive, managing to completely avoid uncertainty over the course of the three years. Statistically speaking, nobody gets through the period without being affected by HIV uncertainty.[18]

The Remarkable Consistency of Uncertainty, 2012–2019

To make one final point about the gravity of HIV uncertainty in Balaka, I emphasize the persistence of uncertainty in the aggregate over the course of a decade: there is an astonishing consistency of uncertain responses to questions about HIV risk over a ten-year period characterized by change. On a personal level, individuals are experiencing marriages, births, divorces, new partners, explicable and inexplicable fluctuations in health, and turns of fortune. As those life course transitions unfold, HIV mortality is declining, treatment options are expanding, child survival is improving, new people are migrating to Balaka, and the town is growing. However, figure 4.6 shows that when examined at four points in time, the story of uncertainty changes only once: as the youngest respondents age out of adolescence. From there, it hardly budges. In 2009 only half of our respondents are married. Perceptions

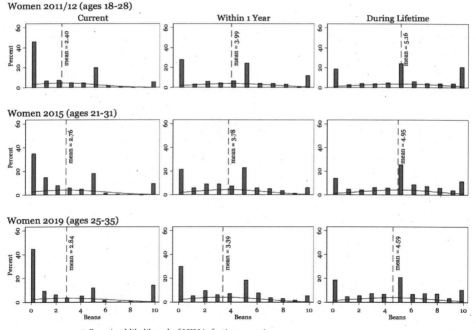

FIGURE 4.6 Perceived likelihood of HIV infection over time

Source: TLT-1 (wave 8), TLT-2, and TLT-3.

of risk currently and in the coming year are fairly low, though mean level of lifetime risk is a little higher than four beans. By the time the first phase of the study has ended, 80 percent are married. Current levels of risk rise to two or three beans, the mean number of beans for infection in the coming year rises to four, and the mean number of beans is five for lifetime risk. Once marriage rates surpass 80 percent, the distribution of responses stays remarkably stable, even as the population ages, over the next seven years. Subjective risk assessments in this sample stay the same in 2015 and 2019.

This underscores the fundamental puzzle of stable rates in a context of change that runs in parallel to insights others have made about fertility. While each and every birth results from a unique set of circumstances for the index woman and couple, the birth rate in any population tends toward stability rather than volatility. So too, it seems, with HIV-related uncertainty in Balaka. The prevalence of uncertainty barely fluctuates from year to year. Despite the facts that testing and treatment have expanded, that AIDS-related mortality and new infections have declined, and that the specifics of Patuma's circumstances are fundamentally distinct from Linda's and from Blessings's, the associated uncertainty has an unexpected solidness—a discernible shape and size. Think of HIV-related uncertainty as the long shadow of the epidemic itself: socially patterned, the product of aggregated personal experiences, but (like other rates and aggregations) a decidedly population-level phenomenon.

Consequences of HIV Uncertainty for Fertility and Health

Beyond this demonstration that HIV uncertainty is prevalent and persistent over time, a key aspect of a demography of uncertainty is the ability to demonstrate that uncertainty is consequential. In fact, I argue that the uncertainty— and not the disease itself—drives much of the chaos and instability AIDS has brought about in affected communities. In Balaka, the consequences of uncertainty are manifest in multiple domains of life. I begin by exploring its impact on fertility and health.

Because TLT was designed and funded to study the relationship between HIV and childbearing, the first phenomenon we examined carefully was the relationship between perceived risk and fertility intentions. Research with Sara Yeatman, published in *American Sociological Review*, showed that perceived risk of HIV influences the intended timing of births for young adults, with people at high risk tending to accelerate their childbearing.[19] In other words, rather than stopping (which is what most of the previous research based on clinical samples had predicted), "at risk" women in the prime of their childbearing years intend to have their babies in a hurry in order to

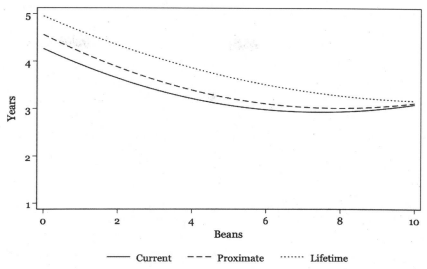

FIGURE 4.7 Desired time to next birth by perceived risk of HIV

Source: TLT-1, wave 1.

Note: This figure is substantively identical to figure 4 in Trinitapoli and Yeatman 2011.

capitalize on an unknown window of good-enough-for-safe-childbearing
health. The central finding of this paper is what led me to turn away from
"perceived risk" and toward uncertainty as the key phenomenon of interest.
This is evident in figure 4.7, which depicts intended time to next birth across
the spectrum of perceived risk (0–10), for men and women combined, net of
a robust set of controls.

The first feature of interest is that the acceleration of childbearing begins
with just one bean—the minimal expression of any uncertainty about one's
HIV status. Second, the acceleration flattens out around peak uncertainty
(theorized between four and six beans). Third, at ten beans, a tiny uptick is
discernible to the eye, but statistical tests tell us not to make much of it as a
"difference." Both conception and infection can result from sex, and these
first analyses were cross-sectional, so the relationship could be operating in
precisely the opposite direction. But this seemed unlikely to us, and as data
collection progressed, I established the causal direction more firmly using
all eight rounds of the closely spaced survey data. Uncertain women want
children sooner, and, indeed, those accelerated preferences are manifest in
actual births one and two years later.[20] Sarah Hayford, Victor Agadjanian,
and Luciana Luz discovered a similar pattern among women in rural Mozambique and dubbed it the "now or never" approach to childbearing. In the face

of uncertain health and an uncertain future, for women concerned with HIV, the best time to have a/another child is right now.[21]

Linking these findings about HIV to an even larger conversation about uncertainty and fertility, the acceleration we observe seems to be part of something far more general. Other studies from around the world have connected existential uncertainty due to other environmental stressors—violence, short life expectancy, and natural disasters—to early or accelerated childbearing. Extremely careful analyses point to fertility acceleration as an uncertainty response among young women in Chicago during the 1990s as a response to violence, among a sample of disadvantaged young women in metro Detroit from 2000 to 2014 (also homicides), in Russia and Eastern Europe during the economic crisis, and in Indonesia in response to the Indian Ocean tsunami of 2004.[22] So while our specific empirical case here is HIV uncertainty and its relationships to childbearing, placed in conversation with a broader literature about fertility, the force of uncertainty seems to be part of a more general phenomenon.[23]

Fertility preferences were the starting point from which to ascertain that uncertainty may be a distinctive state. From these analyses it seems that being uncertain is, in some ways, similar to being HIV positive. In continuing this work, I have become convinced that uncertainty is its own distinctive and consequential state—a state that merits much more attention than it has received to date. Beyond fertility, consider how physical and mental health is patterned along the spectrum of perceived risk. I selected four outcomes health researchers deem important: self-rated health, days of school/work missed due to illness in the past month, a depression measure constructed from three commonly asked questions, and a global measure of overall life satisfaction.[24] Figure 4.8 depicts what we would learn if we took the typical approach of searching for differences in the Balaka population along the lines of known serostatus. For all four outcomes, and this should not surprise anyone, individuals who identify as HIV positive (placing ten beans) are disadvantaged. The results are identical when we use the biomarker data, rather than a self-report, to distinguish the seropositive and seronegative groups.[25] Compared to those who test negative for HIV, people living with HIV have lower levels of self-rated health, miss more days of work and school, have higher depression scores, and perhaps slightly lower levels of overall life satisfaction.

When we center uncertainty in our analyses and design our models around the sizable proportion of respondents who tell us they don't know their HIV status, we gain new insights that are far less predictable. Just as we did with fertility timing, figure 4.9 presents the standardized values across the

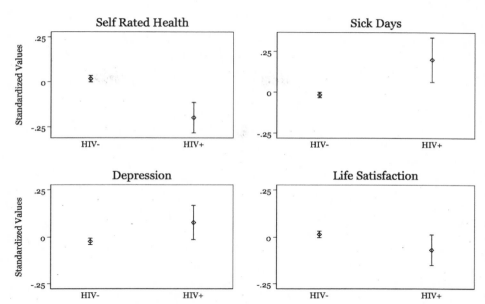

FIGURE 4.8 Predicted values (standardized) for four health outcomes by HIV serostatus

Source: TLT-1, waves 1–8.

Note: All four outcomes are standardized; the y-axis can be interpreted as deviation from the mean.

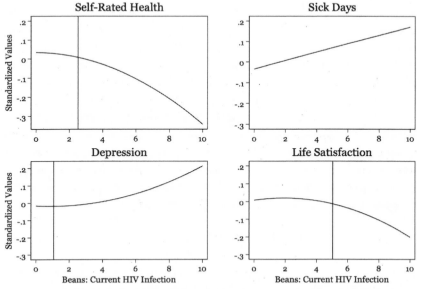

FIGURE 4.9 Predicted values (standardized) for four health outcomes along the HIV-risk spectrum

Source: TLT-1, waves 1–8.

Note: All four outcomes are standardized; the y-axis can be interpreted as deviation from the mean.

spectrum of HIV risk, measured with beans. We are interested here in at least three things: the general shape of the relationship, the severity of the gradient, and the statistical "tipping point"—the threshold at which values begin to diverge in a statistically significant way. The tipping points are generated by the data, rather than by theoretical intuition, and are marked with vertical lines.

Let's take the four panels one by one. Self-rated health follows a downward-sloping curve, with a threshold at about two beans. Respondents who place two or three beans on the plate have significantly worse health than those who assess their risk at zero or one, and the gradient declines precipitously between two and ten. In contrast to the declining curve, morbidity measured by days of work or school missed because of illness follows a strong, linear relationship with HIV risk, with the full difference between one and ten amounting to about one full day of work. Turning to mental health, I follow the conventions of mental health researchers who recommend that positive and negative mental health be measured as independent constructs. Depression follows a steep, positive, J-shaped curve, which turns at one bean—the expression of any uncertainty—and continues to increase along the spectrum of HIV risk. Conversely, overall life satisfaction follows a downward-sloping curve that tips at peak uncertainty (five beans) and declines from there.

One could, of course, enumerate the significance levels at every gradient point for all four outcomes in pettifogging detail. While such an exercise may hold some value for a niche audience of specialists, it is unnecessary for our more general purpose of understanding that HIV uncertainty influences health. The crucial point about the consequences of uncertainty is apparent from the three features: shape, slope, and threshold. If we think about HIV as an individual-level phenomenon, characterized by the presence or absence of a specific virus in one's bloodstream, we neglect the experience of those who don't know their HIV status. Along the lines of fertility and health, a binary view of the relationship between HIV status and health is likely to mislead us by suggesting that there is some kind of real "difference" between those who are knowingly living with HIV and the rest of the population, when in actuality the consequences of HIV manifest independently of the virus and are often expressed at key thresholds of uncertainty.

Not Knowing: A Pervasive and Distinctive State

This chapter uses theories of uncertainty and tools from demography to braid together three views of the epidemic: an ethnographic view of HIV certainty and uncertainty through two examples of population chatter, an epidemiological portrait of rising HIV prevalence, and a demographic analysis of the uncertainty young adults in Balaka experience as the events of young adulthood unfold. The patterns of infection identified in the TLT study align closely with estimates generated by other high-quality studies in the region,[26] and they confirm a fact that has been established for nearly two decades: early adulthood is the most perilous period of the life course for young women.[27] During their peak childbearing years, in particular, women are at heightened risk for contracting HIV. Even though the infection rate has been steadily declining since 2004, new cases of HIV are rising in this population. Stated in proportional terms, we observe a doubling of HIV prevalence (from 6 to 12 percent) in just three years.

The novel contribution here is not the careful measurement of HIV through biomarker data but a population-based view of how the epidemic is experienced. Even in a high-prevalence context and even during this very vulnerable time, most young adults do not have and will not contract HIV. Subjective assessments of risk in this population, however, far outpace even the most pessimistic forecasts for HIV prevalence, and this is true for the present, for the near future (the coming year), and for the long run (one's lifetime). Beyond the distinctions that can be made based on HIV status (infected vs. uninfected), and the accompanying levels of risk in the population, based on subjective probabilities (high, medium, low, or 0–10), this chapter quantifies the experience of uncertainty about HIV within this population. Unlike either being infected or thinking that one is infected (accuracy aside), uncertainty—the state of not knowing one's HIV status—is a prevalent and distinctive state. Linda's words to her nursing baby give us a clear example of what this uncertainty sounds like in everyday conversation. It is neither panicked nor pressing but a bother, one that's entangled with other kinds of uncertainties, addressed at greater length in chapter 6 on romantic relationships and chapter 8 on mortality.

Whether we define uncertainty as truly not knowing one's serostatus (fifty-fifty) or as having some uncertainty about it (perhaps just a shade of a doubt), uncertainty is an overwhelming force in this population. At epidemic levels of just 6 percent, nearly 50 percent experience at least a moment of acute uncertainty about their HIV status, and over 80 percent experience a period of some uncertainty. Not knowing is pervasive. Unlike HIV, uncertainty cycles through the population as a state that people move into and out of, and it is not a condition that afflicts one particular subset of the population (i.e., a "worrier class"). While HIV prevalence and incidence are markedly patterned by age and by sex, the accompanying epidemic of uncertainty affects men and women about equally. And when we prioritize uncertainty analytically, we can begin to see how its consequences are manifest in the real world. In some cases, those who don't know their status are more similar to those who live with a confirmed or suspected infection. For example, with respect to fertility timing and depression, the crucial distinctions begin with any expression of uncertainty. The differences in self-related health are manifest at a slightly higher threshold, with those experiencing peak uncertainty being more similar to people living with HIV than to those who believe they are (probably) negative. Health and fertility are not the only domains of life in which the force of uncertainty has real consequences, but they are crucial plot points in individual lives and essential patterns that structure populations. In both, we find concrete evidence that uncertainty shapes people's preferences and behaviors.

Overall, this portrait of magnitude ignites a series of questions about HIV-related uncertainty: Who is uncertain? What are the predictors of uncertainty? What kinds of changes resolve uncertainty for the individuals who are experiencing it? In the next chapter, I treat uncertainty as the outcome, seeking to establish its correlates both cross-sectionally and dynamically, over time.

5

HIV Uncertainty and the Limits of Testing

Know Your Status

Know your status. Get tested.
Get tested. Know your status.

It sounds so simple. Whether stated plainly in conjunction with the iconic red ribbon; or depicted in cleverer instantiations, such as a play on the British "Keep Calm and . . ." meme, painted on a homemade wooden sign in a dusty African village; or delivered with more artistic ambition, the message is unambiguous, and the expectation is reasonable (see fig. 5.1). If one is willing to learn one's status, all it takes is a painless finger prick, a few drops of blood on a rapid-test strip (with the technologies constantly improving in terms of accuracy and speed of the test result), and a few minutes for the test to develop. All it takes is the desire to know. Counselors working for ministries of health, AIDS-related nongovernmental organizations (NGOs), universities, community organizations, and health departments worldwide can test your blood, deliver a diagnosis along with counseling (to process the diagnosis, regardless of outcome),[1] and refer you to treatment and other support services. It takes just thirty minutes. It's easy. As stated in a related campaign, "The risk is not knowing."

This line of thinking underpins the UNAIDS 90–90–90 targets established in 2014. The stated worldwide goal for 2020 was for 90 percent of people with HIV to "be acquainted" with their status, for 90 percent of people with HIV who know their status to be receiving antiretroviral treatment, and for 90 percent of those being treated to reach a state of viral suppression.[2] In other words, thanks to treatment, the infected person's viral load would be what researchers call "U-U," or undetectable and untransmittable, so low that

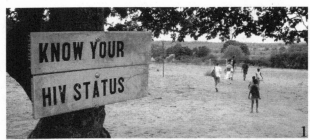
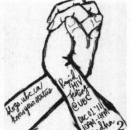
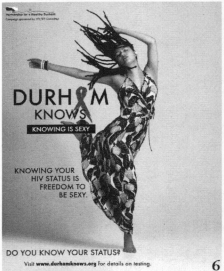
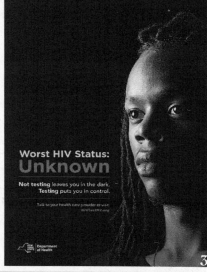
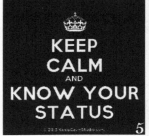
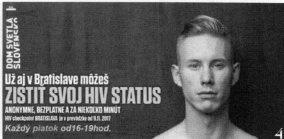

FIGURE 5.1 Examples of "Know Your Status" messaging from five countries

Sources: (1) Photo by Jon Rawlinson, reprinted with permission. (2) Drawing by Paige Zhang, reprinted with permission. (3) Reprinted with permission of the New York State Department of Health. (4) Reprinted with permission of Milos Stefancik on behalf of Lighthouse Civic Association, Slovakia. (5) Reprinted with permission of Keep Calm Studio. (6) Photo by Zach Soberano, reprinted with permission of Partnership for a Healthy Durham.

even unprotected sex does not transmit the virus. The first and most important step toward calm, toward sexiness, toward treatment, toward population health is, by this logic, one and the same: know your status.

The centrality of testing to prevention programs has roots in the health belief model (HBM), a theory developed by US-based public health experts during the 1950s with the goal of better understanding low levels of participation in Public Health Service programs designed to address the issues of the day, especially tuberculosis. The HBM is a value-expectancy theory that seeks to explain puzzles like the following: Why do people avoid screening procedures that detect disease at early stages when treatment is more likely to be effective? Why do they fail to adopt recommended healthy behaviors, such as smoking cessation? For seventy years, the model has traveled far and wide, to other contexts and topics: sunscreen, condoms, seatbelts, pap screening, mammography, and HIV testing. Today, the HBM is the most widely invoked model of health behaviors in the medical literature. It undergirds nearly 200,000 scientific papers on HIV prevention in sub-Saharan Africa and nearly 30,000 papers focused specifically on Malawi.[3] The model predicts that an individual will participate in an action he or she believes will increase the likelihood of a desirable outcome, especially staying healthy or preventing illness. The promotion of voluntary testing for HIV follows this logic: an early diagnosis will link the patient to necessary care and prevent infections to other partners, while a negative result will quell the uncertainty so many people experience and incentivize adherence to prevention strategies. In order to choose the health-promoting behavior, people need to want to know.

For our purposes, "Know your status" raises an empirical question: Does testing eliminate or even abate uncertainty? For anyone looking for a silver bullet, the answer I derive from the TLT data will disappoint: Not really. I come to this conclusion after analyzing the quantitative data in three ways: first, at the aggregate level; second, at the individual level with a focus on within-person change over time (during TLT-1's three-year period of intensive interviewing); and third, by interrogating a period of about forty-five minutes in 2015,[4] during which questions about risk perceptions were asked both shortly before and immediately after HIV testing and counseling had been conducted. Read alongside these quantitative analyses, Gertrude's fieldnotes bring a different kind of evidence to bear on the testing question. What she hears from women who happen to be discussing TLT and testing while going about their morning chores offers more evidence that testing will not resolve HIV uncertainty. While no one piece of evidence should be read as a conclusive answer to questions about the origins of uncertainty, together

these analyses show why biomedical solutions are, and will remain, insuf-
ficient for addressing uncertainty in the context of a generalized epidemic.

Journey to a Culture of Testing

Rapid testing for HIV relies on an ELISA (enzyme-linked immunosorbent as-
say) test, which detects the presence of *antibodies* in blood and saliva samples
(i.e., not the virus itself). Because direct-testing assays are far more expensive
(US$140 vs. US$1 at the time of writing) and take considerably longer to reveal results (two to three days), they are seldom used. The ELISA test is one of
the global health community's most important tools—fast, cheap, sensitive,
specific, and accurate. But ELISA tests are not designed to detect brand-new
infections, so this amazing technology comes with a dilemma clinicians and
HIV researchers refer to as "the window period."

When a person becomes infected with HIV (i.e., *seroconverts*), they are
hyperinfectious, but the virus is not immediately detectable using ELISA as-
say tests. At the outset, newly infected individuals often experience flu-like
symptoms that can easily be confused with malaria or other conditions such
as fever, rash, and body aches.[5] This stage, when the viral load is very high
but antibodies are not yet present, is known as acute HIV infection (AHI). It
lasts for only a few weeks, but during this time the virus spreads extremely
easily through sexual activity. New evidence suggests that as many as 40 percent of new infections are transmitted by persons in the first six months they
are infected. To be absolutely certain of one's status, one needs to get tested
twice—at least twelve weeks apart (though 95 percent of infections can be
detected at four weeks)—and have no exposure to risk in the intervening period.[6] Situated in a generalized epidemic, these facts belie the apparent sim-
plicity of "Know your status."

When we first designed the TLT study, voluntary testing for HIV was still
something of an innovation in Malawi. Tests to detect HIV first became available in the 1990s, but at that time access was severely limited, and a culture
of testing only began to emerge around 2007 or 2008. During the 1990s and
early 2000s, tests could be found in urban areas only, mostly at private health
clinics. Some research centers were able to run assays but clumsily and at great
expense.[7] Around 2005 testing began to expand beyond the large government
hospitals and became available in some rural clinics, but in those days testing
was still a giant hassle. In earlier work about religion and HIV based on data
from 2004 and 2005, I wrote about how testing was a considerable burden on
individuals. A person who wanted to learn their status would have to make
not one but two trips to a testing facility: one to initiate testing and give the

specimen (by finger prick or oral swab), which would then be sent to a lab, and another trip a week or two later to receive their results. For most people in rural areas, this was simply out of reach because of the associated transportation and opportunity costs involved. In a subsistence economy, spending two full days seeking health care meant going without food. In that era of extraordinarily high AIDS-related morbidity and mortality and very little hope of accessing treatment, most testing was conducted as part of antenatal care or initiated by clinicians to confirm with an expensive biomarker what was already apparent from the characteristic symptoms of advanced HIV infection and full-blown AIDS. That blood could be tested was widely known, but testing was thought of as "not easy," and patient-initiated testing was extremely rare.[8]

With the introduction of cheap, rapid-test technologies around 2006, things began to change. An opt-out testing policy for pregnant women seeking antenatal care had been designed as early as 2003 and was finally implemented countrywide in 2005. Symptomatic women living with HIV who were also pregnant would receive lifesaving antiretroviral medicines—both for their own health and for the health of their babies. But these medicines were in short supply and had to be rationed carefully. Universal testing became routine in antenatal care, as part of a highly coordinated national effort to prevent mother-to-child transmission, which was easily accomplished by distributing single-dose nevirapine to asymptomatic HIV-positive pregnant women. In a high-fertility setting, where most adult women are bearing children, women were getting tested at very high rates, primarily through their ongoing contact with these antenatal facilities. Symptomatic individuals who presented at hospitals and clinics with common AIDS-related comorbidities like tuberculosis, skin conditions, and Kaposi's sarcoma were receiving provider-initiated testing and counseling, in accordance with WHO recommendations and treatment when it was neither too early (not sick enough) nor too late (at death's door).

On the heels of opt-out testing for pregnant women and rapid-test technologies for the general public, the national rates of HIV testing in Malawi rose rapidly. In 2004, only 15 percent of adult women and 16 percent of men reported *ever* having been tested for HIV. By 2010, 75 percent of women and 54 percent of men had been tested at least once in their lives.[9] This astounding increase was facilitated by the expansion of what were then called voluntary testing and counseling (VCT) services, now referred to as HIV testing and counseling (HTC) services. VCT occurs when a person voluntarily makes the decision to find out his or her HIV status and seeks HIV testing services (HTS) at sites established for that purpose. Supported by efforts like mobile testing clinics and national testing day, "Know your status" campaigns are not designed to change the practices of experts and health care providers but to spur demand for knowledge among the general population. This new generation of tests was cheap and relatively easy for health providers to administer.[10] Results could be obtained within minutes. The barriers to knowing one's status were being reduced. Traditional authorities (chiefs) and religious leaders began to encourage their communities to get tested; the recommendation was sometimes given as tailored advice to a particular individual, sometimes as blanket advice to an entire constituency, and sometimes as a suggested group activity or part of premarital counseling. One religious leader I interviewed in 2005 proudly recounted having hired a minibus to take his entire congregation on a "field trip" to get tested.[11]

Many writers have anecdotes about people's reluctance to learn their status or the strong urge to avoid bad news. Take, for example, the cartoon featuring Nganga, a beloved character in a national cartoon strip, famous for his good humor and simple-mindedness (see fig. 5.2). In some unspecified, religiously diverse setting of Malawi that could easily be Balaka, a bishop and a sheikh observe Nganga skipping away from a closed VCT center. Nganga is happy, they agree, because he went for testing and found the facility closed. Another common trope about fear of testing features a man just meters away from a VCT clinic, standing behind a tree, trembling with fear, being encouraged (seductively) by a lovely woman to bring her an "all clear" message. Such

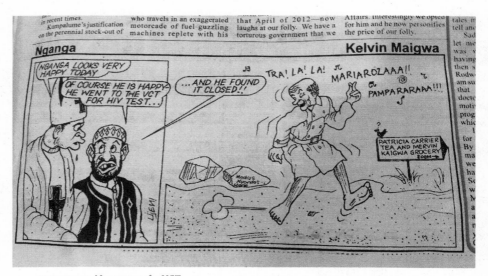

FIGURE 5.2 Nganga goes for VCT

Source: Cartoon by Kelvin Maigwa. Originally printed in the *Nation* (Malawi) newspaper, July 2016.

representations of a comedic failure to do the easy thing abound, usually depicting the reluctance of men, in particular.

A careful reading of the high-quality scientific evidence from the region, however, suggests something else entirely. The demographic data show that across AIDS-endemic contexts the demand for testing and knowledge about one's status is remarkably high. The first study to have offered home-based testing to a population-representative sample in three districts of Malawi clearly demonstrates how high the barrier to knowing one's status really was at that point in the epidemic. In 2004, when respondents could give a specimen in their home but had to travel to a predetermined location several weeks later to receive their results, 90 percent accepted the initial test that was offered and 67 percent returned several weeks later to learn their status. By 2006, when results could be generated immediately by rapid tests administered in the home, 92 percent accepted the test (no statistical difference from 2004) and a full 98 percent of those chose to receive their results.[12]

This background illuminates the environment in which TLT was designed and fielded. Further illustrating the magnitude of the difference between provider-initiated and respondent-driven testing, when TLT began in 2009, testing experience among women who had ever been pregnant was 87 percent and among women who had never been pregnant and/or attended antenatal care, 28 percent. Among men of this same age, 32 percent of those without children reported having ever been tested, and the proportion among men with children was considerably higher (54 percent), though not nearly as high as it was among their female counterparts. If we assume that the testing rate among women without children represents a decent estimate of VCT uptake, as distinct from provider-initiated testing, just shy of one-third of the young-adult population wanted to know their status enough that they got tested and obtained the results of their own volition. Among young men, I find no independent association between children ever born and testing (net of age), but for women the odds of ever having been tested are ten times greater among those who have had at least one pregnancy (compared to none).

With support from the global health community, Malawi's Ministry of Health made truly incredible strides in expanding testing and counseling services between 2000 and 2020. The barriers to testing that characterized the early 2000s—traveling long distances to clinics, long wait times to receive results, and limited information about how and where to get tested—have been eroded; sound policies and new technologies make it easier than ever to "Know your status." Access to testing in Balaka, specifically, went from inaccessible to readily available in just a few years. Today a person who wants to learn their status can get tested for free in a variety of locations within the boma and receive results in minutes. If they test positive, they will initiate care on that same day. Three decades into the epidemic, uncertainty about HIV cannot be attributed to an unmet need for testing or to a lack of demand for knowledge. How, then, does an epidemic of uncertainty persist in Balaka despite this relative ease of access to biomedical knowledge about one's status?

HIV Testing and Counseling Procedures

Before moving to the analyses themselves, let me clarify here what HTC entailed in the 2009–19 period. Those who have gotten tested for STIs in the United States at student health services, Planned Parenthood, or any other health facility may already know the drill. But the difference in timing for receiving results is crucial. Students getting tested at University of Chicago student health services between 2015 and 2019 typically waited three days to receive STI test results, usually over the phone. When I participated in routine screenings for a battery of STIs, including HIV, in early 2020, I received results through an online portal about forty-eight hours after the blood draw. At TLT, on the other hand, respondents always received their test results within minutes.

HTC is organized in three steps: (1) a pretest counseling conversation that covers ten topics, including the importance of HIV testing, HIV risk behaviors, confidentiality, disclosure, and the window period; (2) the test itself; and (3) post-test counseling, which includes a discussion of the results, disclosure strategies, treatment options, and prevention strategies. Notably, the finger-prick component of testing takes up relatively little time in the whole ordeal. The prick is sandwiched between two conversations, both of which HTC counselors are carefully trained to manage in a professional and nonjudgmental manner, with ample assurances of the WHO's essential "5 Cs" throughout.[13] As is the case in other settings characterized by generalized epidemics, testing sites in Malawi are subject to monitoring by the local Ministry of Health, which usually consists of drop-in visits by a district-level health commissioner for quality control. Counselors are certified after taking a rigorous six-week course and participate in periodic refresher training to stay current and improve their skills. The test results develop in about fifteen minutes, during which time the counselor and the respondent occupy the room together, discussing procedures, protocols, and subjects related to counseling. Occasionally other topics come up, but the conversation tends to stay centered on HIV-related issues.

The delivery of results and post-test counseling is the final step. Counselors undergo intensive training to prepare for this part of the job and are encouraged to use their discretion while navigating the conversation, with the following Ministry of Health guidelines in mind:

> Posttest counseling is an integral component of the HIV testing process. All individuals undergoing HIV testing must be counseled when their test results are given to them, regardless of the test results. Posttest counseling should be provided based on the outcome of the test results. Clear and concise information should be provided about:
> - HIV risks and risk reduction
> - The meaning of an HIV-positive and an HIV-negative diagnosis
> - Linkage to other relevant services
> - Disclosure.[14]

In contrast to pretest counseling, which elaborates the more general purposes of testing, post-test counseling covers just four essential topics and is tailored to the respondent's specific circumstances. When respondents test positive, they are connected to HIV care and services. The scope and specifics of those services have changed over time, as elaborated in the earlier discussion of the changing treatment landscape. Today enrollment on ART happens on the same day, but that was not the case before 2016. HIV services in Balaka also include introduction to a support person who has been living positively with HIV for longer periods and can give additional advice about disclosure strategies and recommended dietary changes. Post-test counseling for those who test negative, on the other hand, has been consistent from 2009 to today, focusing on how clients can continue to protect themselves from HIV. Follow-up appointments are recommended along the following schedules: HIV-negative persons with ongoing risk behavior are recommended to retest every twelve months; HIV-negative persons who have had a specific incident of known HIV exposure within the previous three months are recommended to retest after four weeks; and pregnant women with a negative HIV test during antenatal care will be retested during labor or before they are discharged.

Altogether, the HTC process is confidential, comprehensive, and interactive—very different from the simple "+/−" results of something like a self-administered pregnancy test. The required counseling offers a wealth of information about HIV; some of it addresses immediate concerns (i.e., prevention strategies and test result), and some of it addresses technical details about the window period and frank discussion of recent and ongoing risk behaviors, which may in fact plant seeds of doubt about one's vulnerability to the virus. Regardless of their status, people come away from HTC with a lot to think about.

Testing and Uncertainty: Four Views

To learn more about the relationship between HIV testing and uncertainty, we built into TLT-1 an experimental approach to HIV testing. All respondents were randomly assigned to one of three groups and differentially "treated" by the frequency of testing. Group 1 was offered HTC at the end of each interview during all eight waves. According to the initial logic of our study design, these individuals would be answering questions and making decisions about other aspects of life (fertility in particular) in real time with as much information about their HIV status as possible. Group 2 was tested once in the middle of the study at wave 4 and then again at the end. From these individuals, we could learn about how "surprises" about one's HIV status (new information that *changed* perceptions and assumptions) might lead to changes in childbearing strategies and other aspects of life. Finally, Group 3 respondents were tested at the very end of the study.[15] By doing this, we would learn how perceptions (rather than knowledge) of HIV status influence people's decision making. And we could find out how young people in Balaka were navigating the districtwide testing infrastructure outside of TLT. For reasons that will soon become clear, this study design did not reveal precisely what we thought it would. Instead, the HTC experiment taught me to think differently about the resolution of uncertainty in Malawi and illuminated just how fuzzy the boundaries between knowledge and perceptions can be.

THE AGGREGATE VIEW

To begin exploring the relationship between testing and uncertainty, I first take an aggregate view, leveraging TLT's experimental design to detect group differences in the simplest possible way. I estimated hazards of uncertainty separately by experimental condition, just as I earlier estimated these separately by gender.[16] Conventional wisdom suggests that respondents who are getting tested and receiving their results regularly should be more certain of their status than those who are not being given that same opportunity. But this is not what we find—not when we examine the narrow definition of uncertainty (acute uncertainty in the left-hand panel of fig. 5.3) or when we take a more expansive view, defining uncertainty as any uncertainty about one's status (between one and nine beans). Somewhat unbelievably, the intervention of regular testing—a finger prick to detect HIV antibodies and counsel-

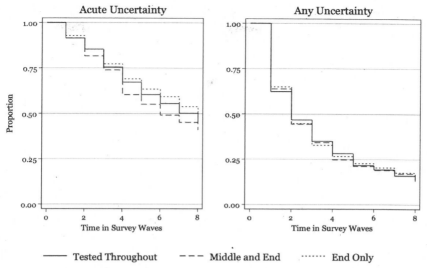

FIGURE 5.3 Incident uncertainty by testing condition

Source: TLT-1, waves 1–8.

ing about the result of that test, repeated up to eight times at four-month intervals—makes no difference in the prevalent experience of uncertainty in this population.

THE DYNAMIC, MICRO VIEW

There are limitations to the aggregate view, and it would be unwise to conclude from these analyses alone that testing does nothing to rectify uncertainty. The hazard models are a great tool for seeing the big picture, but they're not a perfect tool, because uncertainty is not actually an absorbing state the way a death or an HIV infection is. People can move in and out of uncertainty as a state, and they do. Fixed-effects models are ideal for this because they offer the most stringent tests of within-person change over time, isolating all the unobserved heterogeneity (the differences within a population researchers like to control for, e.g., ethnicity, age, personality traits and tendencies, or family-of-origin characteristics) and dealing statistically with each person as his or her own "control." Here I estimate fixed-effects models to identify the forces of change that push people into and pull them out of (un)certain states over time, with an emphasis on testing, time, relationships, and religion. I summarize the results in figure 5.4 using coefficient plots, which depict the magnitude and significance levels of the associations of interest.

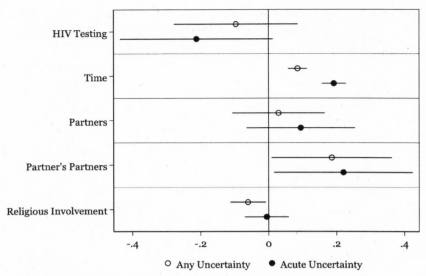

FIGURE 5.4 Predictors of HIV-related uncertainty among all TLT-1 respondents in Balaka

Source: TLT-1, waves 1–8.

Note: Displays unstandardized coefficients and 95 percent confidence intervals based on two fixed-effects regression models. Dots to the right of the centered, vertical line indicate a positive association with uncertainty; dots to the left pull toward certainty.

When I define uncertainty as "any," the fixed-effects model confirms the no-differences conclusion about testing suggested by the aggregate view. Testing does not reduce uncertainty; furthermore, time (measured in survey waves) erodes certainty, and the fact that simply living through this period of life pushes young adults in Balaka into the experience of uncertainty says something important about the accuracy of perceptions. The risk of contracting HIV increases as our respondents age into higher-incidence age groups, making the secular rise in uncertainty fully consistent with the epidemiological reality as documented in the literature. In other words, these objectively very high levels of uncertainty are warranted and should not be dismissed as misperceptions or attributed to bias.

Turning to sexual behavior, relationships within one's control (the acquisition of a new sexual partner) are also unrelated to HIV-related uncertainty, even though such changes get flagged by clinical risk assessments. Young adults in Balaka have tremendous confidence in their own ability to select safe partners. Partnership anxiety, on the other hand, strongly predicts becoming uncertain: knowing or suspecting that one's partner has other partners is the single strongest factor pulling people out of a state of certainty, and it affects both women and men similarly.[17] Although I had studied religion in Malawi for more than a decade (and knew enough to look for this but not enough to expect to find an association), one additional insight surprised me. Relating *change* in religious involvement to *change* in uncertainty over time, the model shows that increases in religious involvement reduce HIV uncertainty when uncertainty is defined expansively.

To test the robustness of these analyses to a narrower specification of uncertainty, a confirmatory model (dark circles) estimates movements into the state of acute uncertainty.[18] From this view, the drivers of uncertainty are slightly different. Testing does push respondents out of acute uncertainty and toward the base of the pyramid. But the effect of testing barely offsets the march of time, let alone concerns about a partner's behavior. Again, knowing or suspecting one's partner of having other partners is the strongest factor pushing people into a state of uncertainty. And again, one's own sexual history (lifetime number of partners) does not alter the equation in any real way, probably because we all make excellent choices in the sexual realm all the time; it is other people we must worry about. While religious involvement assuages uncertainty, expansively defined, it has no significant effect at this threshold of acute uncertainty.[19]

TLT is not the only study that has produced underwhelming findings about the impact of HIV testing on people's lives. Kathleen Beegle, Michelle Poulin, and Gil Shapira designed their Marriage Transitions in Malawi project presuming the importance of testing: "removing uncertainty about one's status may affect expectations of young people about their life expectancy as well as opportunities that will be available to them in the future."[20] Following a cohort of never-married women for more than three years, they were surprised to find no impact of testing on *any* of the subsequent behaviors they examined. The research group concluded, "For many of the respondents it is likely that learning test results did not provide new information that would alter behaviors. . . . Learning a negative test result, as most of our respondents did, provides information only about current HIV status. As these youth reside in a setting with a generalized epidemic, they might still perceive high risk of infection associated with different behaviors and high uncertainty for future status."[21] Likewise, the conclusion drawn from six years of the MDICP study set in three Malawian districts was summarized by Abdul Latif Jameel Poverty Action Lab (J-PAL) researchers as minimal short-term effects on subjective beliefs about HIV and no long-run impacts: "Two years after receiving their results, there were few significant differences between HIV-positive and HIV-negative individuals in propensity to save, amount worked in the past six months, income, or expenditure."[22] Outside of Malawi, the role of testing for reducing incidence has been called into question in a variety of contexts, from Uganda to Australia.[23] Knowing that testing actually does very little to bring about certainty makes findings like these less surprising.

Over several years, I analyzed and reanalyzed these data and presented the findings about uncertainty to many audiences, most of which reacted with astonishment at the fact that test results have negligible impact on the experience of uncertainty. Despite the fact that the TLT-1 study design was more intensive than any other study of this scale, the intersurvey period is long if something as sensitive as perceived risk can turn on a dime. During TLT-1, respondents were asked about their perceptions and then tested minutes later, right after the survey had been completed. But our next measure of perceived risk was then collected a full four months later. Perhaps the lack of resolution came from not believing the test results. Perhaps it was driven by other changes in the respondents' lives, including ongoing exposures to new risks. Or perhaps risks are truly that omnipresent in the intervening period and widely understood as such.

"How I wish we had these measures right after testing too," I mentioned to Sara several times as we poured over these analyses. And when we had the opportunity to reinterview all our respondents in 2015 for TLT-2, Sara astutely pointed out that the only thing preventing us from asking those questions twice was the time burden on respondents and our own priorities. So three years later we asked the three key beans questions twice—both before and after testing.

We adapted the core questionnaire to reflect the passage of time while maintaining consistency across all the core modules. And we administered the survey just as we did during TLT-1, with the beans questions falling in the final third of the survey. All respondents were offered HTC, even if they had tested positive with us at an earlier time or had recently learned their status during antenatal care or some other testing initiative. After the full questionnaire had been completed, after testing and counseling, and without making any big shift back to the questionnaire, the interviewers grabbed their plates and beans and casually pivoted back to the realm of perceptions, asking:

> I know I already asked you these questions, but I want to revisit just three questions now that you've been tested and received your results. How likely it is that you are . . . infected with HIV/AIDS now? Will become infected in the next 12 months? During your lifetime?

These pre- and post-HTC responses to the beans questions were typically gathered within forty-five minutes of each other and always asked within the hour. The second set of responses were gathered in the immediate wake of receiving the test result in the confines of the closed interview room, before the respondent had gone out to meet and converse with other respondents and bystanders and before they had had any new sexual contact. While these measures may not perfectly reflect a person's mind-set at that time, I have been unable to come up with a way to get any closer. The comparison is instructive in many ways and is depicted in figure 5.5, a Sankey diagram that shows the distribution of responses before testing and the distribution immediately after testing, with the magnitude of the flows indicated by the width of the bands.

From this diagram, several statements can be made about the shifts of these distributions over the short, hour-long period and what the flows reveal about the trajectories of individuals. HTC functioned as an intervention in the TLT sample: certainty doubled through testing. Sixty-five women who did not already know they were positive received a diagnosis and then calibrated their post-test responses to indicate they believed the results, but most of the increase in certainty came from individuals who thought they could be, might be, or probably were infected but then learned they were negative. Still, uncertainty remains high. In the immediate aftermath of a test, 28 percent of women and 21 percent of men indicated that they still did not know their status, placing between one and nine beans on their plates. Post-test uncertainty is lower among respondents who test positive than among those who test negative. In other words, in the context of a widespread and generalized epidemic, learning that you are positive brings certainty, whereas learning that you are negative does not. Among men, 95 percent of those who tested positive were then certain of their status, while only 80 percent of those who tested negative felt the same. Among women, the divergence is very similar, but certainty levels are lower in both groups: 88 percent of women who tested positive indicated certainty, while only 75 percent of those who tested negative indicated certainty. Of the 513 women I categorized as experiencing acute uncertainty, 75 percent had their uncertainty resolved through testing, responding after the test with either ten or zero beans.[24] This suggests that acute uncertainty is indeed a resolvable state rather than a trait. But it points to the puzzle of why uncertainty is resolved for some and not for others.

Beyond being overwhelmingly seronegative, who are these women for whom test results fail to bring even a moment of certainty? There is no clear answer to this question. But models predicting *certainty among women who tested negative just minutes before* provide a few hints. I find no differences in post-test certainty by age, education, marital status, or any of the other standard sociodemographic characteristics we typically look to for explanatory

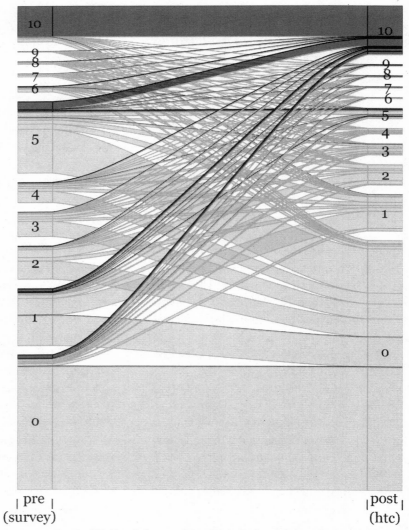

|pre|
(survey)

|post|
(htc)

FIGURE 5.5 Perceived likelihood of current HIV infection (in beans) before and after participating in HTC and receiving a result

Source: TLT-2.

Note: Each line depicts a respondent from the 2015 survey round. Women who tested negative are depicted in light gray; those who tested positive, in dark gray.

power. As with uncertainty before the test, a woman's lifetime number of sexual partners has no bearing on her certainty level in the wake of it. Similarly, both before and after testing, women who are heavily involved in their religious communities are most likely to express certainty about their HIV status.

Could persistent post-test uncertainty be the consequence of a particular mind-set with regard to HIV? Four attitudinal measures intended to gauge the way people think about this disease—avoidable or unavoidable, supernatural or biological in origin—shed some additional light on the epidemic of uncertainty. In 2015, 22 percent of women agreed with the statement, "AIDS is in the flour." The phrase is taken from a popular song lyric and indicates a sense that the disease is unavoidable and omnipresent—like when we jest in the United States that pregnancy is "in the water."[25] Women who think about AIDS as having this kind of omnipresent property are less likely to convert to certainty even after having been told that they are negative. Conversely, the vast majority of women (73 percent) agree with the statement, "Nowadays a man who gets HIV is deliberately choosing death." Three specific elements of this statement merit explanation. Men (less vulnerable than women) nowadays (not early on in the epidemic but today, now that knowledge about HIV is widespread, prevention campaigns are clear, and condoms are widely available) don't just "get" infected but rather become infected through a series of unwise actions. This attitude matters: women who hold this view, that HIV is avoidable, are more certain of their status after receiving their test results. Two supernaturally oriented statements, that HIV can be inflicted by God (15 percent) or by witchcraft (38 percent; "enemies" in fig. 5.6), also indicate a lack of agency with respect to the disease, but these attitudes are statistically unrelated to post-test certainty. In sum, those who view HIV as ambient are uncertain, and those who hold an agentive view of the disease are most likely to have their uncertainty resolved through testing. It is these ideational and epistemological differences, and not particular characteristics, patterns of behavior, or myths about HIV, that sustain the epidemic of uncertainty.[26]

THE VIEW FROM THE BOREHOLE

Gertrude's fieldnotes shed additional light on uncertainty and testing at TLT and help us understand why HTC sometimes fails to resolve a woman's uncertainty. While going about her morning chores, Gertrude happens upon women who are talking about their testing experiences and what they heard from a friend who participated in TLT in the 2015 survey round. She writes at the end of a long day:

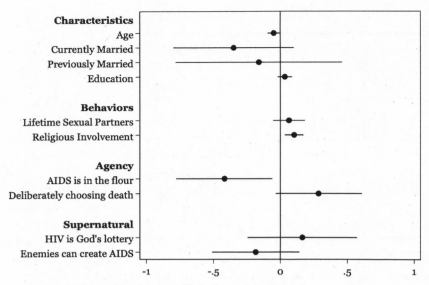

FIGURE 5.6 Predictors of certainty, immediately after receiving test results, 2015

Source: TLT-2.

Note: Displays unstandardized coefficients and 95 percent confidence intervals based on a single logistic regression model. Dots to the right of the centered, vertical line indicate a positive association with uncertainty; dots to the left pull toward certainty.

In the morning when I woke up, I cleaned the house, washed plates, and went to the borehole to fetch water because there was no water at the tap. On the way to the borehole I saw one woman selling groundnut flour and popcorn at her home. And at the borehole I found the sister of my neighbor telling her friend that some days ago she went to TLT and was asked a lot of questions. She said after answering the questions she received 2,000 MK, and she was also asked to test her blood, and she did that. She continued that she was also told to test for pregnancy, but she didn't like that and refused that test. Her friend asked what it was all about. My neighbor's sister said, "I don't know what those people are up to. It's not a clinic for giving ARVs, but I like it because the questions were okay and they were giving money. Otherwise I wouldn't have participated. I went there in the morning and was home in the afternoon."[27]

The woman who was listening said, "Patience also went there to TLT. She told me that she was asked lot of questions and after that she was told to test her blood and also pregnancy. When she reached home she told her husband what happened there. Her husband asked why she tested her blood. And she said she agreed to test her blood because she was doubting him. She told him she thought he might be HIV positive because of the business that he does; he sells some smaller things at the [bus] depot, and he could have girlfriends there."

. . . Another woman asked, "So why do these people give money for being tested?"

"Those people know what they are doing. And we receive money to buy what we want."

After fetching water, the women left. And I also left.

The secondhand story of Patience's experience at TLT and subsequent conversation at home reveals important things about uncertainty, about husbands, about attitudes to testing, and about women's worlds. Even though Balaka residents could get tested at the government clinic and certain private local hospitals in 2015, there was still abundant appetite for receiving the results of an HIV test in a quiet, private space with minimal waiting time. During the TLT-2 survey round, 94 percent of our female respondents and 90 percent of the male respondents accepted the HIV test their interviewers offered. Patience and Gertrude's neighbor's sister were among the overwhelming majority who jumped at this chance to learn their status, and it is noteworthy that the respondent Gertrude found fetching water that morning refused the pregnancy test but accepted HTC. She was not just passively complying with our protocols; she had some reason of her own for getting tested.

Uncertainty despite testing shows clearly in the talk about doubts and more subtly in Patience's mode of interacting with her husband. "Doubt" (Chichewa, *kukakira* [v], *khakira* [n]) is a word many Malawian women use when talking with friends about men.[28] Patience's husband is the root of her uncertainty, as husbands often are.[29] Patience tells her husband that she got tested *because* she had doubts about her own status and his, when she could have simply told him that that TLT was testing everybody, just like they do at ANC. In telling her husband about the test at TLT as part of the happenings of her day, Patience seems to be provoking a conversation about present-continuous uncertainty rather than announcing any sense of relief we might expect her to feel from a negative result. Apparently, her doubts about her husband's business, his behavior, and his serostatus are unresolved by the test and the counseling that accompanied it. In fact, the information exchanged in the counseling portion of HTC—the naming of past and ongoing risks, the technical description of the window period, and information about strategies for staying healthy—may have exacerbated the uncertainty that prompted Patience to accept the test in the first place. Further evidence of uncertainty as a response to testing can be seen in figure 5.5; a small group of respondents actually move from no or minimal uncertainty (0 or 1 bean before the test) to more uncertainty (1 to 9 beans) in the aftermath of a negative result. In the 2015 data, 9 percent of female respondents, 10 percent of random-male respondents, and 7 percent of the male-partner sample *become* uncertain through testing.

Uncertainty as a more general phenomenon also shows in the women's lack of emphasis on the actual test results while gossiping. The women at the borehole ask no follow-up questions about Patience's HIV status or about the neighbor's sister. They are, however, interested in the conversation between Patience and her husband and more curious about the monetary incentives than the diagnoses. Used to uncertainty themselves, they know how to grant it to another woman, how to leave things open. There is neither secret nor scandal here—just an open balance, in between.

A Phenomenon Impervious to Biomedical Solutions

Addressing the correlates of uncertainty through a Western lens, using the tenets of the health belief model, leads to a set of expectations about behavior and knowledge, knowledge and behaviors: "Test! People will know their status. Uncertainty will be eliminated." But this model provides a poor fit for the data from Balaka. In contrast, when we examine the correlates of uncertainty using insights from population chatter as the analytical framework, it comes as no surprise that AIDS-related uncertainty would be impervious to biomedical solutions. As with much of the best research on AIDS in this part of the world, an approach that pairs demographic estimation strategies with indicators tailored to the specific cultural context both "fit" better on the data and are more powerful for generating new insights about how young adults experience HIV—not fundamentally as a virus or a syndrome, but as a phenomenon.

The uncertainty manifest in a generalized but stable and well-managed HIV epidemic cannot be resolved by testing. While testing people at extremely close intervals, we learned that 20 percent of the young-adult population expresses some degree of uncertainty about their status just minutes after testing negative. Test results don't allow these young people to "know" their status at all because exposure is constant and ongoing. Could a more perfect test—no window period—change that? Probably. A better test would almost certainly reduce the prevalence of post-test uncertainty by a few percentage points. But it would not eliminate it completely, and even if it could, the epidemic of uncertainty would persist, because uncertainty is fundamentally about the future. By 2019, HIV prevalence among women in the TLT study (now ages 25–35) had risen to 15 percent. Among the 85 percent who had received a negative result just minutes before, 57 percent expressed a non-zero chance of contracting HIV in the coming year, and 78 percent expressed a non-zero chance of being infected in their lifetimes. To the extent that the test brought them any certainty about the present, it was an extremely short vacation from risk.

The fact of persistent uncertainty within a regime of widespread testing underscores the unique value of a demographic approach. Approaches to uncertainty that are focused on personal perceptions and individual experiences are useful for showing us how individuals move into and out of uncertain states over the course of their lives. But a focus on the population as a whole makes visible the fact that this widespread uncertainty is manifest as something akin to a demographic rate: it is fairly stable over time, irreducible to the individual-level experience, and consequential for the population as a whole. In the next chapters, I address three empirical puzzles that follow from these insights about magnitude: How is uncertainty manifest in romantic relationships? How is it managed and navigated? And how does AIDS-related uncertainty rank relative to other uncertainties young adults face?

Relationship Uncertainty and Marriage Instability

Njemile's Relationship: A Cautionary Tale

During the transition to TLT-2 in 2015, Sara and I presented highlights from TLT-1 to the TLT research team. We focused on the key findings of our published papers: fertility trends, HIV prevalence, and the massive scope of HIV-related uncertainty in Balaka. Among our slides were a series of figures about romantic relationships: HIV prevalence by marital status, relationship instability, and the prevalence of suspicion and gossip in the population. I showed bar charts depicting the proportion of men and women who agreed with the statement, "Most married men these days are faithful," and analogous figures showing the proportion of men and women who said they either knew or suspected that their partners had other partners. We compared these to the proportion of respondents who disclosed that they themselves had partners "on the side." We talked about how these on-the-side partners were almost certainly underreported in our data, and we brainstormed strategies for reducing social desirability bias and encouraging our respondents to be a little more honest about their sex lives.

After that presentation, Njemile, a health surveillance assistant (HSA) who had helped us write and translate survey questions about common STIs based on what she sees day to day, pulled me aside and told me that we needed to talk in private. Born and raised in Balaka, Njemile was orphaned at a young age and raised by grandparents who struggled but did their best to support her. This vibrant mother of three is the breadwinner for her own children and the large, extended family that took care of her as a girl. She is adored for her beauty, her perfect manners (e.g., she never gossips, never loses her cool, and always helps others), and her ability to inject her sharp wit into every conversation and leave her friends rolling on the floor with laughter. Njemile told me:

Jenny, if you are writing a book about what people know and don't know about their relationships, you need to hear the true story about how I came to learn about my co-wife, and you are going to want to put this in your computer.

You see, during our courtship, my husband didn't disclose to me that he was already married. Of course I asked him whether he was married. He said he was divorced from his first wife, and I didn't have any reason to question that. Our relationship happened fast; after a few weeks we started staying together, without ankhoswe, as husband and wife in my village. Two months later, I was pregnant, and as soon as we noticed that I was pregnant, he took me to his parents' home. They are wonderful people. They treated me extremely well and started making plans to do *chinkhoswe* [a traditional marriage ceremony]. My husband is a driver, so he travels a lot—he goes all over Malawi and sometimes to Zambia, Tanzania, or even South Africa. The best trips are when he goes to South Africa because the money is good and he can bring back a lot of nice things. One day he was getting ready for a trip to Mozambique, and he invited me to accompany him on the first part of the journey. This was 2012. I had just found out I was pregnant, and he was being very kind and attentive to me. He was taking good care of me back then.

We planned to sleep in Faraway Town[1] one night, and while we were there, he discovered that he had forgotten his blue book [which shows ownership of the truck]. It was good that he realized this before he had traveled any farther. My husband called his brother, who stays at his home, to get him to bring him the blue book. Early in the morning, my husband told me that he was going to the depot to meet his brother, and I said to him, "Why are you going to meet him at the bus depot? Can't you tell him to bring it here?"

"My brother is in a hurry; he has to go straight back home. I just have to go meet him. I'll be right back."

So my husband went out; he got his blue book and came back to the rest house where we were staying. I thought nothing of it. We spent the morning together. It was a romantic day for us; we didn't leave the rest house at all—not even to eat. In the afternoon I had to return to Balaka to work the next day, and my husband had to proceed with his journey. There had been a transport problem that day, no petrol in town, so the minibuses from the morning had been waiting there for five hours, maybe even six. People at the depot were complaining that they had been waiting since morning, but I didn't see my brother-in-law there.

At Faraway Town depot I boarded a coaster [big bus] to Balaka. We were packed like sardines, and the driver's assistant was giving orders so that everybody could squeeze in. He pointed at me to sit in the back, next to a certain lady who was about my same age, so I took my seat next to this lady. A woman directly in front of us was struggling to take care of her children; she had a baby on her back and another baby in her hands. So I helped her by carrying the baby who was in her hands, and I kept that baby happy during the whole ride. The lady next to me started admiring me for what I was doing. She was saying, "That was so nice of you to help her!" and "You are really good with this baby. This baby loves you."

It was her first time visiting Faraway district so she didn't know the area. This lady was friendly and talkative but maybe a little too talkative. She kept asking me questions like, "Where are we now?" And I was like, "We are at such-and-such place." But then my heartbeat started to race, so I asked myself, "What is happening? I feel like something strange is happening." I prayed through my heart [silently] because I wanted to know this lady much better. I asked her who she was and how she had ended up in a place she was not familiar with. She explained to me that her husband had forgotten the blue book for his truck, so she had come from home that morning to bring it to him so he could proceed on his journey to Mozambique.

I thought to myself, "This is not happening. I am not sitting next to my husband's wife on this coaster." And then I said to her, "How nice that you were able to help your husband. What is his name?" I was shocked when she answered with the name of my hubby. It was so painful. I don't know how I did it, but I managed to control myself. I didn't show any emotion at all. I asked her more about her marriage, whether she was happy. And I said, "Because, you know, some drivers cheat a lot." And she said to me, "Not my husband. He's a good man. We have four children together, and he takes good care of us. But what about you? You must have a lucky husband." I told her my name, that I'm married. Right at that moment we were passing through a road stop, and I said, "Mmmmmm. My husband is a policeman. We're getting ready to do chinkhoswe next month." Remember I was newly pregnant, but I didn't say anything about the pregnancy to her.

When the bus reached the Balaka depot, I got out, and she continued on her way. I thanked the lady—my husband's wife—for the good time we had. Honestly, on that day I liked her. But being in a relationship like mine is really dangerous. It's dangerous because of HIV. Women can cheat too, so having another wife in the picture raises my risk. And it's also dangerous because as women we compete with each other to win the husband. She and I are competing to this day. I still blame myself for having made a mistake like this, but I was young.

When I reached home, I called my husband and told him what had happened. He laughed, and right away he admitted that he had lied when he said he had asked his brother to come with the book. He had actually called his other wife to bring it. And about our marriage he said, "Had I told you that I was married, you wouldn't have accepted me as your husband." I blamed myself. I had so many doubts about him and about the situation. But I was also pregnant with his child, and I loved his family. Realizing that worrying can't solve my issues, I cooled myself down.

We did chinkhoswe with my relatives and his family a few months before my son was born. For almost a year, his other wife didn't know anything. But she's a complicated person. She quarrels with everyone—with her husband, with her neighbors, and even with her husband's relatives. I don't know exactly what rude thing she did, but my husband's relatives grew tired of her behavior, and finally one day someone shouted back at her and said, "At least our son now also has a respectful wife." That ended the secret. Eventually he told her about me—that I am the one she chatted with on the bus from Faraway. She stole my number from his phone and started calling me and insulting me. She was calling me for weeks, saying awful things, but I have never insulted her in return. Her father is a traditional healer, and she was even saying that they would find a way to kill me. I worried about that a lot.

One cannot serve two masters; now that he is older, my husband knows this. My relationship is not easy, and my husband . . . you asked me if he's worth all this, and I have to say, probably not. But his relatives support me. If I get sick, they are the ones who come take care of my children. When our son was in the hospital, they were the ones who visited and brought food. When my husband and I quarrel, they take my side—even if I'm the one who started the argument. They are so loving, so supportive; my in-laws really are my true family.

When I spoke with Njemile five years later to confirm that she still felt OK about sharing her story in a book, we talked at length about her feelings— then and now. She takes her work as an HSA very seriously and also occasionally consults with various health-focused NGOs and research projects like ours. She is still devoted to her in-laws, but after becoming more involved in her church, Njemile no longer worries that her co-wife might harm her: "I just pray for protection from God. Because He protects me, no weapon formed against me shall prosper." Although she is proud—proud of her work, her children, and her ability to support her relatives—and respected in her community, Njemile still carries an amount of pain and shame about her marriage. Yes, she was young and immature and an orphan, but as a smart, educated woman, she feels she should not have been duped by a womanizer. In her roles as a health worker and HTC facilitator, she counsels others to protect themselves from HIV by practicing faithfulness in monogamous marriage, not polygyny. In describing her own moral compass, Njemile says that every act in her life is guided by two principles: prayer and kindness. She never retaliates and would never try to talk a man into abandoning his wife and his children. How would they survive?

Njemile's story is by no means typical of what happens in Balaka; hers is a cautionary tale, and Njemile knew that when she told me to get my laptop. But her story is analytically powerful for a few reasons. She shows us what women in Balaka fear and try to avoid as they navigate romantic relationships. Njemile's story raises thorny intellectual and ethical questions: it implores us to distinguish the vulnerability inherent to all relationships from the physical and emotional injuries particular relationships sometimes inflict, and it stands in contrast to theories that name uncertainty reduction as a driving force in human behavior. Indeed, by staying with her husband and hiding her marriage from her co-wife for years, Njemile sustains and participates in the uncertainty that characterizes her relationship.

Njemile's story also raises a bundle of empirical questions about relationship uncertainty. To the extent that marriage in Balaka is a process, and not a discrete event, what constitutes a marriage? At what point in this story was Njemile "married"? Do the new protections of the MDFRA do anything to assuage relationship uncertainty? What role do ankhoswe play in settling marital disputes? Do mobile phones do more to provide or conceal information in intimate relationships? To what extent do gossip and suspicion actually destabilize relationships? How many steps of the marriage process do most couples complete? And how is HIV prevalence patterned by marriage type? In the rest of this chapter, I provide a descriptive analysis of relationship uncertainty in this population, offer two vignettes that further demonstrate the nature of relationship uncertainty in Balaka, and show how relationships, HIV, and their associated uncertainties are linked empirically. Chapter 7 continues this line of inquiry, addressing related questions about mobile phones, the marriage process, and relationship quality.

The Magnitude of Relationship Uncertainty in Balaka

In chapter 5 we saw that concerns about a partner's other partners are a key driver of HIV uncertainty. This fact was present both in the survey data (fig. 5.4) and in Patience's post-test conversation with her husband. How prevalent are these concurrent (and often covert) sexual relationships in Balaka? How prevalent are women's worries about them? Do men experience these same uncertainties?

Relying on self-reports of sexual behavior, concurrent partnerships are rare and nothing to worry about. About 2 percent of the married women in the TLT study reported to us that they had an ongoing sexual relationship with an on-the-side partner, and among the sample of male partners who enrolled in the study (men in relationships with these same women) the proportion who reported such partnerships was a little higher: about 6 percent.[2] The estimates we gathered in TLT are comparable to those from other surveys in the region that have attempted to measure concurrent partnerships, but I would not bet a whole lot on the validity of these responses—either in our data or in other studies. People may not disclose the full truth about elicit relationships to a stranger in the context of a survey,[3] so I share these 2 and 6 percent estimates with a grain of salt.

Relationship uncertainty is not primarily about what people report doing or even about what they are truly up to despite their reports. Relationship uncertainty is rooted in what people think their partners, their friends, their friends' partners, and everybody else is up to. We specifically designed the TLT survey to measure the phenomena of trust, suspicion, and anxiety in romantic relationships. These were the slides that spurred an animated debate at the research center, and this is the phenomenon that sustains the persistently high levels of HIV uncertainty I documented among young adults in Balaka.

At multiple points in the study, we asked our respondents if they agreed or disagreed—just a simple yes or no, no gradations—with the assertion, "These days, most married men are faithful to their wives." We wanted to get their sense of what they think most people do, and we had not yet asked them about their own relationships. About half the male partners agreed that most men are faithful to their wives, and their reports did not change much from one wave to the next (see fig. 6.1). The TLT women, however, gave a less sanguine view, and their view deteriorated as the study progressed. In 2009, when they were quite young, 38 percent of women agreed with this optimistic statement about *most* men's faithfulness, but as the cohort aged and experienced marriage firsthand, that number dropped to 29 percent. The general consensus about men is that they wander in their relationships. This does not mean that individuals stop expecting or desiring faithfulness in their own marriages, but it captures a sentiment that strongly disputes the 6 percent estimates derived from men's own reports.

What do people think is going on in their *own* relationships? We asked TLT respondents whether they thought their current partner had other partners on the side at any point in the relationship. Using casual vocabulary to reflect the way people talk to each other, we gave respondents four options to choose from: "Yeah, I *know* s/he does," "I *suspect* so," "One can never know what another person does," and "Probably not." "Probably not" is a generous category, and indeed most married respondents gave this response about their own relationships. But the proportion of women who know or suspect their partners have other partners is sizable, and it grows over time. Assessed

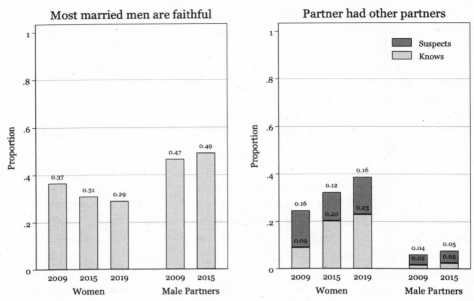

FIGURE 6.1 General and personal perceptions of faithfulness in relationships

Source: TLT-1 (wave 1), TLT-2, and TLT-3.

only for currently married respondents, a handful of men know (2 percent) or suspect (5 percent) that their wives have other partners; in other words, men's responses align pretty closely with what these women say about their own behavior, so if women are underreporting extramarital relationships, their husbands are none the wiser. Married women's perceptions, on the other hand, differ dramatically from what men report about their behavior. Depending on how we combine "know" and "suspect," between 20 and 40 percent of women think their husbands have other partners.[4] Are they overestimating that concern? Perhaps. And we have no way to externally validate whether the men's reports or the women's perceptions are more "correct." As we will see, this perception has real consequences: it leaves a mark on women's lives by shortening the longevity of these relationships.

As with the multiple views of HIV uncertainty we examined in chapter 4, the view from repeated cross sections conceals whether we are viewing mostly women like Njemile who know about a co-wife or paramour who is a stable fixture in their relationship or whether a larger proportion of women are moving in and out of suspicion as a state—either by confronting their partners and navigating the relationship back to a state of faithfulness or by leaving the relationship entirely. Here again, hazard models clarify the difference.

Using just the closely spaced period of the TLT-1 study, between 2009 and

2012, I estimated a pair of hazard models that leverage data from all the women in the study—even those who said they were not currently in a relationship—and all the men who enrolled in the study as partners.[5] At each wave, about 10 percent of women report that they think their primary partner has had other partners in the preceding months. This represents yet another remarkably stable population pattern: suspicion levels never exceed 11 percent, nor do they ever drop below 8 percent. But these are different women at every wave. As with the hazard models shown in chapters 4 and 5, figure 6.2 begins with all women and excludes at each wave those who reported experiencing relationship uncertainty. By wave 8, we see that during the three-year period nearly half of all women reported suspicion about their partner to us at some point during the study period. Men, meanwhile, are not immune to such concerns, but their collective experience of suspicion is roughly half that of women.

I also plotted analogous estimates for a more stringent indicator of perceived faithfulness. Starting in wave 2, we asked whether in the past four months or since their last interview, respondents had *heard rumors* that their partner might be fooling around. Relevant hearsay could come from concerned friends or from people chatting at the market, at the hair salon, or at funerals. It could come from friends or rivals via text message, as in Patuma's experience.[6] As expected, more women than men report being on the receiving side of gossip about their partners, with more than one-quarter

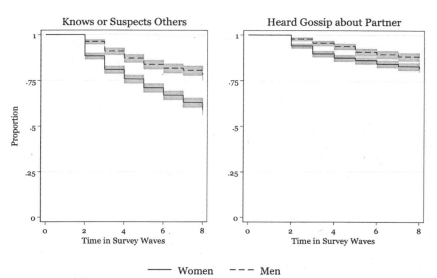

FIGURE 6.2 Hazard of suspicion and gossip in Balaka, 2009–2011

Source: TLT-1, waves 1–8.

of women and about 15 percent of male partners having encountered this kind of gossip. Many men and women feel stable and safe in their relationships. But if we take these levels of suspicion and gossip as a feature of the population—constitutive of a particular relational context—we start understanding relationship uncertainty as a population-level phenomenon.

Population Chatter at the Salon

The survey data show us the prevalent view of relationship uncertainty but cannot adequately convey how relationship uncertainty is manifested and felt in daily life. While Njemile's story clearly demonstrates how a particular woman experiences relationship uncertainty, her story was self-consciously exceptional. In contrast, Gertrude's records of her typical interactions around town show us what relationship uncertainty sounds like in the daily conversations women have with one another. In the following vignette, a group of five women discuss their babies, their pregnancies, and the men in their lives. The cast of characters includes Gertrude; Enid, the owner of New Styles hair salon and mother of a small child; Precious, six months' pregnant by a man she is serious with but not formally married to; an unnamed teenage girl with a newborn; and Tiyamike, Gertrude's closest friend in Balaka. Tiyamike has been in love with a married man for more than a year, and she typically juggles two or three infrequent partners alongside that long-standing relationship.

> I decided to pass by New Styles and say hi to Enid. I found her there with Precious and Tiyamike. I joined them to chat, and they said, "Gertrude, let's change your hair style now. You have stayed for a month now without changing." I said, "No problem, girls." And they helped each other braid my hair again.
>
> Precious had to leave for an antenatal check at Mponda clinic, just up the road. She told us, "I'll pass by after the clinic so that we can all walk home together."
>
> A few minutes after Precious left, the man who is in relationship with Tiyamike came to bring her some lunch. He brought two packets of biscuits and two bottles of juice. He also gave her 2,000 kwacha and said she should use it over the weekend, but he didn't have time to chat. He left, but Tiyamike didn't escort him. I asked, "Why are you not escorting him?" And she said, "I'm afraid his wife will see me. She and I quarreled once, and I don't want that to happen again."
>
> "So his wife knows about you?"
>
> "Yes, she knows. She doesn't like it, but she knows."
>
> "How did she come to find out?"

"It's a long story; I will tell you some other time."

Not thirty minutes later, Precious came back from the antenatal checkup with the new RBF[7] card in her hand. The clinic had no lines, so her visit didn't take long. "I received this card at the hospital; the nurse said it's about maternal health. They want to encourage people to give birth at the hospital, not at home, because when you give birth at home, you can lose a lot of blood. So with this card, if we attend all the visits and collect the stamps, we will receive some money."

"How much are you going to receive?"

"5,300." And Precious showed me the card. It was written: 500 MK transport, delivery-related 2,000 MK, and 2,800 MK for something I couldn't read. Total 5,300. Also noted was the distance (4 km), age 22, and Precious's full name.

Then Enid said, "So you decided to receive the money after delivery?"

And Precious said, "Yes, I will if I have the chance, but I won't count on it because I hear that some people receive the card but still never receive any money."

Then another girl came in, wanting to have her hair washed. She was carrying a small baby, and I asked if it was her child, because the girl looked very young. And she said yes it was her child. I asked her how old she is, and she said 16.

"And how old is the baby?"

"One week old."

Then Enid said to the girl, "Are you going to write your final exams?" And the girl said, "Yes I will. We start on June 17."

Enid laughed. "So your baby came out in time, thinking, 'My mother wants to write her exams!' Good baby. And you can leave the child with your mother."

"What about the father?" I asked.

"Mmmmmm. I am not married, I just got pregnant while at school. I had a boyfriend, and I thought that we would get married, but when I told him that I am pregnant, he didn't say anything. He doesn't take care of me or the child, but my mother does."

"Does he at least come to see the child?"

"No. Not even that."

When I asked the girl where she delivered, she said, "At Mponda Clinic." I motioned to Precious and asked, "Did you receive any money after giving birth?"

She said no, and I asked why.

"I don't know why. I gave the card to my mother. Maybe she didn't go to receive the money."

Then Precious asked Enid to wash her hair. Enid said, "Do you have money to pay?" And Precious said, "Yes I do."

Then Enid said, "Then I will wash your hair tomorrow, because I want to close quickly today."

Precious said, "No, my husband is coming to see me, so can you please wash my hair now?"

"OK, fine, I'll wash you now. Is he going to spend the night here?"

Precious said yes and she looked happy. She had already bought eggs and tomatoes; she wanted to prepare nice food for him.

After washing her hair, we closed up the salon. And as we were ready to leave, the man who gave a child to Enid passed by. Precious started heckling him, shouting, "Look! That's the one who impregnated Enid, but he ignored the responsibility. He doesn't even take care of the child. He just keeps proposing women. Now that he is working and he has money, you girls always accept him, and he doesn't even tell you girls that he has a child."

That man was shuffling away quickly, as if he couldn't hear Precious. We were all laughing, even Enid.

"I hate him," said Enid. "We just had sex one time, and I fell pregnant. He ignored me, and I feel the pain because I'm taking care of the child myself as if I had created her on my own."

"Why didn't you use a condom to prevent it?" I asked.

Enid replied, "Sometimes when you feel love you don't even think about the consequences, but you start regretting it even before you reach home. And you start asking yourself, 'Could I be pregnant?'"

Precious laughed a lot and said, "You see, girls, I am pregnant again because I thought we would get married. But he just comes and goes. He always makes promises, but he doesn't fulfill them. He told me to look for a house, but he hasn't paid for any house."

We all laughed.

Enid said, "That's men. They all make someone cry."

Women sorting hair and doctor appointments while chatting about the men in their lives is a typical scene in Balaka, and it has some more universal resonance as well. The conversation is casual, occurring in public among a group of women with varying levels of familiarity with one another. Gertrude and Tiyamike are close friends, as are Precious and Enid, but across the dyads the women are mere acquaintances, and the teenage girl is encountering these four for the first time. The older women treat this new mother as a child, peppering her with questions and encouraging her, in their own way, to persist in her studies rather than abandon education for motherhood. Engaged in population chatter, the group works collectively to understand the specific carrot of the RBF4MNH policy through the experiences of Precious and the teenager. Precious should receive an amount close to US$6 when she delivers at the hospital, but the fact that the teenager never received any money casts doubt that it will happen. The teenager gave birth just a week ago at the same hospital. Perhaps the program does not extend to her for some specific reason. Perhaps the girl's mother (and solution to her schooling dilemma) received the money and kept it for herself. We don't know. But within the broader economy of Balaka, it is impossible to imagine that the duo simply neglected to claim a rightful stipend. In the register of population chatter, Enid also provides her own explanations for the phenomena demographers study as unprotected sex and unintended pregnancy.

Keeping in mind that this set of interactions occurs in public spaces, we can look more carefully at the relationship chatter and what it tells us about the men. In addition to getting her antenatal checkup, Precious is preparing for a visit from her migrant husband. Her hair is fixed, she has acquired special foods for a nice meal, and she is visibly excited, yet she expresses an underlying disappointment that her marriage remains informal; she is expecting her third child, still without ankhoswe, and still without a house of their own. In articulating this complaint about the husband to whom she is not yet married, Precious underscores the ambiguity surrounding and the importance of marriage in Balaka—a topic I explore at greater length in chapter 7.[8]

When Precious takes it upon herself to heckle the deadbeat father of Enid's child, she injects what might have been a gripe session about absent fathers and untrustworthy men with a dose of comedy that boosts morale and undercuts the profundity of her closing synthesis: they all make someone cry. Even Tiyamike agrees with the statement. Her ongoing relationship with a married man is apparent to the group, relatively discreet, and not particularly scandalous. What Tiyamike will not discuss with anyone beyond her closest friend is the row she got into with his wife; in other words, it is the conflict from the relationship and not fact of it that she attempts to conceal.[9] The specifics of these women's respective dilemmas may be unique, but their collective narration establishes that the hardship is more universal. In discussing the messy reality of family formation with one another, these four women are affirming the collective burden they share as women while also modeling for the young girl how grown women are expected to carry these facts about men and relationships—with excitement and desire, the expectation of tears, tolerance for ambiguity, humor, and perhaps the occasional dalliance of one's own to cope.

Decomposing HIV Prevalence by Marital Experience

The ethnographic vignettes help us understand the paradox of marriage in Balaka. Marriage is crucial for economic security, for status as a bona fide adult, for child rearing, and for enjoying a good life. At the same time, marriage is the most dangerous and riskiest relationship a young adult will have. Here I use the TLT data to show that the experience of relationship instability causes a behavioral pattern of relationship churning, which drives Balaka's HIV epidemic. I show that HIV prevalence rises precipitously with marital experience—a unique process that often gets conflated with chronological time and biological age. In combination with population chatter, the decomposition of HIV prevalence clarifies which patterns are highly visible to ordinary people navigating an epidemic, which patterns remain undetected, and how these patterns get interpreted and discussed in everyday conversation.

Thinking about marriage as part of a life course transition encourages us to think about marriage dynamically—over time for this sample and about the elements that go into it. Recall that this sample transitions from 50 percent married when they are 15 to 25 years old to over 95 percent married at least once ten years later. Not only do most women in the sample get married during the observation period but many of them divorce and remarry as well—some of them multiple times. Recall also that HIV prevalence among TLT women rises from around 6 percent in 2009 to 11 percent in 2012 to 14 percent in 2015 and to 16 percent in 2019 and that prevalence among young, never-married women at the start of the study was around 1 percent (see fig. 2.5). Nearly all the HIV infections that will occur in these women's lifetimes take place during this decade, and these infections happen through romantic relationships (long term and short-lived), not through prostitution or one-night stands.[10]

When we bring marriage into our understanding of rising HIV prevalence in young adulthood, we encounter a common analytic problem: this sample is aging and gaining marital experience at the same time, making it hard to pinpoint which of the two processes contributes more substantially to the rise in HIV prevalence. One way to solve this problem is to truncate the sample at each time period and focus only on women 21 to 25 years old, comparing the reality for women of this age in 2009 to the reality of women of that same age (i.e., different women, same stage of life) three years, six years, or a decade later. Looking at HIV prevalence through the age-standardized lens (as in fig. 2.5), we see that the HIV situation is improving over time: 13 percent of 21- to 25-year-old women tested positive for HIV in 2009, but the proportion bounces between 8 and 10 percent in 2012, 2015, and 2019. Likewise, applying the truncation approach to marital experience, figure 6.3 shows that while the TLT study women gain marital experience as they age—by 2019 almost 40 percent of TLT women have transitioned out of their first marriage to being divorced or in a second or third marriage—among women between the ages of 21 and 25, the proportions of never married, married, divorced (not remar-

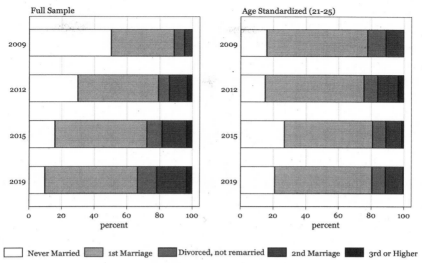

FIGURE 6.3 Marital composition of TLT sample, 2009–2019

Source: TLT, all waves.

ried), and remarried women are quite stable. In other words, the marriage patterns themselves do not seem to be changing; the women in our study are simply moving through the marriage regime that characterizes Balaka—one that features a high divorce rate and rapid remarriage.

Is HIV prevalence patterned by marital experience? Yes, to a great extent. Indeed, the patterns depicted in figure 6.4 are crucial for understanding the epidemic. Starting in 2009, the difference between never-married women and those who have been married one time is almost identical to the difference in birth cohorts we saw in figure 2.5, because those two categories (age and marital status) were almost perfectly overlapping. But a big jump in HIV prevalence is evident in the sizable minority (about 10 percent) of women who in 2009 had already transitioned out of a first marriage. Of about one hundred women who had divorced or separated but not yet remarried, nearly 30 percent tested positive for HIV. Among those who had already gotten married for the second time, prevalence was lower—about 15 percent— but these confidence intervals are large, meaning that it would be unwise to draw strong conclusions about a true "difference" between divorced women who had married a second time and those who had not.[11]

There are some salient points we must grasp from this first panel from 2009 before moving to the dynamic view. One is epistemological. Recalling the key principles of causal reasoning, a marriage cannot truly *cause* an HIV infection; after all, marriage is an institutional arrangement. Marriage is, however, crucial because it is simultaneously the context in which large numbers of new infections occur and a serosorting process—who gets married, when, who stays married, and who remarries—through which HIV is either being contained within a relationship or spreading to new ones.[12] The epidemiological patterns are striking: between the never-married group and the first-married women, prevalence increases two-and-a-half-fold, and from there HIV prevalence is five times higher among divorced women than it is among women in their first marriage. That is a surge, and it happens through marriage rather than due to marriage. This is not to say that no women were infected in their own extramarital partnerships (or divorced for that reason). Some were. But the vast majority of the HIV infections we identified in 2009 originated with the first husband through a mix of actions, accompanied by perceptions and suspicions that, in combination, also led to the divorce. This is clear from the responses to our survey question, "reason marriage ended," from the marital histories, in which the two most common reasons given by women were "partner unfaithful" and "partner took another wife." In contrast, the male partners in the TLT study collectively attributed their divorces first to their own unfaithfulness and second to their partners' by a margin of about four to one.[13]

A final point from the first panel of figure 6.4 is that women proactively leave relationships they think are putting them at risk of contracting HIV. Whether they leave before or after becoming infected is less clear. Divorced and separated women will have new relationships and remarry, and this is consequential for HIV transmission.[14] Of the one hundred women who were divorced but not yet remarried at the time of their first interview, just seven had not remarried by 2019.[15] When people living with HIV know their status, are receiving antiretrovirals, and are responding well to treatment, they will be "U-U"—having viral loads that are both undetectable and untransmittable. Recall, however, that antiretroviral availability was limited in 2009. So if a divorced woman living with HIV did not serosort (i.e., re-partner with another person who has a known infection), in the absence of treatment, new infections would likely result.

The initial relationships between marriage and HIV prevalence shift over time, as the TLT women age and a greater proportion of them have married. By 2015, the women are between the ages of 18 and 28; only 16 percent had never married, and just 3 percent said they had never had sex. In other words, six years later we had a sexually active sample that was mostly married. By this point HIV prevalence was about the same (around 10 percent) for women who never married (a select group of women who are marrying later than is typical in this setting) and those who were in their first marriage.

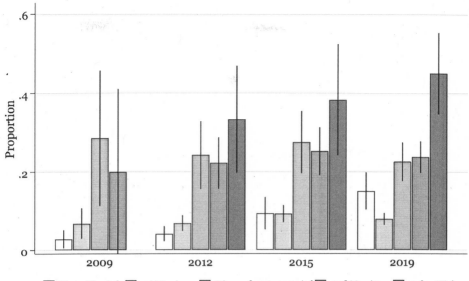

FIGURE 6.4 HIV prevalence by marital experience for women, 2009–2019

Source: TLT, all waves.

The evidence of negative selection out of a first marriage remains: HIV prevalence is far higher among those who left a first marriage than among those
who are still in it. And the light evidence of positive selection into a second
marriage has disappeared. HIV prevalence is essentially bifurcated, with very
low prevalence among the never- and onetime-married and very high prevalence among all those who ever divorced or remarried.

By 2019, only 5 percent of women had never married and HIV prevalence was higher among these women than it was among women who have
been married once and only once. It is at this stage of the life course that
we observe what some refer to as the "protective" quality of marriage in an
HIV epidemic.[16] The pattern helps us understand Njemile's dilemma from a
slightly different perspective. Although she is in a difficult marriage and although divorce is common and widely accepted in Balaka, she stays. Through
population chatter and her own view of the demographic terrain, Njemile
understands her position (see fig. 6.4)—as a woman in her first marriage—as
perhaps the safest one she can occupy. And given the overall sentiment about
men's faithfulness, Njemile is not optimistic that a different husband would
be any safer. HIV prevalence among divorced women and those who have
entered into a second marriage is a little over 20 percent, and among women
who have had more than two marriages, nearly half are living with HIV.

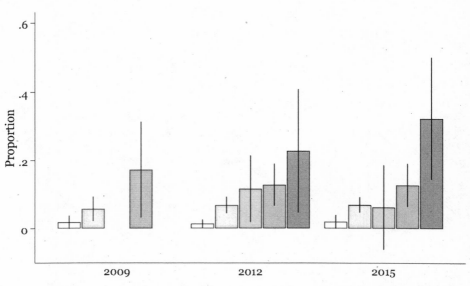

FIGURE 6.5 HIV prevalence by marital experience for men, 2009–2015
Source: TLT-1 (waves 1–8) and TLT-2.

Among the male partners who enrolled in TLT, the relationship between marital experience and HIV prevalence is quite similar (see fig. 6.5). HIV prevalence rises from 6 percent in 2009 to 8 percent in 2012 to 10 percent in 2015, and the marital-experience gradient at all three points in time is extremely strong, stretching from less than 2 percent of never-married men to over 30 percent of men in their third or fourth marriage.

Changing marriage composition and HIV prevalence by marriage presents a classic demographic puzzle. The amount of HIV in the population depends on both the prevalence that characterizes each marital state and the proportion of people in that state. HIV prevalence among the thrice married may be very high. Indeed, it is. What that means for the whole population depends on how many thrice-married women there are; that number can be low or high, and it can be stable or variable over time. Using a tool called decomposition, I apportion the observed increase in HIV prevalence to these two forces: changing marriage composition and changing marriage-specific HIV prevalences. Is the increase being driven primarily by an increase in the proportion of women married multiple times? Or by rising prevalence within in each (or most) of those categories? For women, HIV prevalence increases by 8 percentage points between 2009 and 2015 (the common end point in our data for both men and women); 45 percent of that increase is due to changes in the marriage composition, and 55 percent of it is due to differences in the marriage-specific HIV prevalence rates themselves. For male partners, however, 85 percent of the observed rise in HIV prevalence (4 percentage points, from 6 percent in 2009 to 10 percent in 2015) is due to marriage composition and just 15 percent to the HIV rates.

The stakes of choosing well when entering into a first marriage are extremely high. Relationship churning—moving through marriages during young adulthood—puts young adults at risk of contracting HIV; it also increases prevalence for the population, and the process is gendered. Not only is HIV prevalence higher for women than it is for their male partners, but it is also patterned differently, which has implications for uncertainty. Increasing HIV prevalence for men is overwhelmingly attributable to the fact that, over time, more of the group occupies the high-prevalence states on the spectrum of marital experience. The 85/15 decomposition split for men conforms to a clear pattern that can be perceived in everyday life, even without specialized demographic data and methods. In contrast, the 45/55 split for women is equivalent to a perpetual coin toss: about half the increase is due to rising HIV prevalence within each marital state and half to the rising proportion of TLT women who have gotten divorced and remarried. This combination of forces creates a reality that may, in fact, appear quite random to the population experiencing these rates. Population chatter offers some clues to what ordinary people perceive about these patterns, specifically, whether HIV is understood as within or outside one's ambit of control.

Patrick and the Tragicomedy of Marital Shopping for Men

Based on the survey data and ethnographic vignettes presented thus far, the gendered nature of relationship uncertainty is strong. Measured by suspicion, gossip, a characterization of how "most men" behave, stated grounds for divorce, and common complaints, women are extremely concerned about their partners' faithfulness; men, on the other hand, are less so. The men of Balaka come across as a real problem. But men's experiences of courtship, marriage, and relationship dissolution are worth our attention as well, and when we listen to the population chatter produced by men, their stories illuminate a distinct set of concerns about relationship uncertainty. Recall that the earlier vignette from the salon was written in May. By October, Precious had given birth to her third child; the child was vomiting and running a fever, so Precious took the child to the hospital for tests and treatment. In a show of friendship, Gertrude and Enid trek to the hospital to check on Precious, bringing her refreshments and moral support. Along the way, they meet

Patrick, who amuses them with a story that gives us a taste of the distinct flavors of relationship uncertainty from a man's perspective.

In the morning when I woke up, Enid knocked on my door and told me that Precious was at the hospital with her child and that we needed to go see her before the visiting time is over. I said, "No problem." And we agreed to leave in the afternoon at 4 o'clock. On our way, Enid complained that life is a bit tough because she is not working much. She couldn't pay rent for the salon, the landlord changed the lock on her kiosk, and she doesn't know if they will let her open it again. These days she is just braiding people's hair from home. We ran into a man—a friend of Enid—who joined us. He said he wanted to see the child too.

Enid introduced the man as Patrick; they had met in Zomba while Enid was visiting her grandparents, and he now stays with relatives in Balaka. As we were walking, Enid asked Patrick if he is still married, and Patrick said he is not. He added, "Nowadays if a man doesn't have money, that means there is no marriage at all."

Enid asked Patrick why he would say that. He replied, "If you have married and you have some money, the woman loves you a lot. But if you don't have money, just know that the marriage is over. There will be no love at all." Patrick said he often asks himself why he isn't already dead after having been lied to by so many women. "With my first wife, I was doing business and could find money. I was paying school fees for her while she was in secondary school; I even bathed without using soap so that everything could be hers. But then when I started lacking money, she left me for another man. After that one, I fell in love with another woman, but that marriage ended when she started prostituting at our local bar."

I asked him, "So what's the main reason marriages don't last long these days?"

"The main problem is that women lie and say that their marriages were in the past," he said.[17] Patrick explained that after his second marriage, he fell in love with another woman whose family brews beer. They were in relationship; he was in the process of marrying her, and she fell in love with another man who had a big radio that people hire for activities in the community. "Even her family preferred the man with the radio because he had more money than me. So I ended that relationship.

"And I didn't stop there. After that I fell in love with a girl who was in form one. And from my past experiences, I didn't want to send her to school and pay for her education. I just wanted to marry her as quickly as possible. So this one was my fourth wife. After a few months of seeing how we were staying together [getting along], I decided to pay for her school fees. I gave her the school fees, and instead of going to school she used the money to go to Lilongwe to meet her aunt. After a few days, I called her and asked her to please come back home. At first she said she was on her way—she was about to leave. She would depart the next day. Then after calling her for the third day, some man answered her phone and warned me never to call that number again. He said, 'That girl is now married here in Lilongwe.'" Enid and I laughed at Patrick's bad luck. He said, "I don't have any appetite for women anymore. They can kill a man, and they can also make him poor."

By then we had reached at the hospital. We found Precious and her child; the child was recovering, and Precious said they would be leaving the hospital the next morning. We praised God for that and gave Precious the soft drinks I had bought. We didn't stay there long. We just turned back to get home before dark.

Then Patrick said he wanted to finish his story. Enid and I laughed, and said, "Oh?! Is there more? OK. We should give you a chance to finish." Most recently, Patrick's parents found another woman for him to marry. He said his parents introduced them, and he liked the woman so much that he completely forgot about all the women he had been married to before. "She was beautiful and lovely, and within a week we were engaged." Again, he didn't send her to school because he was afraid to repeat those past experiences. Then one day they decided to have a walk at Majiga 2.[18] As they were walking they saw a certain man, and the woman whispered to Patrick, "Do you see the man in front of us? He was my boyfriend before your parents told me about you." The man saw the girl and stopped her. And he said to Patrick, "Stay away from this woman. And know that this girl is beautiful because I am the one giving her money. Last year she was pregnant, and she has my child, and her mother is keeping the grandchild so that the girl has a chance of finding another man to marry, as if she were not already a mother. We met at church, we were in the choir, we were singing together, and I ended the relationship when she got pregnant. Now she has given birth, and I want her back. So stay away from her." Enid and I couldn't help laughing at poor Patrick.

He said, "Enid, I don't have any appetite or sexual feelings for any woman. I have learned a lot of lessons."

Enid said, "I think marriage is a gift from God. Some were made for marriage, while others were not."

Patrick and Enid thanked me for letting them join me on the walk to the hospital. And I said, "Thanks for keeping me company." Patrick took my telephone number and said, "Let's keep chatting."

When Patrick summarizes his history with the women he almost married and those he was married to briefly, he illustrates a bundle of related and distinct concepts that could have been lifted directly from the scholarly literature: marital shopping, relationship churning, impulsive marriages, serial monogamy, fragile unions, and the semiotics of support. The epidemiological and demographic acuity of Patrick's tragicomedy is remarkable. Still in his early thirties, Patrick's "bad luck" has taken him through five "marriages," and although he claims to be done with women completely, the fact that this vignette ends with him hitting up Gertrude for her phone number suggests that his hiatus from the romantic sphere may not last for long. Granted, not all of Patrick's relationships were true marriages, but that detail is key to understanding Patrick's relationship history. His narration shows that ambiguity surrounding the marriage process—the definitional issues woven throughout Njemile's reveal and the complaints Precious and Enid exchange at the salon—affects men too.

In particular, Patrick's insights underscore a key point from the decomposition analysis: the legibility of a marital experience gradient is strong enough to be perceived from within the population for men but not for women. Within the TLT study, Patrick would be located at the highest end of the marital experience spectrum, where HIV prevalence is almost 50 percent (see fig. 6.5), and he shows an awareness of this pattern when he wonders why he is not already dead. By casually remarking on the deadliness of relationships to Gertrude and Enid, Patrick is assuming common knowledge of the epidemiological milieu they all inhabit, not speaking with the insight of a specialist or disclosing a deep personal fear. This clarity on the relationship between men's marital experience and their HIV risk stands in contrast to the population chatter Gertrude captures in women's spaces, where men's infidelities and the gossip and suspicion that accompanies them is spotlighted, conveying a perpetual sense of vulnerability regardless of whether the relationship is a first or an nth marriage.

Importantly, Patrick is not womanizing; he is looking to marry and start a family. In an important but little cited paper, the economist Jeremy Magruder uses simulation models to show that a pattern of serial monogamy and rapid re-partnering is sufficient to sustain a generalized HIV epidemic—even without any concurrency (i.e., overlapping partnerships) attributable to infidelity or polygyny. Magruder formalized this process of "marital shopping" with a model that basically mimics Patrick's story, only with fewer partners, reflecting the distribution of sexual experience for never-married young adults in South Africa. From the simulations, Magruder concludes that the very process of becoming married is dangerous: "A simple search and matching model of serial monogamy is capable of generating high prevalence with relatively few partners because short periods of high partner turnover coincide with a brief window of high infectiousness immediately following infection."[19]

The dangers of marital shopping for HIV prevalence have been elaborated by a handful of scholars but typically with a focus on the experiences of women, in large part because we only occasionally have detailed data on men's relationships and rarely a glimpse of their feelings about those experiences.[20] In her study of the sex-money relationship among unmarried young adults in Balaka, the sociologist Michelle Poulin elaborates the semiotics of support and argues that the salience of money is highest when it is hard-earned or "nearly all one can give."[21] In Patrick's case, the sacrifice of washing without soap was still not enough once he slid into a period of unemployment. Ethnographic research from across the region further underscores the tremendous pressure men are under to provide in order to get and stay married, confirming Patrick's observation that love abounds for the employed but evaporates when work is scarce.[22]

One final note about the larger significance of Patrick's story as emblematic of the kind of gossip and rumor that constantly circulated in and around Balaka: Deception by a young wife who insists she wants to further her education and then flees to her aunt's house is noteworthy because it is a cliché. The episode must be understood both as a hurtful, humiliating, and expensive experience for Patrick personally and as a prototype of rumor that depicts men's anxieties and their collective experience of relationship uncertainty. Recall from chapter 2 the adolescent in Mudzi who tricked her suitor into making bricks alongside her for months and then vanished once the house was complete. Gertrude captured versions of this trope almost a dozen times, referencing different individuals and variations on the general theme: sometimes the young woman left with the school fees; sometimes it was money she said she would use to start a business; in one case she helped her husband save for and buy a motorcycle and then rode off on it herself. Often the young wife escapes to stay in a big city with her aunt, or she goes to relatives in a distant district; one went as far as Zimbabwe. In every instance, the credulous husband is both shocked and heartbroken. The duped men in these stories illustrate that the vulnerability of relationships is a mutual rather than a one-sided phenomenon. Relationship uncertainty looms large in men's lives too; it is inseparable from the economic sphere, overlapping with livelihood uncertainty—its own subject of inquiry. When one listens to population chatter about relationship uncertainty, what emerges is structured like a call-and-response song, sung as a battle of the sexes metanarrative that connects love, support, mischief, and betrayal to HIV. The women call, "That's men. They all make someone cry," and the men respond, "A woman can kill a man, and she can also make him poor." The song is beautiful, funny, and cathartic because it captures both the comedy and the painful truth about relationship uncertainty in a context of persistent, endemic HIV.

The Consequences of Relationship Uncertainty

The data presented already in this chapter make a few things abundantly clear: relationship uncertainty (suspicion and gossip) is widespread, unions are unstable, divorce is common, remarriages happen quickly, and aggregate-level HIV prevalence tracks strongly with marital experience. To say that these phenomena are gendered does not mean they are experienced exclusively by women; indeed, both men and women are responsive to these uncertainties and subject to the HIV prevalence rates they produce. Looking below the surface, at the subjective realm, I show how personal uncertainty drives the differences in prevalence. Figure 6.6 elaborates the iterative process of relationship and HIV uncertainties with marital transitions and HIV infections in a conceptual model. Below marital experience, three dimensions are located on their own "plane": relationship uncertainty, HIV uncertainty, and HIV status, with personal HIV status as a micro-analog of the aggregate prevalence measure at the top. Note that the story of uncertainty as a driver of the epidemic has to be understood through both the presence of arrows connecting key phenomena to others and the absence of arrows between other pairs. Here the arrows indicate that a strong empirical relationship can be confirmed in the TLT data, using models designed to assess whether and how a change in one status or state is associated with changes (positive or negative) in another.

Patuma's story (and Njemile's) is manifested at the center of this diagram, where all the action is. Relationship uncertainty—operationalized here as suspicion that a partner has other partners—plays a powerful role in this constellation of HIV uncertainty, actual HIV infections, and marital instability.

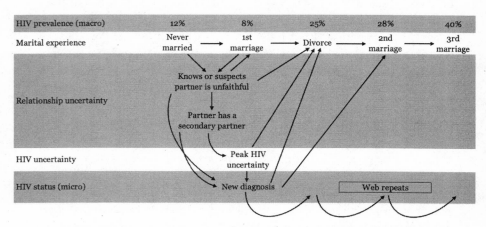

FIGURE 6.6 Summary of associations clarifying the process by which relationship and HIV uncertainty perpetuate the spread of HIV

For married respondents, knowing or suspecting that one's partner has other partners is positively related to two HIV-related phenomena measured at the next wave: moving into a state of peak uncertainty and getting a new HIV diagnosis.[23] Beyond the relationship with HIV-related phenomena, relationship uncertainty manifests in two other, tangible ways. Not surprisingly, suspicions of a partner's other relationships are positively associated with divorce in the subsequent two waves. Many men and women leave the relationships that may be putting them at risk, even without meeting the "caught red-handed" threshold of evidence Patuma so bravely managed to collect. The more epidemiologically complicated consequence of relationship uncertainty is that these suspicions are positively associated with women's reports that they themselves acquired secondary partners in a subsequent wave. In network terms, we might call this a leveling of an imbalanced sexual network within a relationship. Linda Tawfik and Susan Watkins observed something similar when they pushed back against simple narratives about survival sex, arguing that women in Balaka also pursue relationships for passion, pleasure, and revenge, with a special emphasis on revenge.[24] Consistent with the findings reported in figure 5.4, the acquisition of a secondary partner has no relationship to HIV uncertainty or to a new HIV diagnosis. Thoughts of a partner's partner trigger HIV uncertainty, while one's own partners do not.

Both new diagnoses and uncertainty about HIV strain relationships. While married people living with HIV are not, when studied as an undifferentiated group, at increased risk for divorce, married respondents *are* at increased risk for divorce during the two waves that follow a new diagnosis, and the odds of divorce are also elevated for those who hover or move in a state of acute uncertainty about their HIV status. In other words, both HIV uncertainty and the stress of a new diagnosis (arguably its own uncertainty) predict divorce, while HIV, as a simple serostatus, does not.

Relationship and HIV uncertainty have a unique relationship to the transition to first marriage. While the process of uncertainty between marriage and divorce and remarriage is consistent for men and women, the process I describe here is specific to never-married women. Knowing or suspecting that one's boyfriend has other on-the-side partners may not seem like an obvious predictor of first marriage, and it is definitely not an idyllic one. Empirically, however, women experiencing relationship uncertainty are more likely to get married in the next wave—perhaps as a strategy for solidifying and formalizing that relationship and perhaps with the specific objective of eliminating any lurking secondary partners from the picture. Compared to those who express certainty about their HIV status, women who experience acute HIV uncertainty are more likely to have gotten married by the time of their next interview. While counterintuitive, these are not anomalous findings. In fact, in the domain of marriage, HIV uncertainty plays the very same role we observed for fertility: it acts as an accelerator, pushing never-married young adults who may feel adrift into the project of marriage and family formation. It is a stage of life governed by strong scripts, clear expectations, tangible goals, and the bestowal of adult status and respect in the community.[25] Jens Beckert suggests that many people respond to acute uncertainty by setting themselves on paths that impose rigidity, limit their flexibility, and reduce the set of choices they will face in the future.[26] Unlike the myriad ambiguities of extended young adulthood for single people in Balaka, the project for a couple is admittedly difficult but perfectly clear: marry, build a house, have babies, provide for and educate those children. In that sense, accelerated marriage and childbearing can be understood as strategies of uncertainty reduction, despite the fact that they also lead straight into a different set of uncertainties.

Demographers usually study romantic relationships in terms of "nuptuality," with a focus on events and the goal of quantifying marriages, divorces, and their consequences in a population (especially for fertility and migration), but have far less to say about what these patterns mean for those who experience them.[27] Analyzing romantic relationships in Balaka with traditional demographic tools and an ear to population chatter, I find that, like HIV uncertainty, relationship uncertainty is widespread, that it should be thought of, measured, and understood both as a personal experience and as an ambient force at the population level, and that it has concrete consequences for marital patterns and for HIV. Consensus positions about what "most men" do reflect and inform personal experiences with romantic relationships. Gossip is ubiquitous, fueling both suspicion and actual relationship instability. Relationships are both dangerous and essential, and relationship uncertainty is central to the decisions and actions that constitute the dense eventfulness of young adulthood. At the individual level, relationship and HIV uncertainty work in tandem, pushing and pulling young adults into and out of relationships, raising the risk of contracting and spreading HIV, and generating a phenomenon of relationship churning that aggregates into a particular marital regime by which the HIV epidemic is strongly patterned. In this sense, the consequences of relationship uncertainty are as real as education, socioeconomic status, and all the other phenomena social scientists routinely consider as predictors of relationship quality, divorce, and HIV status.

Call the Ankhoswe

With what tools do young adults navigate relationship uncertainty? Are they completely at the whim of a partner and luck? Or are there strategies that shore up relationships, forge trust, and ensure their durability? Chapter 6 made it clear that there is a lot of relationship uncertainty in Balaka. Indeed, readers may come away with the sense that young adults in this community are adrift in a sea of total chaos in the romantic realm, starting with their earliest relationships. But there are patterns within the chaos, delineated by both the age-old traditions that govern marriage and the new technologies that facilitate relationships. Of course, these institutions and technologies are never perfectly stable; just like policies, they change over time, and the patterning of relationship and HIV uncertainty changes along with them. This chapter is devoted to analyzing relationship uncertainty alongside changes in two domains of life: marriage traditions (ankhoswe and chinkhoswe) and communication technologies (mobile phones).

At first blush, mobile phones and marriage mediators may seem to have nothing in common. What links them conceptually, with relevance for uncertainty, is how they influence the pace of relationship formation and dissolution. While intimate relationships are indeed navigated by a couple, that couple is never truly alone.[1] Lovers communicate with one another directly, but they also often send messages through friends and via phones. In centering salient others in the analysis of relationship uncertainty, I look outside the couple, spotlighting the best friend, the mother, the gossiping neighbor, and the marriage mediators. With an emphasis on the speed at which relationships are forged and dissolved, I point to the proliferation of mobile phones as a likely accelerator of relationship processes and to the secular decline of ankhoswe as an erosion of what has historically been a decelerator of nuptial events. With relationship trajectories unfolding ever more quickly, relationships in Balaka seem uniquely uncertain.

Writing about women's expectations and experiences of marriage in northern Malawi, the folklorist Anika Wilson notes the widespread use of the phrase "marriage is endurance" and elaborates an important insight into the diverse connotations of what it means to endure—thriving, coping, surviving, and adapting.[2] The strategies Wilson identifies for how women cope with marital insecurity[3] include storytelling (lore), aggressive public confrontations with romantic rivals, monitoring and surveillance, and the invocation of elders and other go-betweens for advice and intervention.

The therapeutic role of storytelling is evident in the conversation from the salon presented in chapter 6 and the intensity Patuma and Njemile brought when telling their stories. Public confrontations, such as the one Tiyamike referred to with a bit of shame, are regular events around town but only occasional in any one person's life. Gertrude summarized a typical fight, which did not involve any of her regular interlocutors. During fieldwork periods, I typically witness a confrontation like this one about once a week.

> Then I left and passed by a shop where a large crowd had gathered. I asked, "What happened?"
>
> A women explained that the shop belongs to a certain man at Majiga 2 who is married. He invited his girlfriend to collect some money at the shop. And because the woman who was married to the owner of the shop heard some rumors that her husband has got girlfriends, she just went to the shop without telling her husband. She wanted proof. As that woman was collecting the money the wife appeared and started beating the girlfriend. The man didn't do anything to end the fight because the wife came with her friends and they were helping her to beat the other woman. Instead, the man just ran away and left them fighting. Then other people took advantage, stealing things from the shop as the fighting was happening. Two policemen who were nearby came and took all the women—six total—to the police station. People laughed and said, "This is what men are doing nowadays, leaving you at home while coming to town to meet other women."

Surveillance can take dramatic forms, as in Patuma's adventures in the bush, or subtler ones, like this simple observation from Gertrude about the presence of the electrician's wife in her home.

> Due to a faulty socket at home, I've been charging my laptop at the tailoring shop when I chat with the guys. They usually charge 50 MK, but I am charging for free since I have earned "regular customer" status. The landlord finally sent a man to fix the socket in my house. I asked if he is an electrician, and he

said, "Yes." He came with his wife. His wife just sat there watching while her husband was working. She watched him for three hours.

As a strategy for managing relationship uncertainty, mediation and advice link back to Susan Watkins's insistence that "socially salient others" are crucial for understanding demographic patterns and changes, specifically with respect to marriage. In Balaka, when a couple experiences trouble or conflict, they are expected to call on their traditional marriage mediators—their ankhoswe—for help. Ten years ago, the word *call* in that phrase had the clear connotation of summoning in some physical way. Increasingly, calling the ankhoswe involves a literal phone call or series of SMS messages that initiate a variety of conversations among appointed relatives who will descend to offer clarity, advice, and help resolve the conflict, which may happen through peace and conciliation or through a condoned dissolution. One bike taxi driver beautifully summarized to Gertrude the importance of ankhoswe for stabilizing relationships in a context of widespread uncertainty.

> The ankhoswe are like poles that make the house strong. The ankhoswe help to bring peace in the family. When people have disagreements in their family first of all you talk to your partner yourself. But if some weeks later you see that the problem is still going on, that's when you go to ankhoswe so that they should help you solve the problem. If the ankhoswe fail to help you solve the problem, then you take the issue to the police or the chief's court. Or you may just have to leave.

The Marriage Process and Relationship Quality

To do chinkhoswe in Balaka is to hold a traditional marriage ceremony—small or large, with minimal or considerable fanfare. When a couple decides to get married, the families of the bride and groom each appoint a relative (usually a maternal uncle, sibling, or cousin) or close friend to act as their *nkhoswe* (noun, sing.); though male ankhoswe (noun, pl.) are typical, female relatives can and do fill the role. The ankhoswe are the marriage guardians who facilitate communication between the two families, officiate the traditional ceremony, and commit to supporting the marriage should difficulties arise. They serve as counselors when the couple needs advice, support, or mediation—much as a godparent commits to supporting the spiritual formation of a godchild. When marital problems are serious enough to be escalated to court, ankhoswe are expected to be present for the hearing. And when a couple divorces, the ankhoswe from both sides meet to authorize and witness the dissolution as well.[4] A good nkhoswe has more life experience than you do, will show up when you need them, and is a person whose advice you respect, especially when it comes to matters of the heart. An ideal nkhoswe is someone whose advice your spouse will also heed and can be trusted to look out for your best interest if the marriage ever starts to crumble.

The marriage ceremony is seldom mentioned in Gertrude's conversations, but the ankhoswe are a regular topic of population chatter, and because Gertrude is from a different region, her genuine lack of familiarity with the particular norms in Balaka provides a foil for questions that draw out explanations and examples of how ankhoswe (and the lack thereof) factor in young adults' lives and relationships. *When do you call them? Will they actually help? Mine came and set my husband straight! Lucky you, mine are useless; they don't even bother to call me back, and his doesn't even have a phone!*

Talk of ankhoswe raises questions about the marriage process: the level of formality or informality that characterizes a relationship. Njemile did chinkhoswe with her husband after her pregnancy and before her son was born. Therefore, in addition to her supportive in-laws, she has ankhoswe she can call when disagreements intensify. Patrick regales us with a story of five "marriages," at least three of which are near-marriages or informal marriages. In none of these relationships did he have anyone to call. Most demographic studies in the region collect data on marital status and ask about co-wives and mobility to assess polygamous versus monogamous patterns of marriage or differentiate matrilocal from patrilocal groups. But few studies attempt to collect complete marital histories or detailed data on the forms of marriage. Using the TLT data on marital steps, I link the institutional status of marriage, which ranges from informal consensual unions to white weddings and outcomes like relationship duration, relationship satisfaction, suspicion and relationship uncertainty, and HIV prevalence. Considered in light of the MDFRA policies (see chap. 2) designed to formalize and stabilize unions, regulate terms of their dissolution, and improve vital statistics, these data suggest that marriage is not the binary state social scientists often presume it to be and that treating it as such in quantitative analysis might be a mistake.

Consensual unions, cohabitation, living together: the various terms for informal marriage are widespread in the literatures on sexual behavior, union formation and dissolution, and HIV in Malawi.[5] But when we asked married respondents in 2015 and 2019 about the steps they had gone through the last time they had gotten married, we learned that only 5 percent had never paid the chief. This is a function of the MDFRA, which gives chiefs wide latitude to impose fines on couples who have not paid to record their marriage in the village registry. About 30 percent of respondents got married informally, by simply moving in together, but most of them organized to pay the chief

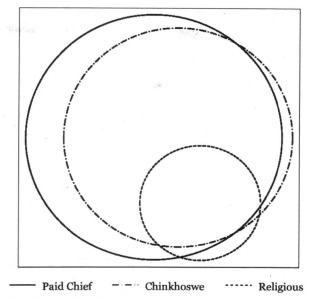

——— **Paid Chief**   — · —·· **Chinkhoswe**   ······ **Religious**

FIGURE 7.1 Venn diagram of marriage steps

Source: TLT-3.

Note: Square represents all ever-married women interviewed in 2019, including the refresher sample
(N = 2,364 women). Circles are proportional to size.

soon afterward rather than accept the inevitable fine. Overall, the steps in the
marriage process range from no ceremony at all (i.e., just moving in together
or consensual union) to having engaged in three different ceremonies to formalize the relationship within one's community. Depicted as proportions, the
relationships between these steps basically take the shape of concentric circles
(fig. 7.1): most people have paid the chief; among those who did that, a majority also did chinkhoswe; but only a small proportion of married women—20
percent—also had any kind of religious ceremony.

In Balaka, there is considerable variation in what constitutes a marriage
and, as illustrated by Patuma's response to the marital status question, occasional ambiguity about the status itself. Naturally, this ambiguity contributes
to the high levels of relationship uncertainty revealed by everyday conversation and present in the TLT survey data. Interrogating our couple-matched
data sets from 2009 to 2015, I found that only 80 percent of the informally
married couples we interviewed even agreed about whether they were married, and in a full 20 percent of those cases one partner described the relationship as a marriage and the other as a cohabitation, an engagement, or a dating
relationship. Among those partners who had gone through multiple steps in

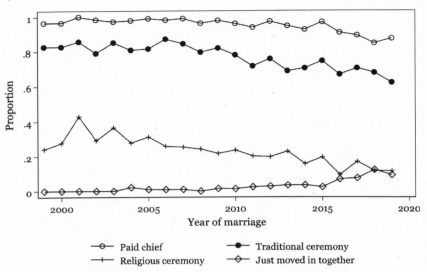

FIGURE 7.2 Trends in the marriage process, 1999–2019

Source: TLT-3.

Note: Graph summarizes 2,342 most-recent marriages reported by 2,617 women in 2019.

the marital process together, however, agreement on the basic fact of whether they are married was nearly perfect.

A few decades ago, chinkhoswe was synonymous with marriage. As recently as 2002 Mike Mthambo Mtika and Henry Doctor wrote, "No one in rural Malawi is without *nkhoswe*."[6] Read in that light, figure 7.2 shows that payments to the chief, chinkhoswe, and religious ceremonies have been in decline and informal marriages on the rise since 2015. The exact reasons for this trend are unclear, and since marriage is a process, it is possible that these recently married couples may still go on to do chinkhoswe or have a religious ceremony. The decline in payments to chiefs is particularly noteworthy as a response to a law that mandates its enforcement. To the extent that fees to register a marriage with the chief have been transformed from small and symbolic to steep and standardized, it seems to have had the unintended consequence of creating a larger class of partially married couples, that is, more uncertain relationships. Although the MDFRA of 2015 was intended to stabilize marriages by improving the vital registration system maintained by chiefs (which covered nearly 100 percent of young-adult marriages in Balaka from 2000 to 2011), it may have contributed to the erosion of forms of support that actually matter to those navigating relationship uncertainty and marriage.

Table 7.1 provides evidence that the steps of marriage process depicted in figure 7.1 sustains relationships in tangible ways. From subjective assess-

TABLE 7.1 Relationship outcomes by marriage type

	Informal	Paid chief	Chinkhoswe	Religious
Relationship quality				
Overall satisfaction	0.75[a]	0.84[a]	0.87[b]	0.87[b]
Partner cares	0.76[a]	0.80[a,b]	0.80[a,b]	0.82[b]
Suspects infidelity	0.39[a]	0.31[a,b]	0.34[a,b]	0.30[b]
Relationship duration				
Still together in a year	7.78[a]	8.13[a,b]	8.29[a,b]	8.57[b]
Marriage lasts to 2019	0.46	0.68	0.68	0.88
Safety and security				
IPV last year	0.22[a]	0.14[a,b]	0.10[a,b]	0.08[b]
HIV prevalence (all)	0.29[a]	0.11[a,b]	0.13[a,b]	0.08[b]
HIV prevalence (first marriages)	0.20[a]	0.10[a,b]	0.11[a,b]	0.06[b]

Source: TLT-2 and TLT-3.

Note: Still together in a year is measured with beans. All other variables are represented as proportions, ranging from 0 to 1.

[a] Difference from couples who had a religious ceremony is statistically significant ($p < 0.05$) in a multivariate model.

[b] Difference from informal partnerships is statistically significant ($p < 0.05$) in a multivariate model.

ments of relationship quality to divorce, HIV prevalence, and violence, women in informal marriages are disadvantaged in comparison to those with chiefs, ankhoswe, or religious communities to support them. Indeed, in Balaka, the "most married" enjoy high levels of relationship security, while the relationships of the informally married are characterized by layers of uncertainty and hardship. The table contains predicted values for eight outcomes by marriage type, based on regression models that control for respondent's age, socioeconomic status, education level, and relationship duration. The values can be interpreted as group means, and the significant differences between groups are denoted with letters, to differentiate statistically meaningful differences from those that are minimally different or could be an artifact of chance.

Taking the outcomes one by one, overall relationship satisfaction is highest among those who have completed traditional or religious ceremonies and lowest among the informally married. Strong agreement with the statement, "My partner shows that he cares for me," follows a similar pattern. When asked whether one's partner has other partners, more women in informal marriages suspect infidelity than do women who have gone through additional steps in the marriage process, by a difference of about 10 percentage points (39 to 29 percent). Asked (with beans) how likely they will still be together with this partner a year from now, most respondents are optimists. Even in this context of high divorce rates, respondents place, on average, eight beans on their plates, and their responses follow a light positive gradient across the spectrum of marital steps. Considering the relationship outcomes, marital longevity tracks closely. Among respondents who were in a first marriage in 2015, half of the informal first marriages and 68 percent of marriages registered with chiefs or officiated by chinkhoswe survived to 2019, compared to 88 percent of marriages that had been blessed by some kind of religious ceremony.

Experiences of intimate partner violence (IPV)—whether the partner has hit, slapped, pulled the hair of, or thrown things at the respondent (or engaged in another violent behavior in the past year)—tracks with the marriage process by a magnitude of three: 21 percent among the informally married and 7 percent among those who completed multiple steps. Finally, within first marriages, HIV prevalence is strongly patterned by marriage type, and although the relationship may not be causal, the differences are stark and significant: 25 percent prevalence among the informally married; 12 and 13 percent among those who have paid the chief and done chinkhoswe, and just 7 percent among those who also had a religious ceremony. That infidelities would be more prevalent in relationships where commitment levels are underspecified and expectations tacit, rather than explicit, is not surprising. Ankhoswe do not ensure a stable marriage in Balaka. Neither do white weddings. However, the differences in IPV and HIV are especially striking and suggest that the process of formalizing a marriage—and in doing so, designating a salient other to support your relationship—may bring a modicum of stability in an uncertain environment.

Mrs. Samosa

Old and young, male and female, married once and married five times, Gertrude's interlocutors have plenty to say about marriage as endurance and the importance of ankhoswe in their relationships. Advice about how to find love and stay married abounds in Balaka, and since Gertrude is unmarried she receives a lot of it. This short vignette about "Mrs. Samosa" is less colorful than the others. She is a happily married chef-entrepreneur who sells her goods and has few complaints about her husband. Nonetheless, the vignette is instructive because this content woman in her early thirties also experiences the stressors that sink many marriages and endorses the ankhoswe as an important resource for staying together and staying in town.

On my way, I met a woman who was selling samosa near the railway. She was alone, and I jokingly asked her if I could help her sell the samosa. She said, "Please do. I feel lonely here."

"Are people not buying?"

"They are buying. I always make about 2,000 MK; at 11 a.m. or 12, you will see that I have sold out. I also give a bucket to my daughter who sells them on her way to school. And she sells all of hers too."

I asked, "What does your husband do?"

"He was selling secondhand clothes at the market, but he stopped because he was never making a profit. Lucky enough, we stay in our own house. At first we rented for five years, and that was very tough. Landlords. But my husband worked hard until we built our own house, and now we stay there in our own house. Some time ago things became tough, and we thought of going back to the village. But now I'm used to staying in town: we eat nice food here, we dress well, my daughter is studying. I don't think I could bear to go back to village life. If we went back to the village, my kids would not go far with education and we would just be stuck there. So I decided to start this business."

"Who gave you the capital to get started?"

"My husband did. We also have a field where we grow maize. Last year we harvested twenty-four bags, but this year I know we will not have as much because the rain was not enough."

"So you stay well with your husband?"

"We stay well together. We understand each other, we always forgive each other when there is a misunderstanding. When we quarrel in our family—for the first time, we don't go directly to ankhoswe. But if we quarrel for a second time about the same issue, that means it's something we cannot solve on our own. Then we go to ankhoswe to ask for advice. If your husband is not taking good care of the family, if he is spending all his money on beer, you have to talk to him. But if he doesn't listen, you'll get tired of his behavior. Go to the ankhoswe for help. If it is your first marriage, you are young. You don't have the experience; you are impatient. You lack wisdom. You don't know what it means to quarrel or resolve it, and you might be afraid to go to the ankhoswe. But they need to help you with the marriage. Once you get older, you won't need your ankhoswe as often. You can sort out the problems yourself."

Mrs. Samosa and her husband have managed what many seek and few accomplish. They moved to town, built a house, are sending their children to school, and have grown enough surplus maize to start some small businesses. They are working together in a committed way and have called on their ankhoswe to help them navigate disputes. From subsequent conversations with Gertrude and others in the months that follow this initial exchange, Mrs. Samosa's relationship with her husband is indeed a low-drama partnership in which the couple farm together, wrap dough together, pay school fees, and make small improvements to their home. Although their business ventures are not always successful, the couple exchanges what Mrs. Samosa refers to as "support" in myriad ways: money, practical help, and encouragement. They succeed as companions and as business partners. When Gertrude's friends gossip about the Samosas, they repeat two key observations: Mr. and Mrs. Samosa frequently bathe together, even though they are no longer young lovers; and they spend all their time together at home "making budgets," a habit that impedes the formation of strong friendships with peers. The substance of this gossip underscores the complete lack of privacy in Balaka, the delight with which residents gossip about other people's relationships, and the Samosas' enviable ability to manifest the ideals of companionate marriage—an ideal that many hold but few achieve given the obstacles of the existing gender structure and the impossibly difficult economic terrain.[7]

Mrs. Samosa unapologetically desires the good things in life—good food, nice clothes, and better opportunities for her children—and those desires are supported by a combination of skills in the domains of farming and cooking and some business acumen, generating small profits on a regular basis.[8] She rarely complains about her husband and divulges no appetite for having additional men in her life. Theirs is a relationship of quiet and calm, unusually high levels of trust, and few worries about the relationship itself. Mrs. Samosa's analysis of marriage generally, not just her own, is that ankhoswe support is most important during the early years when relationships are especially fragile, and she is astute in this regard, as the claim is strongly supported by the TLT survey data and the high-quality literature on marriage in southern Malawi and nearby contexts. Impulsive marriages, informal marriages, and consensual unions are common, and these relationships are fragile. In relationships that last, the probability of divorce declines as each additional year of marriage accumulates.[9] This is a tautology, but it still means something. Rather than try to understand the role of marriage—duration and type—with a style of analysis that obsesses over causality, I have begun to think about union formation and dissolution as a selection process or a filter, where the process of filtration, rather than the outcome of the process, is the most analytically important piece of the puzzle.

Like Sophie (discussed in chap. 4), Mrs. Samosa belongs to the small club of insulated individuals, and because there are fewer than twenty such women to analyze in the closely spaced survey data (only three of these married at the time of their baseline interview), it is impossible to quantitatively assess what sustains a long-run sense of certainty about being and staying HIV negative in the context of a romantic relationship. A simple analysis of the cross-sectional data from 2015, however, provides one additional clue. Net of a standard set of controls for key background variables, the only strong predictor of feeling "insulated" (see fig. 4.2) on three time horizons is having ankhoswe to call. Population chatter from Balaka reveals an acute awareness of the fragility of marriage, a wealth of wisdom about common pitfalls, and a set of strategies for maintaining and sustaining a loving relationship in a context of uncertainty. Like the poles that support a house, ankhoswe play a key role in supporting marriages; in the next section I summarize the kinds of calls they field, describe how they help, and assert that the presence of ankhoswe reduces relationship uncertainty.

Ankhoswe as a Counterweight to Relationship Uncertainty

The ankhoswe are mentioned in almost every story about a marriage that has been shared so far in this book. Patuma, Njemile, and Mrs. Samosa all mention calling for help when describing what it means to leave or to stay in a marriage. The population chatter and the ethnographic data make it clear that ankhoswe provide a crucial counterweight to widespread relationship uncertainty. But how do ankhoswe factor into the larger trends of union formation and dissolution? Who calls their ankhoswe? For what reasons? And what kind of help, if any, do they get? I leverage the TLT data to answer these questions and show that the ankhoswe process reveals a great deal about conflict, uncertainty, and HIV risk within marriage.

Figure 7.3 walks through the steps that determine who can call on ankhoswe for support. The bars represent, as a proportion of all respondents, the currently married subpopulation, the subset of married respondents who married by doing chinkhoswe, and those who reported in TLT that they ever called for support in their most recent marriage. Assessing the gaps between *married* and *married with ankhoswe*, women are more likely than men to be informally married and lacking the support of designated kin they should be able draw on in a time of need (25 percent of women compared to 14 percent of men). Among those with ankhoswe, however, women are 20 percentage points more likely than men to report having relied on their ankhoswe to mediate a dispute.

In Gertrude's fieldnotes, the men of Balaka frequently remark, with regard to marriage and ankhoswe, that "everyone knows that women complain more than men." Indeed, that impression is validated by our survey data: 1,048 married women in the 2015 sample produced 3,720 complaints (with one reporting that she called her ankhoswe 50 times), while 715 married men produced about 600 complaints. Theories of gendered power help explain why women may leverage ankhoswe as a resource for navigating relation-

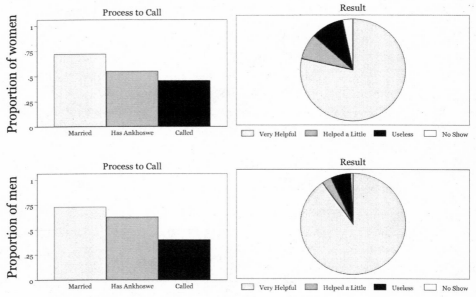

FIGURE 7.3 The process of getting help from ankhoswe

Source: TLT-3.

ships and address problems in their relationship indirectly, relying heavily on kin mediation for problems big and small. At a very basic level, the sheer quantity of complaints can be read as evidence of widespread relationship uncertainty and reliance on salient others to help navigate this rocky terrain.

Shifting from a view of the individuals who call to an analysis of the complaints they make, table 7.2 summarizes the reasons our respondents sought help from their ankhoswe, using the specific example of their most recent dispute. Stated here as list of top tens, there is considerable overlap between the complaints men and women bring forth, and the categories are not totally independent from one another; for example, domestic violence is often linked to drunkenness, which may reflect an ongoing dispute about resource allocation, or "not providing." Housing disputes are often related to extended family conflict, and calls to ankhoswe can stem from an intertwined bundle of reasons rather than a singular cause. Nevertheless, these data set the basic parameters of typical marital conflict in Balaka and allow us to situate and weigh the ethnographic evidence from within those parameters. The next section unpacks Stella's extended-family conflict (with in-laws) and housing dispute, which resulted from a combination of land pressure and economic need. Patuma's discovery of infidelity may be more colorful than most but is certainly not unique. A notable inversion here is that women call most

TABLE 7.2 Top ten reasons for calling the ankhoswe, by gender (%)

Women	N = 688	Men	N = 392
1. Unfaithful	30.24	1. Rudeness	31.51
2. Money disagreement	10.78	2. Suspicion	15.76
3. Suspicion	10.33	3. Money disagreement	12.54
4. Rudeness	9.13	4. Unfaithful	7.40
5. Not providing	8.68	5. Laziness	6.11
6. Beatings/cruelty	7.93	6. Drunkenness	3.54
7. Drunkenness	7.34	7. Extended-family conflict	3.22
8. Refusing sex	2.25	8. Not providing	3.22
9. Housing dispute	1.80	9. Child-rearing dispute	2.89
10. Extended-family conflict	1.35	10. Housing dispute	2.57

Source: TLT-2.

often about known infidelities and to a lesser degree about their suspicions, whereas men call about suspicions far more often than about known infidelities. Taking suspicions of a partner's other partners as our key indicator of relationship uncertainty, this suggests that women tolerate more uncertainty than men. Money disagreements and a failure to provide further attests to the crushing weight economic precarity places on marriages, which are already built on a terrain of livelihood uncertainty.

Linking this process of calling the ankhoswe to resolutions, the right-hand panels of figure 7.3 represents callers' assessments of the result: whether their ankhoswe helped a great deal, helped a little, showed up but didn't help, or never even showed up. The definition of "help" here does not presume a particular outcome. This deliberate ambiguity allows for two kinds of resolutions: one in which the ankhoswe help the couple sort out a problem and maintain the marriage and another in which the ankhoswe support a partner's decision to leave a relationship that is beyond repair. In this case, for example, the ankhoswe "helped a lot" by supporting this respondent's decision to end the marriage and priming the chief to prioritize her needs in the allocation of property and custody.

> I divorced because my husband was having an affair with another woman while we were married, and I went to complain to our ankhoswe about what was happening in my family. The ankhoswe said I should continue to stay with him, and they advised him to change. But after some time my husband didn't change, so I went to complain to our ankhoswe for the second time. My ankhoswe agreed with me that he would never change, and they went to tell

the chief to dissolve the marriage. The chief called me and my husband, and when he asked my husband about what is happening in my family, my husband said, "I don't know this woman, and I don't love her, and I am already engaged to another woman." Then the man left. Our ankhoswe—mine and even the ones from his side—said that it is not good how he was treating me. So we divorced. I was thinking of going to the court to complain, but the ankhoswe told me to just let him go. And the chief told me to save my energy because going to court would not change anything for me. My husband should leave without taking anything from our home aside from his own clothes.

Among callers, the overwhelming majority reports that their ankhoswe showed up when needed and that they helped a lot (see fig. 7.3). This is consistent with the bike taxi driver's summary of ankhoswe as house poles and Mrs. Samosa's advice that it is normal for young couples to rely on the wisdom of their ankhoswe early on in a relationship. Of course, some ankhoswe are less effective: they helped just a little or were useless. Ankhoswe rarely shirk their duties completely, simply failing to show up when called upon, but when they do, it tends to be the women who miss out on this important form of support. Not every ankhoswe intervention is successful, but as a social structure, the ankhoswe do a lot to reduce relationship uncertainty and mitigate its consequences. So it matters that an increasing number of married young women do not have ankhoswe to call.

The Perils of Bypassing Mediators

The mobile phone and the marriage mediators are noteworthy details in the stories both Patrick and Njemile shared, and the stark juxtaposition of the "traditional" marriage guardian with the "modern" innovation of the mobile phone captures the essence of social interactions in Balaka today. The proliferation of new information and communication technologies (ICTs) across sub-Saharan Africa has been an important topic of inquiry for scholars focused on development, the measurement of socioeconomic status, social networks, and information diffusion. Like access to education, to a radio, or to a bicycle, the mobile phone, it seemed, would soon represent a new dimension of stratification in Balaka—a digital divide that, though outside our focal topics of HIV and fertility, should not be overlooked in a study about social change.[10] The empirical questions at the center of this literature on ICTs encompass a variety of outcomes related to livelihoods, health, and family, for example: Might phones facilitate stable employment opportunities? Or are they an expense that drains family resources with constant demands for purchasing data units, accessing electricity (at great cost), and cultivating an appetite for upgrades? Do women with mobile phones have better access to information about contraception and health services than those without? These questions are interesting but irrelevant to our goal of understanding uncertainty in everyday life. Phones matter for uncertainty because they are used to facilitate relationships, relay gossip, and transmit money and because they have changed the flow and structure of many established social interactions that inform relationship formation and maintenance.

While I was observing and documenting the rapid proliferation of cellular phones in the TLT catchment area, population chatter clued me in to the fact that our study was uniquely positioned to address some of the relational consequences of phone ownership. In 2015, I was drafting a paper on the relationship between mobile phone proliferation and declining fertility, making graphs like figure 7.4 to depict this major transformation—alongside so many others—over the study period.[11] Fewer than 20 percent of TLT respondents owned a phone in 2009, but phone ownership increased to 53 percent in 2019; among women who had completed secondary school, the proportion of phone owners exceeded 90 percent. As I was taking a break from graph coding to read yet another batch of Gertrude's riveting fieldnotes, a passage struck me.

While staying at her husband's home, Stella, the landlord's adult daughter, had been fighting excessively with her in-laws. She returned to her family's

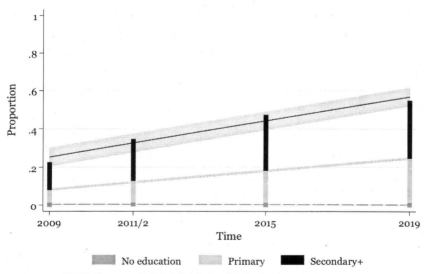

FIGURE 7.4 Mobile phone penetration in Balaka by education level

Source: TLT-1 (waves 1 and 8), TLT-2, and TLT-3.

compound to take a break from that conflict, and since her younger sister had also moved home (pregnant) from secondary school, the main house was crowded. Gertrude suddenly found herself with a rent discount and a room-mate. Two weeks into their unexpected cohabitation, Gertrude and Stella were spending a lot of time together, cooperating on errands and domestic duties, but their social circles had only just begun to overlap.

> Stella and I were browsing the kiosks just outside the main market at dusk, just looking for something nice in the bales of secondhand clothes. While we were sorting and showing each other the nicer garments, a police car pulled over onto the side of the road, slowly. He drove almost all the way into the market, dispersing the crowds of people engaged in market activities at dusk—the bus-iest time of day. The car stopped next to us, and the officer in the car motioned our way. Stella turned to me: "That's my boyfriend; he works at the police sta-tion, and he gives me a lot of money. But I told him that I am married, so he shouldn't call me at home because my husband will get suspicious. When he wants to give me a call, he calls me on my mother's phone."

I knew from Gertrude's earlier fieldnotes that Stella's marriage was difficult, so I was not shocked to learn she had a partner in town. But the policeman calls her mother's phone! I certainly did not anticipate that Stella's mother would be in on the ruse.

Beyond the fact that new technologies typically unsettle things by virtue of their newness, I had not yet made a clear link between phones and uncer-tainty.[12] But I became more attentive to phones and their roles in everyday life. I began reading Gertrude's fieldnotes with an eye to how phones factored into a wide variety of exchanges; I started paying attention to when phones were conspicuous or hidden in my own interactions; I studied the economy of phone units and their currency as gifts between friends, relatives, and lovers; and I supervised Hannah Furnas's excellent dissertation on mobile phones and social networks.[13]

Two years later, I encountered ethnographic research on mobile phones and social worlds in African and diaspora settings. This literature made the links between phone ownership and uncertainty abundantly clear.[14] In her exploration of the intimacy and romantic lives of young adults in Inhambane, Mozambique, the anthropologist Julie Soleil Archambault focuses on the role of the mobile phone in experiences of everyday uncertainty. She writes, "In Mozambique, like elsewhere, mobile communication has transformed how people express love and affection, how they argue, and how they sleep."[15] In contrast to Wilson's work, which focused primarily on how women tried to resolve uncertainty within their marriages, Archambault wrote about uncertainty as social practice and social resource, pointing to the fact that uncertainty is often deliberately produced in order to keep options open and avoid negative information. According to Archambault, the phone has allowed young people to "cruise through uncertainty" and manage the "hermeneutic of suspicion" that characterizes daily life in Inhambane, where, as in Balaka, work is scarce, livelihoods are managed through a combination of piecework and patronage, and privacy is an illusion. While "cruising through uncertainty" using mobile phones, some young adults move a little too quickly, bypassing important steps in the relationship process.

Salient others everywhere play important roles in facilitating romantic relationships. And because Balaka is densely populated and rural life fundamentally communal, salient others are especially visible in the romantic lives of the young adults TLT followed. Friends and relatives play a variety of supporting roles, and these roles are crucial rather than ancillary. They make introductions, tease to indicate their awareness of a relationship, signal their opinion by expressing approval or distaste of particular partnerships, and may eventually endorse the marriage as guests at a wedding. As mediators, friends and relatives relay relevant gossip and background information to help their friends discern the safety of a relationship while simultaneously helping other friends conceal illicit affairs. Salient others provide a fount of advice on which people draw to navigate complaints and conflicts. They mediate in formal and informal ways, sometimes injecting information that reduces the uncertainty surrounding a relationship. At other times salient others exacerbate uncertainty, for example, by asking a question that draws attention to the unknown, rendering a latent uncertainty visible.

Years ago, young people in Balaka would have indicated a romantic interest by sending an inquiry through a friend or relative. A confident Lothario may have rehearsed a proposal and delivered it in person, either publicly in a display of courage or through a careful plot to bump into the object of his affection privately. With the rise of literacy, love letters became an especially popular genre for educated adolescents and young adults.[16] Today young people flirt and banter in pursuit of one thing, a phone number. Archambault points out that mobile phones allow young people to bypass kin mediation and move toward intimacy without the watchful eyes of quite as many salient others. The mobile phone allows more privacy for sharing feelings and making plans; an extraordinarily complex ecology of SMS messages, calls, and "flashes" (missed calls to indicate the intention to communicate) has evolved to signal and sustain affection. In contrast to the heavily kin-mediated interactions of years past, mobile-mediated exchanges facilitate intimacy at an accelerated pace, allowing for particularly frank conversations about sexual desires and requests for money.[17]

Phones facilitate communication and access to particular types of information, but they may not necessarily lead young people to the kind of information they need most. In fact, bypassing kin mediation eliminates a crucial step of the marriage process—what the historian Nwando Achebe calls "the investigation period." Writing about love and courtship in Nigeria, Achebe emphasizes the questions family members ask to ensure that a potential spouse's family has a reputation for being hardworking and honest. In previous research about Malawi, I wrote about the "social background check," specific to the assessment of character traits like honesty and fidelity.[18] Skipping over kin mediation can deprive young people of key data points about a partner—in Njemile's case, for example, the detail that he was already married.

The links to Magruder's relationship churning (see chap. 6) and to population-level HIV prevalence are abundantly clear.[19] Summarizing the twin phenomena of fast marriages and early divorce in rural Malawi using the term "impulsive unions," the sociologists Anaïs Bertrand-Dansereau and Shelley Clark describe something similar.

> Contrary to traditional practice, in which families and friends help evaluate a potential spouse, [young women] rely on their own assessment of a man's character, achieved primarily through individual verbal exchanges. Such unions often do not involve friends and family because the potential spouses do not share a community and cannot access public information about potential character flaws. The result is a remarkably fragile form of union in which two people who do not share a community start living together as a married couple a few days or weeks after their first meeting. In many cases, the newlyweds find out about each other's minor and major faults over the course of the first year of acquaintance. Without a strong emotional bond and with little family support, divorce is swift when a young woman discovers that her husband is violent, abuses alcohol, is sexually unfaithful, or has another wife. However, divorce is not so easy when family members are involved in the marriage.[20]

Impulsive marriages in Balaka constitute much of the "informal marriages" category summarized in table 7.1 and the "just moved in together" group in figure 7.2. Although these unions are far from widespread, they are rising coterminously with mobile phone proliferation and the loosening of a cultural norm that once equated marriage with ankhoswe. Informal unions are marriages; they are associated with a host of negative individual-level outcomes, and they are extremely uncertain.

Mobile Phones and Friends in Four Acts

Throughout Balaka, phones are widely discussed as being dangerous for relationships. One man from the tailoring shop—the one with a crush on Gertrude—generalizes comedically on men's behalf.

> Tell me if I am wrong. If you are on the phone and you laugh with the one who gave you a call, your wife always asks about who you are laughing with. Every time.

While chatting outside the hospital, a married woman warns Gertrude about where marriages go wrong, mentioning phones as a common source of conflict.

> Maybe you ask your husband about how the business went that day, and instead of answering you properly, he snaps at you saying, "Why are you asking me so many questions when you know I am tired?" Then the wife gets tired and thinks, "Maybe he has another woman that he shares his money or his ideas with. . . ." Eventually you will get tired and divorce. And those people who have phones will see that the husband is just busy playing with his phone instead of discussing with you how to take care of the family. Maybe you think of another business, but you can't share it with him because he is just busy playing with the phone. You'll also get tired of this and divorce.

In contrast to the development literature, which emphasizes the mobile phone primarily as a communication technology, ethnographic research depicts the phone as a notable gift, as a means of cash transfer, as a tool for surveillance, and as a totem for mistrust. The giving and taking away of phones has become a trope in the metanarrative of adolescent and young-adult romance. This can be seen while Gertrude is passing the time with a woman and her teenage niece selling cassava.

> A teenage girl passed by; the girls I was chatting with gossiped that the girl is in relationship with a certain boy from town who bought a cell phone for her. But yesterday that boy took back the phone after seeing that she was communicating with her ex-boyfriend.

The aforementioned dangers notwithstanding, phones are deemed essential for relationships, particularly among young people. Phones are tools that can be used to cultivate, conceal, and monitor romantic relationships, yet their uses and meanings extend far beyond the messages users send one another. To illustrate, I offer four brief scenes from Gertrude's fieldnotes. These scenes weave together the lives and activities of the salon coterie and the landlord's complex family. The first scene takes place at the salon among

Gertrude, Enid, and Tiyamike. The next two scenes unfold quickly: Gertrude meets a new friend on her walk home from the salon, and Tiyamike visits at a strangely early hour the next morning. In the fourth scene, the three women meet again at the salon. These interactions show phones as gifts, phones being used to send cash, phones as facilitators of illicit relationships, and phones being used for flirtation, seduction, and rendezvous.[21] These scenes unfold within a period of about twenty-four hours and precede by six weeks the salon vignette in chapter 5, when Precious went to ANC and heckled the father of Enid's child. While the key events in each act—giving gifts, arranging romantic trysts, passing messages through third parties—are possible without a phone, phones allow them to unfold more quickly and with greater frequency. As demonstrated in chapter 6, the population-level consequences of relationship churning—through accelerated processes of relationship formation and relationship dissolution—are epidemiologically real. It also heightens the overall, population-level sense of uncertainty about the romantic realm.

Scene 1: New Styles Salon

I went to visit Enid at New Styles, and I found Tiyamike chatting there. There were no customers, so the three of us enjoyed watching a film. After a while, a certain man came in the salon; he greeted us and bought soft drinks for the three of us, and he gave a brand-new phone to Tiyamike. A nice one. I asked him, "Brother, how much was that phone?" He said, "14,000 MK" [about US$22]. To Tiyamike, he said that he would give her a call later to tell her where to meet. And Tiyamike said, "No problem."

When the man left Enid exploded. "Not two months ago, he bought a phone for you, and now he has also bought this new phone for you. What is going on?"

Tiyamike said, "Obviously. We are in a relationship. I told him I really wanted a newer phone, so he bought it for me."

I asked her where they were going to meet.

"Mavuto Lodge."

"Hmmmmm."

A few minutes later, the man gave Tiyamike a call, and she took off, telling us that she would find us later. I stayed with Enid in the salon until somebody else showed up to get her hair braided.

Scene 2: A roadside kiosk where a girl (age 19) is selling sweet potatoes

On my way home I stopped to buy sweet potatoes from a girl who seemed to recognize me.

"Do you know that I stay near where you stay?"

"No! Really?"

"Yeah, I know you because I saw you there with Stella one day."

"Indeed, I am renting there."

Then she said, "Stella was my friend, but we've stopped talking because of something that happened."

"What happened?"

"Well, about two weeks ago, a certain man asked Stella to help find a wife for him. Stella told me she knew a good man for me and asked if I wanted to meet him. Then she gave me his telephone number so that I could be communicating with him. At first I thought, '*No, I can't take this man's number without ever meeting him. . . .*' But then I started communicating with him. Just calls and texts. He told me that he had been married but was divorced. After talking more, it was clear that he is married, he just doesn't like his wife. Now he is pursuing me. Well, I went to Kasungu last week to visit my friends over the weekend. I didn't have enough money to get back home, so I gave this man a call. I asked him for some money; he sent me 2,000 MK through Airtel, and I used the money to get back home. But when I reached here, I realized: *I cannot keep on with this guy—he is married, and I don't even know him.* So I refused him. I just stopped taking his calls, stopped answering his texts.

"Stella got angry with me; she shouted at me and made a big scene, and she said I need to give him back his 2,000 MK. I guess he updated her at some point. I'll pay him back because, fundamentally, I don't like him. He was kind to help me. But I'm done with Stella because . . . Couldn't she manage to find me a man who isn't married? Well, that's why Stella and I aren't speaking."

"That's bad," I said. "Stella should have introduced you to an unmarried man."

We greeted each other by name, and I told her it was nice to know her. I said that I was sorry to hear that she and Stella were on bad terms, but that it would probably be OK in no time.

Scene 3: At Gertrude's house with Tiyamike and her photographer boyfriend

When I woke up in the morning Tiyamike was arriving at my house. It was 5 a.m. I greeted her and told her that she is welcome. And she said, "Sorry for coming early in the morning, but I went to see my boyfriend, and I found him with another woman. I have just left a message for him with the child I found sweeping there. I went to knock at his door, then the young girl who is the young sister to my boyfriend told me that I should not go in because there is another woman inside, that she came on Thursday, and that this is her fourth day here."

I asked, "Is he the one you said pays rent for you?"

Tiyamike said "No, that's another one."

I said, "Or he is the one who gave you capital last time?"

She said, "Not that one."

I laughed and said, "So who is he?"

"He is a photographer. We met some time ago, and we have been in a relationship for about a month now. I just wanted to visit him without giving him a call. I wanted to see if I am the only one, but I have seen that it's not only me, and some other women staying around there told me that the girl came four days ago. And that there are different girls who sometimes spend nights there. So I am not the only one."

I asked, "So what are you going to do?"

Tiyamike said, "I need a favor, Gertrude. Let me meet him here at your house so that we have a place to talk."

I said, "No problem. You can do that."

Tiyamike gave him a call and told him where she was. The man showed up at my house immediately.

Without even greeting us properly, he said, "I just lied to my girlfriend and told her that I need to take pictures for someone. That's why I have my camera with me."

I laughed, and we all greeted each other. He asked how I knew Tiyamike, then I said, "Tiya is the first friend I made when I moved to Balaka." Then Tiyamike told the man, "I am so sorry for what happened yesterday. The man that you saw with me at Mavuto Lodge is not my boyfriend. We were just there chatting." And the photographer said, "I am sorry. I have another girlfriend, and she is at my home right now."

"That means you were in a relationship already, when we met?"

"Yes, I was."

"So what can we do?"

"Go. You continue on with the man you were with yesterday, and I will continue my relationship with the other girls that I have. I never expected you to be in affairs with other men, but there is no need for you to apologize." Then the man left.

When he left I asked Tiyamike, "Well, what happened yesterday?"

Tiyamike said, "I was with the other one, and I didn't know that this one would also be there. Today I wanted to meet him, so that I could apologize, but it seems that he is not interested, so I'll just let him go. He'll come back to me sometime."

"Will you accept him when he comes back?"

"Yes, I will. You know, at this time, I am not doing any business. I don't have capital, so I want to beg money from my boyfriends so that I can start the business again."

"You mean when you were doing hair, you were not saving any money at all?"

"I couldn't save. Plus I knew that the men would each provide a little."

I said, "Sorry for that."

Then Tiyamike begged me for some maize flour and Irish potatoes. I gave her some and she left.

Within ten minutes of her leaving, I saw the photographer coming to my house. He was on the motor bike, and he said, "Sorry for coming back. Is Tiyamike still here?"

"No, she just left."

"I just wanted to let you know that I am a photographer, and I like you. So I have stolen your number from Tiyamike's phone. Don't get surprised when I give you a call."

I laughed and said, "Sorry. I am engaged to someone."

"That doesn't matter. You will see for yourself the difference between me and the one that you have." I laughed again and said, "I am sorry, but I am not interested." Then he left.

A few minutes he gave me a call and said, "I am the photographer who came to your house, and that's my number, I will call you later."

I said: "Sorry, wrong number."

He said, "No. You are Gertrude. I will call you later today." So I just left the phone in my bedroom and went about my day.

Scene 4: Back at the salon

At around 1 p.m. Tiyamike found me again and said we should head back to New Styles like we had promised. Just as we had settled into a chat, Tiyamike's married boyfriend came—the one who bought a 14,000 MK cell phone for her. He didn't look happy. When he arrived, he didn't even greet us, he just walked into the salon and told Tiyamike to give him the phone. She gave it to him, and the man stepped outside and started checking her call history and the SMS messages. Tiyamike got angry and said (to me but loudly so that the boyfriend could hear, even from outside), "Gertrude, imagine this man being jealous with me! He is always checking my phone. Yet he is married with two kids, and I am just his girlfriend."

Enid laughed and said, "Well, it's understandable. He wants to know if you have another boyfriend."

Tiyamike said, "I do have one, and I will meet him this evening. I am in a relationship with this man. And I am grateful that he bought me this phone. But I know that we can't get married. And I have another boyfriend who really loves me, only he is not working."

Enid sighed, "Of all of us, I think only Tiya has found the answer. She plays with three or four men, and one always comes through for her."

The married boyfriend left, taking the phone, including the SIM card. Tiyamike borrowed my phone so that she could communicate with her un-employed boyfriend about where to meet. She told him not to call at that old number again but to use instead her neighbor's phone.

These scenes convey the density of social networks in Balaka, the impor-tance of the mobile phone for navigating sexual relationships, and how distinct forms of mediation—kin and mobile—have become intertwined. Whether accidentally or knowingly, Stella has disappointed her friend with the sweet potatoes by brokering a relationship with a married man. As a mediator, she has proven herself untrustworthy. Other forms of mediation are also evident here: the children outside the photographer's home spill the beans to Tiyamike about his other relationships,[22] and the photographer surreptitiously obtains Gertrude's number. Meanwhile, Tiyamike's neighbor can be counted on to keep her relationship with the unemployed boyfriend alive while she is temporarily phoneless (much like Stella's mother fielding calls from the policeman on Stella's behalf).[23] The romantic realm is full of mischief; these women know a lot about each other's intimate lives, and they are not exceptional in this regard.

In Patuma's story, we saw how women sometimes alert a friend to her husband's escapades—a phenomenon that is also clear in the survey data on levels of gossip reported in figure 6.2. From within Gertrude's network, we see that women also sometimes broker and protect their friends' illicit relationships. At the population level, one does not need to doubt one's own partner to be uncertain about a relationship. This combination of gossip about and shielding of others' illicit relationships fuels the phenomenon of widespread relationship uncertainty. Likewise, we can appreciate (even admire) Tiyamike's unflappable ability to skate by on her charm. Tiyamike is unusual in her openness about her boyfriends; Stella's quiet disclosure to a close friend and reliance on her mother to guard a secret is more typical.[24] Understood against the broader backdrop of resource scarcity, we would be wise to interpret both Stella's and Tiyamike's concurrency through the lens of Enid's analysis. These are not indulgences of promiscuous urges but strategies for navigating the web of uncertainties they live within—uncertainty about money, uncertainty about men, and uncertainty about other women. About a week after scene 4, the three women are together again at New Styles. Enid is braiding a customer's hair and Gertrude is assisting her.

> As we were braiding the client's hair, Tiyamike showed me the message that she received from the ex-boyfriend of Enid who gave her a child. He propositions Tiyamike by phone, writing, "I think we deserve to be in love." Tiyamike laughed but did not reply to him.

Other women, even friends, can pose a grave danger.

Female Friendship and Relationship Uncertainty

A question like, "How widespread are secondary partners among married women in any given population?," is difficult to answer, because it calls for us to estimate something most people share only with their closest friends. Aware that self-reports of sexual behavior in surveys seldom produce good estimates,[25] we built into TLT a few levers for better estimating the prevalence of concurrent partners in Balaka and assessing its contributions to relationship and HIV uncertainty at the population level. Concurrent sexual partnerships are absolutely underreported in our survey data: only 2 percent of our female respondents reported either concurrent partnerships or two nonoverlapping sexual relationships within the past month. The TLT data did suggest that multiple partnerships are more prevalent among phone-owning women than among those without them (3 percent vs. a fraction of one percent).

Handled with appropriate levels of quantitative humility, even imperfect data like these can be valuable when put to use with indirect estimation strategies. Better estimates of concurrency can be generated from the questions TLT asked respondents, male and female, about the behavior of their best friends—questions designed specifically for the purpose of improving population-level measures of sensitive behaviors. Presuming (even loosely) that most women have a person in their life they would identify as a best friend, that best friends trust each other with secrets, that the best-friend relationship is often a reciprocal one, and that social desirability bias should have a weaker influence on reports about the sensitive behavior of a friend than about oneself, we asked our respondents ten quick questions about their best friend's private life.

The benefits of this approach are immediately clear in figure 7.5, which relies on the data from the 2015 survey.[26] Overall, just 4 percent of TLT women reported having two or more partners in the past year, but 16 percent said that their best friend had at least two. Separated out by marital status, comparing married women with multiple partners to married best friends and single women to single best friends, the discrepancies remain in proportion to one another—a three- or four-to-one difference between self-reports and best friend reports. How do our respondents know about these relationships? The same way Gertrude knows about Stella's police officer: they have been entrusted with information as confidantes. In relatively few instances, women know about their friends' dalliances from observations ("saw her coming and going") or from rumors they heard around town.

Mobile phones are communication devices and cannot themselves bring about anything genuinely new. But phones can be used to facilitate intimacy, and the proliferation of phones is changing the scripts of how young people meet and marry and how they access, arrange, and conceal their secondary and casual partnerships. Likewise, ankhoswe neither arrange nor dissolve relationships in Balaka; they merely "support" by helping a couple negoti-

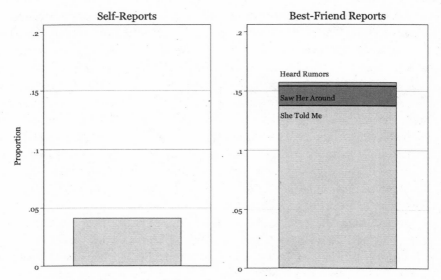

FIGURE 7.5 Women's reports of multiple sexual partnerships, 2015

Source: TLT-2.

Note: I defined multiple partnerships here as two or more partners in the past year.

ate conflict and in some cases bearing witness to and authorizing a divorce. Against a backdrop of widespread relationship uncertainty, rampant gossip, and collusion with friends to keep secret relationships under wraps, the proliferation of mobile phones and the erosion of the ankhoswe tradition seem to destabilize the terrain on which young adults in Balaka build their romantic relationships while accelerating the relationship process. In Swidlerian terms, these are decidedly unsettled times.[27] The strategies for how to act under relationship uncertainty in Balaka all tend to point in the direction of acceleration: accelerated union formation and childbearing and quick dissolutions of romantic relationships that feel dangerous, creating a cycle of relationship churning that aggregates into a stable HIV epidemic that is strongly patterned by marital experience. In combination with an evolving policy context, these examples of quiet, non-AIDS-related macro-social change have an unsettling effect, with tangible consequences within the intimate sphere, including the spread of HIV.

Braiding Together Phones, Friends, Ankhoswe, Relationships, and HIV

The population chatter from Balaka makes a clear link between phones, relationship uncertainty, and union instability. Perhaps more surprisingly, these impressions about the association between phones and relationship instability are borne out in our survey data. Phone ownership is positively associated with heightened levels of suspicion of one's spouse.[28] Figure 7.6 shows that women with cell phones report far higher levels of suspicion than women without, but that pattern does not hold for men.[29] The same pattern of exacerbated relationship uncertainty is also present for women who told us during their first interview that their best friend has multiple partners. As depicted in figure 7.7, both suspicion of one's partner and knowledge of a best friend's extramarital partnerships predict divorce among married male and female respondents, though the relationship is slightly stronger for women. Again here it is not just the possibility that holding secrets for a friend contributes to a culture of relationship uncertainty—manifesting specifically in suspicion about a spouse's behavior—but that this matters for how HIV becomes patterned within a population, concentrated along the spectrum of marital experience.[30]

When I met Stella, I asked her how long she had lived in Balaka and told her what she already knew about the TLT study: we were conducting a research project focused on the lives of young adults in Balaka, specifically, their marriage and childbearing experiences. The following thumbnail sketch of Stella's life conveys the uncertainties of men and marriage, female

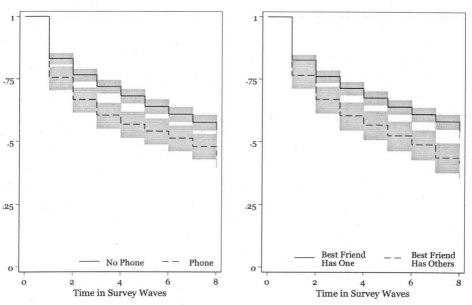

FIGURE 7.6 Women's relationship uncertainty by phone ownership and best friend's number of sexual partners, 2009–2011

Source: TLT-1, waves 1–8.

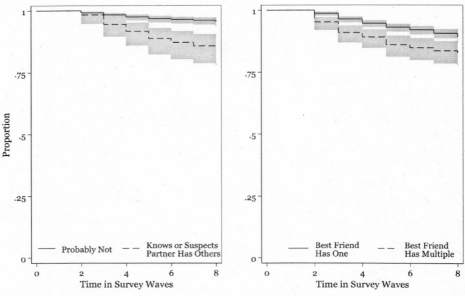

FIGURE 7.7 Divorce among married women in Balaka by phone ownership and best friend's number of sexual partners, 2009–2011

Source: TLT-1, waves 1–8.

friendship, and HIV status in the ART era in fewer than four hundred words from my own fieldnotes.

> I was born here in Balaka. I am married, and I have three kids. The first two are from a certain man—not the one that I am married to now. I divorced that one without a proper reason. My second husband had already been married somewhere else, and his marriage had ended. He and I started staying together, here in town, and things were nice. But after we had our child, my husband changed his behavior. He started having affairs with other women. I got angry and went to our ankhoswe to complain, but even though the ankhoswe came to counsel us, my husband didn't change. One day, while he was out, I took all the chairs that he bought for our house and also the television, and I sold them. I took that money and started living alone in town. My friend asked if she could move in with me, and I agreed to that, to help her. My friend was HIV positive, and she had been collecting her ARVs at Mponda Clinic. The ARVs were working, so she looked normal. Beautiful, even. And each time she went to refill, she would give me her medication to keep so that her boyfriend, when he came over, would not see them. One day my boyfriend came to spend a night at my home. I left him at home with my friend while I went to the market to buy some things, and my boyfriend had sex with my friend while I was out buying the charcoal and relish. Of course I got angry

and ended that relationship right away. When I asked my friend if she had slept with my boyfriend, she said she didn't do it. But my neighbors saw them in the bedroom; they told me they'd seen it for themselves. And I don't know whether they used a condom or not. Shortly after that, I decided to go back to my husband. He had been calling me and begging me to return, and he actually has changed. His behavior is better now. But we don't have our own house anymore, so we started staying together with his family. I quarrel constantly with my in-laws. They are difficult, and they mistreat my older children, and I just couldn't stand it. At the moment, I am back at my mother's house. Well, my kids are at my mother's house and I'm staying next door, in the small house with Gertrude.[31]

Malawians often say, "There is no secret under the sun." Some say the phrase reflects aspects of Bantu cosmology; others point out its Christian origins: a hybrid of verses from Ecclesiastes and Luke. Beyond any kind of spiritual meaning, the saying contains a demographic insight: it is an acknowledgment of the simple fact that the kind of population density Balaka residents experience today seriously undermines privacy. The elicit relationships of husbands, female friends, and boyfriends often come to light. Through a combination of gossip, sleuthing, and serendipity, some uncertainties transform into certainties. Stella's movements between states of suspicion and states of certainty are accompanied by decisive and consequential actions: the liquidation of household assets, a separation, and a subsequent reunion with her husband. I argue that, instead of bringing about certainty, these instances of discovery actually undermine it. Any particular uncertainty about a specific man (the husband) might be actionable: confront him, call the ankhoswe, leave him. But Stella's uncertainty about men actually deepens as the story unfolds, and Stella decides she is better off with her second husband, whose mode of philandering she finds less egregious. Layer on top of this the fact that in the era of ART people living with HIV look well, that they often conceal their status and their medicine from lovers, and that they do this with the help of family and friends.[32]

While this story of hidden ARVs and betrayal by a close friend may seem sensational, bear in mind that it was disclosed to an outsider, without probing, in response to an inquiry about number of children and marital history. In a parallel story from Gertrude's fieldnotes, a woman named Chisomo is newly married to Nelson, who ends the relationship upon finding a packet of ARVs among Chisomo's things. Chisomo tells him that these are not her ARVs; she is keeping them for her sister who wants to wait just a little bit longer to disclose her status to a new boyfriend. In a context of radical uncertainty, the question about who owns these ARVs constitutes an irresolvable issue. Chisomo and Nelson end their relationship, and each re-partners within the year. Thought of as particular instances, each uncertainty about the faithfulness of a friend or lover or about any particular person's HIV status may be knowable and discoverable through facts. Collectively, however, they constitute an environment of collective uncertainty that is latent, perpetual, and irresolvable. This is what it means to navigate an epidemic of uncertainty.

Ultimate Uncertainties and the Mortality Landscape

Lightning Strikes and Uncertainty

Good afternoon, Members,

Lightning has killed 5 people and seriously injured 8 others. The incident happened this afternoon at Kayerekera. Victims met their fate when they were attending Prayers at Pentecostal Holiness Association Church. We reported the matter to DCPC and Karonga Police. All the teams rushed to the scene for assessment. Casualties have been referred to Kayerekera Health Centre for treatment. Some members of the Area Development Committee will attend the burial ceremony of the deceased tomorrow.

Regards,

Fwasani Silungwe Chairman, Mbande Area Development Committee

Early in the morning of February 7, 2021, I woke up, grabbed my phone, and started scrolling through the Whatsapp messages from the TLT research team's group chat to see what news I had missed while sleeping. I gasped when I read the above message. A lightning strike in the northern district of Karonga had killed five church members who were gathered in prayer. My phone kept dinging, with messages of shock, condolences, and prayers. More dinging. Questions about names. Had the families been notified yet? More condolences. May their souls rest in peace. Shaking my head, I opened my laptop and found that the information had already been confirmed by Malawi's national paper. In fact, the original Whatsapp message had understated the toll: five dead and twelve gravely injured. The Department of Disaster Management Affairs spokesperson, Chipiliro Khamula, added that at least thirty-eight people had been killed nationwide by lightning since the onset of the 2020–21 rainy season, with sixteen districts reporting.[1] Utterly unbelievable. Not six weeks later, another lightning strike was reported on our

Whatsapp group chat, this one also confirmed by the papers: Jones Yamikani Chadza, an independent candidate for political office in Lilongwe, was struck by lightning while sleeping in his home. Of all the factors swirling in this syndemic context—HIV, malaria, food insecurity, and now COVID-19—Chadza was struck by lightning at the age of 38.[2]

Previously unaware of the scientific literature on consequential lightning strikes (CLS), I discovered the work of Leonard Kalindekafe of Malawi University of Science and Technology, who leads a research group that tracks and analyzes lightning-related deaths and injuries in Malawi. Viewed from a global perspective, Kalindekafe's group estimates that lightning fatalities in Malawi are about fifty times higher than in the United States.[3] After reading more, their estimates seem conservative. The stunningly high rates of lightning fatalities in Malawi have been noted by other research groups as well: of an estimated 4,000 annual lightning-attributed fatalities globally, 1,008 take place in Malawi (pop. 18 million); between 100 and 150, in Zimbabwe (pop. 14.5 million); 30, in Uganda (pop. 44 million); and 30, in the United States (pop. 330 million).[4]

What do lightning strikes have to do with Malawi's HIV burden? Probably nothing. But do lightning strikes contribute to an environment of widespread uncertainty? Absolutely. Might lightning strikes shape people's perceptions of what lies within the ambit of one's own control versus outside it? Definitely. What about their sense of longevity?

This chapter is devoted to examining the mortality conditions that have characterized the lives of TLT respondents since their births and demonstrating the social salience of these conditions for every dimension of this cohort's lived experience. Coterminous with the HIV epidemic, this thirty-year period is characterized by unusually dramatic changes in Malawi's *mortality landscape*. I advance the idea of the mortality landscape as a concept that pairs what demographers know about mortality in a given setting—the volume of deaths, the age distribution of those deaths, the most prevalent causes, and fluctuations in each—with how ordinary people perceive and make sense of the mortality conditions that surround them. I begin by providing a macro-level view of changing mortality using the gold standard data sources demographers and global-health researchers regularly rely on. I then describe the weight of the mortality burden in young adults' immediate families— parents and siblings—to show that despite recent improvements in every standard mortality metric, this cohort has lived through perhaps the most crushing mortality burden in the contemporary world *while* experiencing a full doubling of the population during their lifetimes thus far. I situate the phenomenon of *changing* causes of deaths within the realm of perceptions by emphasizing net risks, showing that HIV has unique features as an existential threat when compared to other fatal maladies. Through Gertrude's descriptions of the events surrounding three burials, the ethnographic data relay the mortality narratives that circulate when death strikes, show how mortality is connected to other life events (marriage, in particular), and provide evidence that uncertainty accelerates many life course events for young adults in Balaka.

The mortality landscape is a central concept for advancing a demography of uncertainty. In a foundational demographic text from 1878, Wilhelm Lexis transformed mortality research by studying the age distribution of deaths and advancing the notion of "normal mortality" as a concept distinct from average length of life. Noting that deaths at or around the *normal* age could be differentiated from premature adult deaths and deaths to children, Lexis innovated statistically, showing a normal (i.e., random) distribution of deaths around the modal length of life. Normal mortality could be understood, for Lexis, through three values: the identification of the normal age at death, the concentration of deaths around that age, and error. Beyond the breakthrough in data and measurement this represented, Lexis advanced an important idea, a natural law of mortality that revealed something important about "the nature of things." He cautioned, however, that the laws would never be self-evident to observers or residents because in most societies the problems of child mortality and error obscure the underlying, law-like pattern.[5]

Mortality research has come a long way since Lexis, but his basic insights still hold. Formal demographers have tools for thinking about the unpredictability of life and death beyond the matter of sheer volume. These include concepts like thanatological age (remaining time until death) and mortality compression (how the deaths are distributed across age groups).[6] In an outstanding 2010 dissertation, Sarah Marie Zureick provocatively described mortality compression, often thought of as a purely technical subject, as a matter of certainty: "Not only are humans today living longer than their ancestors on average, they also experience greater certainty about the eventual timing of their death. This greater certainty is due to the considerable compression of the distribution of ages at death, which characterizes the mortality transition and results in lower life span disparity at the population level."[7] Although tomorrow is never guaranteed to any of us, the probability of a tomorrow for many Balaka residents is fragile, and the promise of a full decade of good health seems especially elusive—not only because of HIV, but also because of childbearing risks, food insecurity, malaria, accidents, and lightning strikes.

Thought of in this way, mortality is not about the dead at all; the mortality landscape structures the decisions of young adults *living* in Balaka, regardless of whether HIV remains the community's leading cause of death or becomes a genuinely chronic and manageable condition. Combining insights from formal demography with ethnographic and survey data on mortality perceptions, I conclude that the situation in Malawi from 1990 to 2020 can be characterized as mortality decline without legible compression, leaving questions of basic survival extremely uncertain.

Macro-Level Mortality Trends in Malawi

One of the first things a demographer teaches university students is the shape of the classic demographic transition: a shift from the high birth and death rates that characterized historical populations and kept population growth to a minimum for thousands of years to the new low-fertility/low-mortality equilibrium that characterizes much of the world today (see fig. 8.1).[8] Between these two states of negligible population growth is the demographic transition—not *a* demographic transition, but *the* transition. About this transition, demographers know several things: it will only happen once, it is irreversible, mortality falls prior to fertility, and the process kicks off a period of rapid population growth and a wide variety of social transformations in the society experienc-

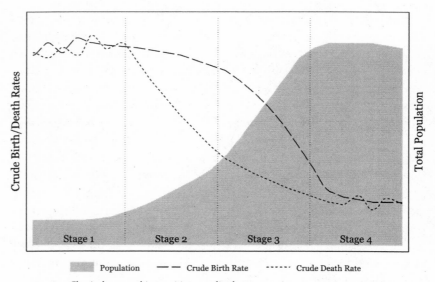

FIGURE 8.1 Classic demographic transition: a stylized representation

Note: Author's depiction, based on dozens of representations in the demographic literature. Stages are differentiated with dashed lines and enumerated 1–4.

ing it. A useful phrase for thinking about daily life amid such a transformation comes from Ann Swidler's work on culture: *unsettled times*.[9]

When teaching the demographic transition, a demographer will emphasize, among these other facts, one hallmark feature of demographic rates: they tend to be stable over long periods. In other words, across human history, large-scale mortality changes are the exception rather than the rule. Furthermore, the low-mortality environment that people in the United States, Italy, and Japan enjoy today is atypical of most of human experience.[10] To understand young adulthood in Balaka, we must situate the experience within a larger story of demographic change, in which residents are living through the shift from extremely high mortality to substantially lower but still high mortality. Although the mortality shifts of recent years are positive, this cohort has been living through a period of change. Change is unsettling, and change is uncertain. Changes in a society's mortality regime, in particular, may be among the most unsettling of all social changes. When mortality changes trend in a negative direction—as the result of war or epidemics—the causes of uncertainty are obvious. But even when changes trend in a positive direction, a changing mortality landscape can be characterized by confusion because familiar patterns have been disturbed, making mortality less predictable, causing rapid population growth, and imposing a cascade of related changes on other institutions, including land tenure systems, burial practices, pension schemes, health care systems, and marriage.[11]

Figure 8.2 provides a sixty-year view of Malawi's transition—from 1950 through the worst of the AIDS epidemic (1995–2010) to today. The shape of the curve reinforces messages about the arc of the thirty-year AIDS epidemic discussed in chapter 2.[12] High mortality in the 1950s and 1960s was largely attributable to extremely high infant and child mortality rates. Infant mortality began to decline during the 1930s, and the improvements continued throughout the twentieth century, raising life expectancy overall and facilitating population growth.[13] This increase in life expectancy at birth for Malawi from 38 in 1950 to 64 in 2020 represents nothing short of a total social transformation. But with the onset of HIV, rising adult mortality threw the entire region into a state of social and economic upheaval. The scale of adult mortality it took to offset the earlier declines in infant mortality was massive. High levels of infant mortality are tragic for a society, but losing income earners in their prime is a completely different phenomenon. If a naive analyst tracks life expectancy at birth over time as the key metric of mortality, these important differences can get washed away.

Malawi's overall burden of mortality dropped precipitously once ART became widely available (ca. 2010). The positive trends are clear in the stan-

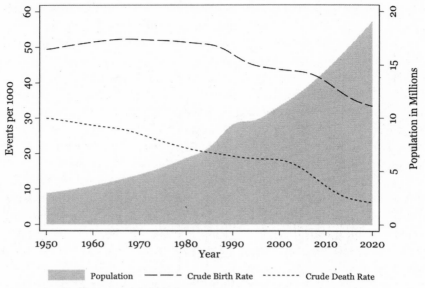

FIGURE 8.2 Population growth in Malawi, 1950–2020
Source: World Population Prospects.

dard demographic measures: the declining crude death rate (from 15 to 10 per 1,000), the jump in life expectancy (from 47 to 55), and the decline in adult deaths due to HIV.[14] Despite all these improvements, in terms of life expectancy, Malawi currently ranks 155th on a list of 183 countries.[15] Despite these high mortality rates, both Malawi and Balaka Boma specifically are characterized by rapid population growth. In the course of TLT respondents' lives, Malawi's population has doubled, and through a combination of natural increase and migration, the population of the boma is estimated to have increased from 9,000 in 1987 to 37,000 in 2017.[16]

The changing mortality landscape is inadequately summarized by sheer quantities; distributions are also crucial. Young adults living in the United States may or may not be aware that they have lived through a modest lengthening of life expectancy over their lifetimes. This story of relative stability is evident in the overall age distribution of deaths for 1990, 2000, and 2019, shown in the first panel of figure 8.3. The graph will be familiar to demographers, but those confronting the age distribution of deaths for the first time need to know that these data come from a life table for a particular country at a particular time and that $_nd_x$ represents the number of deaths (out of 100,000) that occurred between exact ages x and $x + n$, where n is the length of the age interval (e.g., 0–1, 5–9, 50–54). Because the deaths are calibrated to

100,000 in every life table, these measures are not designed to depict differences in the volume of deaths between settings (either geographies or historical periods) but to show how the deaths that happen within a given period are patterned. Examining this dimension of the US mortality landscape, a few features stand out: more deaths in infancy than in childhood, a light increase in deaths between ages 20 and 40, and a sharp increase in deaths at every age beyond age 40. Between 1990 and 2019, deaths became more heavily concentrated at the oldest ages, but overall this is a story of stability, wherein mortality in this society (and others like it) primarily affects the old.

Of many measures of mortality inequality, I find the C-family ("C" for "compression") of indicators useful and intuitive for comparing mortality distributions over space and time. Following Väinö Kannisto,[17] I summarize and compare the concentration of mortality by finding the shortest age interval containing 50 percent of all deaths. In the United States during 2019, 50 percent of deaths occurred to people between the ages of 81 and 95, so the C_{50} interval for this year is 81–95, and the distance is 14 (the length of the interval). Compared to the United States, mortality in Italy and Japan was distributed similarly in 1990 but became even more heavily concentrated over this same

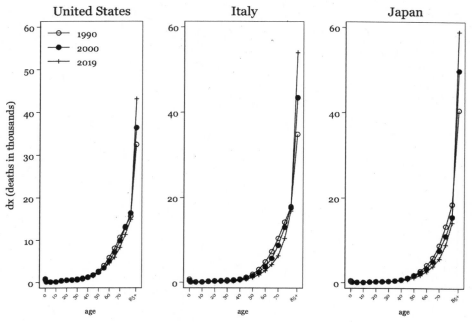

FIGURE 8.3 Death distributions from life tables in three low-mortality countries, 1990–2019

Source: World Population Prospects.

period, making the compression Zureick noted tighter and increasing the overall predictability of mortality. C_{50} for Italy before COVID-19 was 13, and for Japan—the country featuring the world's most compressed mortality structure—C_{50} occupies an even narrower interval (12) between ages 87 and 99.

The age distribution of Malawian mortality over this same period provides a stark contrast to the low-mortality scenarios, both in terms of the shapes observed and in terms of the momentous transformation that occurs during this relatively short time span. I present the age distribution of deaths in five-year intervals, combining the data from 1990 and 1995, when AIDS first began to alter the mortality landscape (see fig. 8.4). Infant deaths in this period declined, while the proportion of deaths in early adulthood bulged, becoming almost as common among adults in their prime as among the elderly. In the year 2000, nearly half of all deaths occurred in adults between the ages of 30 and 59—a span of thirty years (compared to twelve in Japan) placed in the middle of the age distribution rather than at the end. From 2000 to 2005, infant mortality was in decline, and early-adult mortality continued to swell, compressing to $C_{50} = 24$. Beginning in 2010, the age distribution of deaths in Malawi started to resemble the basic shape that students in the United States, Japan, and Italy are accustomed to, a "Stage 4" society (see fig. 8.1), with the

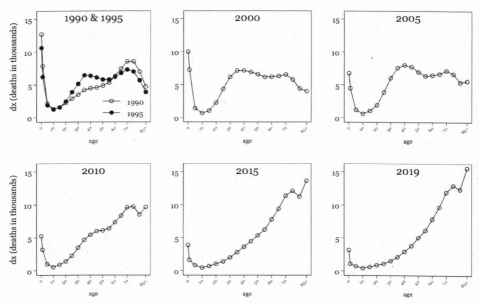

FIGURE 8.4 Death distributions from Malawi life tables, 1990–2019
Source: World Population Prospects.

left-hand tail that represents infant mortality shrinking in every panel and the right-hand tail representing mortality at older ages becoming more pronounced. Even so, keep in mind that the y-axis for Malawi only reaches to 15, whereas the graph for the low-mortality countries extends all the way to 60. After shifting to the right-hand of the age distribution in 2010, Malawi's C_{50} interval capturing half of all deaths has been declining—from a 65-year interval in 2015 to a 40-year interval in the most recent life table. This cohort has not only lived through rising and falling mortality levels but also through a radical and ongoing transformation of mortality patterns—one that may not ever be repeated in history. In contrast to a society with fairly stable patterns of "background mortality," the patterns in Malawi have been too volatile to be read as stable. Therefore, even though the recent changes represent unqualified improvements to the mortality landscape, trending in the direction of longer life expectancy and higher mortality at older ages, the mortality landscape may continue to feel capricious and unpredictable.

Nondemographers seldom pay attention to macro-level mortality trends; indeed, the distance between a country-level mortality rate and decision making at the household or person level is vast. However, mortality is intimately connected to other vital events (including fertility, migration, and marriage) in ways that have been previously overlooked. Measured at the individual level, mortality perceptions—how ordinary people assess their own longevity and think about the conditions that might cut their lives short—constitute a valuable tool for linking macro-level mortality trends and the force of existential uncertainty to a better understanding of day-to-day interactions.[18]

The Mortality Landscape as a Drumbeat

Demographic rates pattern everyday life, and this is true even if ordinary people do not describe patterns and rates in the same way demographers do, referencing doubling times, life-table elements, and mortality compression. Data that might indicate how ordinary people's lives change through mortality shifts over long stretches of historical time are extremely hard to come by. Nevertheless, available survey measures on funeral practices combined with ethnographic insights from across the region offer a few clues for translating the scale of mortality into human terms.

FUNERAL FREQUENCY IN THE SURVEY DATA

How do the mortality statistics collected and disseminated by the global community square with the experience of mortality in everyday life in Balaka?

Village life is organized around vital events and seasonal labor: births and deaths, planting and harvests, initiation ceremonies and weddings. Participation in these rituals used to be universal and expected. Describing funeral behavior before HIV in Nkhata Bay (a lakeside district in northern Malawi), Griffin Manda captured the norms of universalism and the spirit of community: "People are generally very cooperative at funerals. The cooperation may be said to stem from fear that if one does not attend neighbour's funerals, the neighbours will retaliate by neglecting him when he has one. Of course others attend on humanitarian grounds."[19] With the onslaught of AIDS and a growing population, funerals became too numerous to remain universal. Ceremonies that had lasted for multiple days and nights of singing were curtailed to an hour: a prayer and just a few songs. Malawians couldn't grow enough food to feast for every deceased person and had to start being selective about which funerals to attend and contribute to.[20]

Data from the Malawi Diffusion and Ideational Change Project fielded between 2001 and 2010 show that married women under age 30 reported attending four funerals each month during the 2001 and 2004 survey rounds. In 2006 and 2008, the number was about three and a half, and among adolescent women (comparable to the TLT sample), the number was a little smaller, just under three in the past month. Throughout the entire TLT study period, young adults reported attending, on average, one funeral per month. The most recent measures (from the 2019 survey round) show that 62 percent of the sample attended at least one funeral in the preceding month, 40 percent attended two or more funerals, and 70 percent of women agreed with the statement, "I go to every funeral in my village."

Although mortality has been falling, by any standard, it is still extremely high in this corner of the world. High mortality means frequent funerals; bodies need to be transported and buried swiftly. Long-standing rituals of gathering, celebrating, mourning, and feasting have been abbreviated since the AIDS epidemic began to take its toll, but there are no shortcuts in grave digging or preparing to receive and feed a crowd of mourners.

FUNERAL READINESS THROUGH POPULATION CHATTER

The labor associated with attending to the dead looms large in Balaka and can interrupt everyday activities unexpectedly. While walking back from yet another visit to a friend at the hospital on a Wednesday afternoon, Gertrude—dressed in slim jeans, blouse, and smart handbag—bumps into Blessings, who is clad in traditional attire and hauling goods from the train station. Although the two are just ten years apart in age, they are socially distant:

Gertrude is a city girl temporarily stationed in a hinterland, unmarried and childless; and Blessings is a migrant to Balaka from a nearby village, with deep traditional sensibilities and know-how, widowed at an early age and already a grandmother.

On my way back from the hospital I ran into Blessings, who was hauling goods from the train station. "Gertrude, do you know of any kind of business I could do to make money after selling this stuff? I want to look for a job that pays well."

"What kind of job are you looking for?"

"I want to be a cleaner."

"A cleaner? Where?"

"I want a job at TLT because I heard that they pay better than the government hospital. Those people who work at the hospital—they don't receive a lot of money, but I admire the uniforms they wear. I'd like a job with a uniform."

[We laughed.]

She was loaded with bags and baskets—tomatoes and charcoal for selling, more than you can imagine. I helped her by taking one bag and one basket. As we walked together, Blessings received a call: there was a funeral taking place near her house and she should rush home to help. When a person dies, the family and neighbors need to move everything out of the house and find a place for the dead person's belongings. They need to transport the dead body and find places for the mourners who gather to stay. They need to start preparing food for the mourners, which could be a few or hundreds. Blessings asked me to come along and help her. The place wasn't more than 1 kilometer away. She pulled a *chitenje* [wrapper] out of her bag and gave it to me to wear over my jeans. She said, "Gertrude, when you are out and about, remember to always have a wrapper in your bag—just in case you receive a message like what I received. You never know when you will get called for a funeral by the elders. For these occasions you have to wear a wrapper just to show respect."

When we reached Blessings's home, we found just a few people in the area, sitting outside the deceased's home. Blessings asked me to go inside the house with her to help her pack the things so that there would be enough space for guests to sit. Blessings asked what happened to the one who died—her neighbor, more acquaintance than friend. They told us that the woman poisoned herself after hearing that her husband had been cheating on her. She added, "That man did not take good care of his family. He kept saying that he didn't have money. But he was a truck driver, and truck drivers always have money. He used to come home every day; he used to be attentive and supportive, but about a month ago he stopped doing that. Then some days ago people around here saw him taking a woman to Mavuto Lodge. A friend—the one who saw the husband—went to her home and told her what she'd seen. She asked her husband if it was true. He didn't deny it; he just ignored her. She kept hearing those stories about her husband around town, and she got tired. She even told her husband she was thinking about poisoning herself. He did nothing."

Another woman had begun to help bring chairs to the area for mourners. She started to weigh in, saying that this woman shouldn't have killed herself. "She should have thought of the kids. Tired of her husband's behavior, sure. But that's the case for many of us. She could have easily just ended the marriage and found another man to marry."

"You're right. That's true. It is not difficult to find a man, even if you are divorced. Some men have got problems too, and they need other women who have problems."

I helped arranged the chairs and listened to them debate the sin of taking one's own life. There weren't two sides to the debate, just lamentations and disbelief about this woman's decision to poison herself. Her friends knew she was upset about the husband, but they didn't expect this; the close friends stayed quiet and seemed to be in shock.

After packing we took a break, sitting in the chairs where the mourners would be sitting. One friend asked us to find out if the chief was aware of the dead woman. The other woman said, "Yes. We have already sent her brother to tell the chief." The funeral was under way. The songs would be sung here, but the burial would be held at her home village, some 30 kilometers away. And the husband? He hadn't returned any texts.

Always have a wrapper in your bag. At all times, be ready to drop what you are doing to help with a burial. This small detail about how to live a good life in a high-mortality context gets revealed through a subtle moment of population chatter. From Blessings's point of view, perpetual readiness to enter into such a space, and to do so with respect, is a key piece of advice she has to offer a younger friend—an instruction for how to be respectful and cultivate status as a good woman in Balaka. Gertrude is never instructed to ditch the skinny jeans so as to inhabit the world in a different way; she should just carry a wrapper and be ready to transition into a respectful mode—funeral mode—without much notice.

In contrast to the quiet comment about the wrapper, the circumstances of this burial are conspicuous and related to several analytic elements elaborated in earlier chapters: relationship uncertainty, gossip, divorce, and serosorting. That relationship uncertainty, stress, gossip, or HIV uncertainty could lead to suicide cannot be verified with TLT survey data.[21] The quality literature on mortality in Malawi indicates that suicide is uncommon, but alongside this death there has been a spate of high-profile stories about individuals who killed themselves on having discovered either an infidelity or a secret ART supply belonging to their partner.[22] Clinically speaking, these deaths are not classified as HIV-related deaths. In cause-specific mortality tallies, they would

be filed as death by suicide or death by accident and later bundled by most analysts into the broad, umbrella category "externalities." HIV-adjacent deaths
like this one are, however, discussed and understood within the community[23]
as related to both HIV specifically and to the intimate sphere broadly; deception is just one way that men and women in intimate relationships can hurt,
even kill, one another.[24]

Adam Ashforth and Susan Watkins analyzed the form and content of the
death narratives that were circulating in Malawian towns and villages between 1999 and 2012, describing them as "emplotted," that is, situated in a
coherent, logical sequence of actions, organized and recounted so as to generate a collective response to the question: "Who is to blame?"[25] Their verac-
ity notwithstanding, death narratives perform a crucial social function and
can be thought of as a special case of population chatter. This kind of gossip
(captured in fig. 6.2) has population-level consequences typically manifested
as private arguments, breakups, and calls to the ankhoswe (as in the case of
Patuma). Occasionally public confrontations ensue (as with Tiyamike and her
boyfriend's wife or the fight and looting at the market shop), or separations
and divorces follow. But death and suicide are unanticipated outcomes of this
kind of gossip. The good intentions of the informants are never called into
question—not in this exchange or in related conversations in the aftermath.

HIV need not be directly mentioned for the threat to be clear. That men
and women "with problems" need to be able to find each other and live
happy lives was abundantly clear to the women arranging the chairs, and although they never invoke the technical term "serosorting," their awareness
and endorsement of the process reflects both a set of empirically verifiable
population-level patterns and a normative consensus on how people living
with HIV lead a normal and moral life in the era of ART.[26]

THE PERSONAL BURDEN OF MORTALITY

How else is this backdrop of high but declining mortality manifested in the
lives of TLT respondents? Motivating the TLT study design from the very
beginning was the fact that this cohort is the first to have never experienced
life without AIDS. Born between 1984 and 1994, this cohort experienced
extremely high rates of orphanhood because their parents were subject to
the peak adult mortality rates that characterized the period 2000–2005.
Figure 8.5, based on our respondents' retrospective reports of their kin networks, depicts the proportion of our sample that was orphaned at each age.
A full 30 percent had lost a father before age 18 and about 11 percent were
double orphans at that age. For comparison, the Institut national d'études

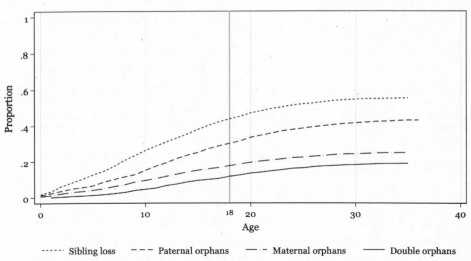

FIGURE 8.5 Family mortality in the TLT sample

Source: TLT-3.

Note: Estimates are based on retrospective reports collected in 2019. About 2 percent could not estimate the year of a deceased mother's death, and 4 percent could not estimate the year of a deceased father's death. Rather than impute an age, I exclude these respondents from the curves represented here and believe these estimates to be between 2 and 5 percent shy of the true rate of orphanhood in the sample. Sibling-loss estimates mark the death of any sibling throughout the respondent's life and do not include children born to the same mother who died before the respondent's birth.

démographiques published a portrait of "orphanhood" in France in 2015 and found that less than half of one percent of French 18- to 24-year-olds would be classified as double orphans.[27] Beyond parents, we can understand this cohort's relationship to mortality through the lens of sibling survival: the proportion who have experienced the death of a sibling of any age. Based on full sibling rosters collected in 2009 and 2019, respondents have an average of five siblings each (a total of six children). Sixty percent had all living siblings in 2009, and that number declined to 44 percent by 2019. In other words, mortality in the immediate family is practically ubiquitous still today.

The combination of sustained population growth and high mortality creates a looming anxiety in Balaka Boma and the nearby villages: labor migration streams from villages to town, a dearth of space for burials in town, and teeming graveyards in surrounding villages combine to create new uncertainties about where Balaka residents will be laid to rest when they die. With few exceptions, the consequences of population change on mortality perceptions and burial space has not attracted much scholarly attention. However, evidence of conflict and consternation around burial procedures is widespread in local news sources and the population chatter from Balaka.[28]

Recall the tailors at the shop, chatting about money when Gertrude first got to town: "If you also quarrel with your friend about witchcraft, the chief asks you to pay money. And if you don't go to attend funerals, the chief asks you to pay three chickens. And if you deliver at home, the chief will ask you to pay." If you don't attend funerals, you will be fined. Furthermore, if you deliver a baby at home or if you fail to register your marriage, you will be fined. What incentive do Balaka residents have to pay such fines, especially those with no resources to support their immediate needs or buffer the consequences of an emergency? What sanctions could they possibly receive for outstanding debts to their village?

To illustrate the basic expectations of the burial process, Gertrude grills one of the secondary school teachers in town about what would happen if she were to die in Balaka.

> "If I die here what can be the processes of my funeral?"
>
> "Do you really want to know before you are dead?"
>
> I laughed and said, "Yes!"
>
> "OK. If you are married, and you paid money to the chief to register your marriage, there will not be any problem. But if you are married, and you didn't pay money to the chief? In that case they will not bury you unless you pay."
>
> "And if I am dead, how will I pay?"
>
> "Gertrude, your family wants you to pay the chief while you are alive. Tell your future husband."

Here is a second insight (of fourteen) from Gertrude on the same topic.

> My friend from Andiamo came to visit. He said he didn't have anything to do, so he decided to pass by and say hi. So as we were chatting I asked him about the burials. I asked, "What happens if someone from your village dies here in town? What happens, and what are the processes that you take?"
>
> "If someone dies here in town, your relatives will decide where to bury you—either here in town or at the village where you are from. If someone dies in the house or at the hospital, here is what has to happen. Before you start crying that you have lost one of your relatives, you are supposed to go to the chief and tell her or him. The chief needs to know who died and what caused the death. The chief will always ask you about the program that you want to do, either a burial in town where you are staying or at your village. After talking with the chief, that's when you start crying. Also the chief arranges for the boys to announce in the village that someone has died, and the boys also tell the people the day of the burial. After the chief has been told, then you can start crying. But if you start crying before telling the chief, the chief will ask

you to pay a fine because you didn't respect the traditions. You have just done it on your own without respect."

"How much is it that the chief would ask me to pay?"

"There is no set amount. It depends on what price the chief decides."

"And what happens if I fail to pay those fines?"

"Next time there is a funeral for one of yours, the chief will tell the men who work at the cemetery not to dig. If you want to be buried at your village, if you want to be buried near your relatives, don't have a debt in your village."

The registration of vital events at the village level is serious business. Chiefs are responsible for maintaining a record of births and marriages, for ensuring compliance with health programs, for granting divorces and making the settlements fair, and for distributing land and settling land disputes. Ultimately, chiefly authority is tied to chiefs' responsibility for maintaining the village burial grounds and assuring a proper burial to all residents, with the caveat that they are residents in good standing. The perpetual threat of mortality and the presumed need for burial assistance are sufficient to enforce the chief's entire agenda—the details of which may change as policies like the RBF4MNH shift with the national and global policy winds.

A context of high mortality is one in which young adults are acutely aware of their own mortality, one in which the threat looms large enough to deter behaviors that will result in fines, and one in which the need to remain in good standing to be eligible for burial (without burdening your family) constitutes a social pressure like no other. The stakes of being a resident in good standing are nothing less than a proper burial for oneself and one's loved ones. Mortality, funerals, and burials do not constitute a distinct domain of life (i.e., the death sphere); the rituals surrounding death and burial provide a constant drumbeat in the background of daily life, with connections to migration and to marriage. They motivate acceptable behavior in the mundanity of the day to day (such as maintaining good relationships with neighbors) and impel adherence to traditional practices around all other vital events, especially marriage, pregnancy, and the birth of a child.

Net Risks and Mortality Perceptions

Understanding HIV demands clarity about the other dangers and maladies Balaka residents live with. Not all of Balaka's heavy mortality burden is attributable to HIV and AIDS. This simple observation relates a notion Alex Weinreb and I referred to in earlier work on the relationship between religion and HIV as living in a "richly risky environment."[29] The argument—that for people living in the epidemic, HIV often takes a backseat to the pressing and urgent problems that characterize daily life in many African contexts—was grounded in a puzzle contained in the cross-national public opinion data from sub-Saharan Africa. When adults in HIV-endemic contexts are asked, "How worried are you about HIV?," they almost always respond with answers like "Very." But when asked in open-ended ways about the problems they are facing in their daily lives, few mention HIV or AIDS—even in very high-prevalence contexts.[30] How can both be true? How can AIDS be a crushing concern, a massive uncertainty, and a footnote? The answer to these questions is not singular but emerges from three analytic moves: a shift from gross to net risks, a focus on mortality perceptions, and an ear to population chatter concerning death and burials.

In her work on the political economy of sex and HIV risk among Mexican migrant workers in the United States, Jennifer Hirsch points out that migrant workers face deadly risks at work on an ongoing basis and situates HIV in light of a much broader set of concerns. She writes, "Working as a roofer without a harness, using a nail gun to hang sheetrock without eye or ear protection, or seeing one's co-worker impaled on a piece of steel at a construction site, also shape how men think about the comparatively remote risk of HIV infection."[31] In an examination of patterns of sexual behavior in fourteen high HIV-prevalence countries during the early 2000s, the economist Emily Oster posited an explanation for "limited behavioral response" to the epidemic: low expectation of life due to non-HIV causes. She measured "risky sexual behavior"[32] and found it was more prevalent in countries where HIV was accompanied by high burdens of maternal mortality, child mortality, and malaria. The basic insight—that people who do not expect to live very long anyhow have no incentive to use condoms to prevent a distant death (or wear sunscreen, for that matter)—likewise communicates the salience of relative risks in a context of existential uncertainty.

HIV IN A RICHLY RISKY ENVIRONMENT

Working within an econometric framework, many scholars have estimated the probability of risky behaviors in x, y, or z domain as a function of expected longevity. A body of research focused on adolescents in the United States leverages the vocabulary "anticipation of early death," "futurelessness," "future certainty," and "fatalism" to show that adolescents who anticipate a short life span are more likely to engage in violent delinquency, nonviolent delinquency, drug use, and risky sexual behavior.[33] Some of this work extends beyond the psyche of the individual, linking fatalism at the level of the school or the friend group to the self-destructive behavior of individual adolescents.[34] A demographic approach raises a different set of questions, many of which are more compatible with ethnographic sensibilities than econometric approaches. Here I follow a set of questions posed by Elísio Macamo in his phenomenological exploration of how residents of a Mozambican community cope with disasters and climate events: "What is it like to live a life of material uncertainty and insecurity? Are the concepts uncertainty and insecurity themselves appropriate to describe such a life?"[35]

To understand HIV as a biological force and as an uncertainty, I move away from studying HIV in isolation and instead position it within the larger set of issues, concerns, and dilemmas that govern daily life. As eloquently stated by John Blacker and Basia Zaba in 1997:

> When discussing lifetime risks, it is necessary to distinguish between gross and net risks. A gross risk is the probability of a person contracting HIV, *assuming that no one in the population dies from any other cause*. A net risk is the proportion who will die of AIDS when allowance has been made for mortality *from other causes*. The difference between the gross and the net risks will of course depend on the level of mortality from causes other than AIDS; clearly the higher the mortality from other causes, the more likely will people be to die of something else first.[36]

Simple facts for communicating the scope of HIV abound: three transmissions per 1,000 acts of coitus, 14 per 100 adults currently infected, 50 AIDS-related deaths per 1,000 adults in a calendar year. Popular understandings of HIV are heavily informed by clinical perspectives on individual case progressions. Represented in the left-hand panel of figure 8.6, this view takes HIV as a sequential phenomenon in which an uninfected individual progresses through stages: infection with the virus, to which a specific probability is assigned ($p1$), then progression to an immunocompromised state that leads to related illnesses ($p2$), and, eventually, to an AIDS-related death ($p3$).

A demographic approach deviates from this sequential view, insisting on a comprehensive view of risk, vulnerability, and death in which HIV is just one of many dangers and hardships people face. When we seek to understand how factors like prevalence, gravity, and urgency are configured and balanced in people's minds as they navigate an uncertain world, we are implementing a net-risks view. This shift in thinking is represented by the right side of figure 8.6. For our purposes, the risk contained in $p1$ (probability of seroconversion from a negative state to a positive state) is uninterpretable as a stand-alone number. Its weight must be assessed in relation to the magnitude of $p4$, the age-specific probability of death from all other causes for the HIV-negative population at this age—an estimate that contains the combined

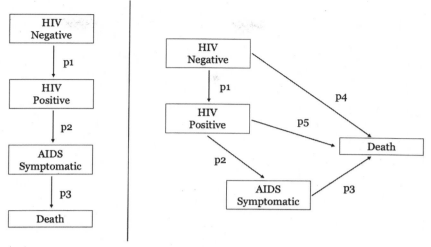

FIGURE 8.6 Gross (clinical) versus net (population-based) views of risk

weight of malaria, motor vehicle accidents, maternal mortality, malnourishment, other infectious diseases, and lightning strikes.

Situating HIV in relation to other dangers and exploring mortality perceptions—by likelihood and by cause—I continue mapping Balaka's mortality landscape in a comprehensive way. Using data from waves 2 through 8 of the TLT study, I adapt the incidence-based tools used already to model HIV-related concerns to shed light on two other major issues endemic in Balaka: food insecurity and malaria. I first calibrate the estimates of HIV incidence established in earlier chapters to the incidence of these other problems as experienced by this population. This offers a sense of scale in experiential terms. Only then do I extend this same style of analysis to model and compare vulnerabilities and mortality perceptions. How large does the threat of HIV loom, really?

For this analytic lens to work, I impose a few false equivalencies. As with mortality, HIV infection is an absorbing state—a state from which one cannot return. The same does not hold for food insecurity and malaria, which are often experienced recurrently (especially among the most vulnerable). So the models I present here are not the kinds of models epidemiologists would use to estimate need for courses of malaria treatment or to project the severity of an anticipated famine. Still the comparisons are instructive. Remember that HIV kills on a fairly long time horizon; absent treatment, new infections result in illness approximately eight years later and in death about two years after that. Hunger, on the other hand, is experienced immediately, in the belly, in the head, and throughout the body; the effects of poor diet and malnutrition manifest quickly (though not immediately) in small children, with signs of stunting, hair discoloration, sleep deprivation, and cognitive decline within only a few weeks.[37] In reporting that they have experienced food insecurity, TLT respondents are not telling us that they needed to manage their monthly food budget carefully or eat nonpreferred foods (e.g., beans rather than goat for protein) to get through the week. They are telling us that they have been skipping meals because they had nothing to eat and putting their children to bed hungry.

Normally written about as a major source of infant and child mortality, malaria afflicts young adults too, though it kills fewer adults than it does children. The symptoms of malaria typically manifest two or three days after the mosquito bite, taking the forms of fever, disorientation, and achiness. Like food insecurity, malaria is endemic, follows some seasonal patterns, and causes acute suffering. Though malaria only seldom kills healthy adults, it often prevents them from working and going about their daily business, and it has serious, negative consequences for household well-being, including nutrition, sanitation, and schooling.

As events, as hardships, as illnesses: HIV, food insecurity, and malaria are neither similar nor comparable. However, the standardization of hardships into a singular framework that adjusts the numerators (the events) to the appropriate denominators (the population at-risk) over a known and consistent period of time is useful conceptually because it provides a portrait of actual incidence and perceived risk across three conditions that assail Balaka residents and disrupt daily life and health for young adults. Although HIV is acute, generating a particular epidemic of uncertainty, it is simultaneously overshadowed by malaria and food insecurity. Though most clinicians would characterize HIV as a condition of far greater gravity, the latter are more prevalent and often more urgent in day-to-day life.

The portrait of incidences shown in the first row of figure 8.7 instantly puts HIV in its place. Asking people whether their household had experienced a shortage of food since their last interview, 20 percent reported in waves 2 and 3 that they had.[38] In subsequent waves, that number dropped to 9 or 10 percent, which (in addition to the seasonal cycle of harvest and hunger for subsistence farmers) may indicate that TLT respondents used the modest incentive they received for participating in the study (about US$3 at each interview) to stabilize their households' food supplies. Like food insecurity in Malawi, malaria incidence follows some seasonal patterns. Wave to wave, many respondents reported having been infected between surveys, with low points (17–20 percent) during the dry season—primarily recrudescence rather than

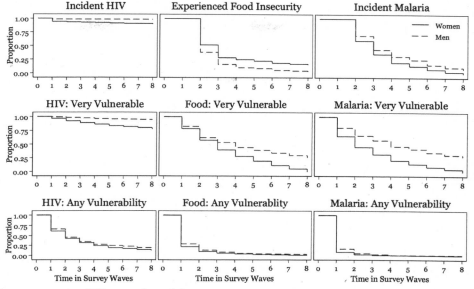

FIGURE 8.7 HIV among other maladies

Source: TLT-1, waves 1–8.

new infections—and an extremely high burden of disease during the most vulnerable seasons, nearing or exceeding 30 percent.[39] In comparison to the HIV infection rate of about 6 per 1,000 observed during the first phase of TLT-1, more than 700 of about 2,000 respondents (58 per 1,000 person-waves for women; 73 for men) reported having experienced food insecurity in at least one wave and 1,300 (140 per 1,000 person-waves for women; 122 for men) reported at least one bout of malaria.

Why and how should "other things" matter for HIV? When more urgent needs and hardships constantly overshadow HIV, which unfolds on a far longer time horizon, prevention will take a backseat.[40] Consider Njemile's dilemma with her husband (see chap. 6), and imagine that the costs of leaving a spouse who puts you at risk of contracting HIV and getting sick eight years from now may seem lower than the costs of severing a livelihood and an extended family that provides love, care, and practical forms of support in a pinch—things like medicine for your sick child or an extra pair of hands in the garden during harvest time. Thinking about "other things" forces a confrontation between the treatment of AIDS as an exceptional disease—the consensus among academics and policy makers—and the lived experience of affected populations (e.g., Linda and Blessings; see chap. 4) for whom it might be one of a trio (or more) of dangers they are juggling at any moment.

This matters both for grasping the relative standing of AIDS vis-à-vis other risks from population-level data and for understanding the fact that perceptual distortions can be condition-specific. Is the distance between incidence and perceptions (minimized vs. paranoid) less accurate, more accurate, or simply different for HIV than for other deadly risks? Alternatively, if the distortions of perception that characterize HIV are pretty much the same as the distortions that inform all kinds of things, is the epidemic of uncertainty we observe in the wake of HIV unique in any way? Or is it simply manifesting a particular appetite for uncertainty that, if eliminated, would be filled by something else? Does HIV uniquely elevate the overall amount of uncertainty this population experiences?

Moving from recent experiences (proximate past) to anticipated hardships (near-future), I again use the beans data. The second and third rows of figure 8.7 depict vulnerability to HIV, food insecurity, and malaria in the coming year according to two thresholds that can be indexed to the incidence measures presented directly above. In the middle row, very vulnerable individuals—those who chose six or more beans (i.e., it is more likely than not that they will be affected by X condition in the coming year)—are differentiated from those who feel less susceptible (e.g., their risk level in the coming year is less than or equal to a coin toss). Both for men and for women, malaria is the most salient risk, food vulnerability is a close second, and vulnerability to HIV trails much further behind. The bottom row models vulnerability more loosely—as any perceived risk in the coming year, where the placement of even one bean in response to questions about a malarial episode gets counted. While there are small differences in the shapes of these curves, generally speaking, all three hardships saturate the entire young adult population with a sense of vulnerability, even though there is far less HIV in the population.

Compared to other conditions, HIV has a particularly powerful ambient effect; this perceptual distinctiveness is important, and the scholarship on HIV exceptionalism provides an explanation. Consider first some of the unique characteristics of HIV the virus: the roulette nature of infection; the long latent period during which time it is detectable by scientists but often unknown to the infected person and certainly not yet visible to friends, family members, or sexual partners; the fact that transmission is almost always sexual, while sexual relationships are often kept secret. Add to that the message that HIV is everywhere and that it is often invisible, that it is impossible to detect with the ordinary senses. A popular Malawian song reminds people that "AIDS is in the flour," conveying a sense of inevitability, since nearly everyone in Malawi subsists on flour.[41] On the international stage, public health campaigns loudly proclaim that "HIV can happen to anybody" and that "everyone is infected or affected."

Consider also the community response: because of its gravity, because of the gruesomeness of late-stage AIDS, and because of its networked qualities, HIV is talked about more than other maladies.[42] HIV's exceptional status is not, however, just about the virus itself, the gossip that flows through an affected community, and the exceptional kind of suffering people living with HIV anticipate and endure. Consider also the political economy of AIDS, the fact that it has been met with an exceptional response from the global community.[43] Adia Benton argues that HIV programs have, for decades, cannibalized the primary health care systems of African countries, subsumed a whole range of priorities, and crept into nearly every type of health and development program on the African continent—from malaria to anticorruption efforts to gender equality to "development."[44] Because of its position on the international stage, even when there is not terribly much of it, HIV weighs heavily on a population.

ASSESSING MORTALITY PERCEPTIONS WITH SURVEY DATA

Having weighted the relative burden of these three conditions in terms of what harms people most gravely and what they most fear in their day-to-day lives, I take this avenue of analysis one step further—to mortality, assessing perceptions of what might kill a person and when. I leverage a set of truly morbid questions, asked again with beans. We asked our respondents to assess their likelihood of mortality in the coming year, within the next five years, and within ten years. And then we asked about causes of death.

> No one likes to think about the end of their life. But we want to ask you about the most serious health risks you will face during your lifetime. Of all the reasons you might die, please tell me how likely you think it is that you might die from . . . malaria, a vehicle accident, AIDS, cancer, childbirth.

These questions were harder to ask than anything else we inquired about. Our interviewers hated asking these questions, and during the baseline survey, 12 respondents (of over 2,000) altogether refused to answer them. We imposed no mathematical or logical constraints on these questions, but only about a dozen respondents answered in implausible ways (placing, for example, eight beans for each cause).

I selected this particular array of causes based on what was known about the mortality burden in Malawi from the best estimates published by WHO, the Global Burdens of Disease Studies conducted by the Institute for Health Metrics and Evaluation, and Malawi's long-standing demographic surveillance study (DSS) in Karonga. Since 2005 the overall top four causes of death for Malawian adults has been pretty consistent: HIV/AIDS and pneumonia account for almost one-third of all deaths; lower respiratory infections are a distant second, primarily affecting children; diarrheal diseases are the third leading cause and malaria the fourth for the population as a whole. Among women ages 20–24, maternal mortality accounts for nearly 17 percent of all deaths, and while road traffic accidents have still never risen to the top of a list of primary contributors to death and disability, they have leaped in recent years (to no. 13) among the young-adult population. In other words, motor vehicles are a new problem and have affected this cohort more seriously than earlier ones.[45]

Given these facts about mortality, the TLT data on perceived cause of death, displayed in figure 8.8, offer several surprises. For each of the five causes of death (just four for men), the triangles represent the mean number of beans (the average level of perceived risk for that cause) placed by women and the circles represent the same for men. Despite the fact that HIV is by far the number one cause of death for young adults in Malawi, malaria, vehicle accidents, and childbirth all receive heavier probabilistic weight than AIDS,

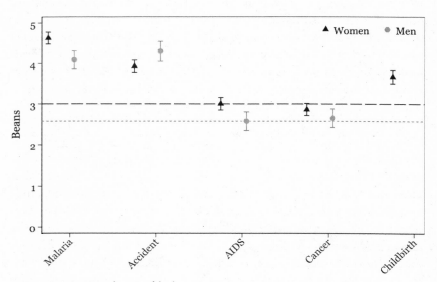

FIGURE 8.8 Anticipated causes of death, 2010

Source: TLT-1, wave 3.

Note: The dashed lines anchor the mean value (by gender) for anticipated mortality due to AIDS.

which falls closely in line with the perceived danger of cancer.[46] These data on anticipated causes of death introduce a profound paradox: uncertainty about HIV saturates daily life; HIV is deadly; yet HIV is not perceived as the greatest mortal danger these young adults face. In fact, of the conditions we named that might kill a person, AIDS consistently ranks lowest (basically tied with cancer). Referring to the notation from figure 8.6, the demographic approach situates estimates of $p1$ and $p3$ relative to the $p4s$ (the probability of survival for uninfected persons) and $p5s$ (the probability a person living with HIV will die from some completely unrelated cause) that characterize this context. Academic demographers focus on the empirically generated rates to calculate relative risks. Extending this logic to the analysis of ordinary people's mortality perceptions (accurate or inaccurate) stands to inform how demographic phenomena are consequential for the patterning of human behavior in other domains of life.

To assess mortality perceptions using beans, we asked each respondent about the probability that he or she will die in the coming year, in five years, or in ten years. In other contexts, this measure has been validated as a strong, positive predictor of actual mortality.[47] When asked about the likelihood of death from any cause in the next year, in five years, or in ten years, TLT respondents grimaced but answered the questions. HIV-positive individuals are, accurately, less optimistic about their longevity than people who do not have the virus. Figure 8.9 summarizes the answers TLT women gave in the 2019 survey round, separated by the results of their HIV test during that round (wherein 90 percent of those who tested positive for HIV already knew their status). HIV-positive individuals placed between one-half and one full bean more than those that tested negative when assessing their likely mortality, and the differences are highly significant on each time horizon. Again here, the binary approach to HIV status conceals key insights about how mortality perceptions are actually distributed in Balaka. When viewed with an emphasis on experiences, rather than along the line of serostatus, uncertainty is the key distinctive and disadvantaged state. On one- and five-year time horizons, uncertain individuals are more similar to those who are HIV positive than those who test negative, and they express an even higher likelihood of their own mortality than those who are HIV positive. When measured as any uncertainty, the uncertain are similar to the HIV-positive population. When measured as acute uncertainty, the uncertain are far more likely to think that death is near than those who have already received a diagnosis.

It is not difficult to imagine how believing that you will not live for very long might have all kinds of consequences on decision making in daily life, from sex to smoking to savings.[48] Insights from evolutionary demography

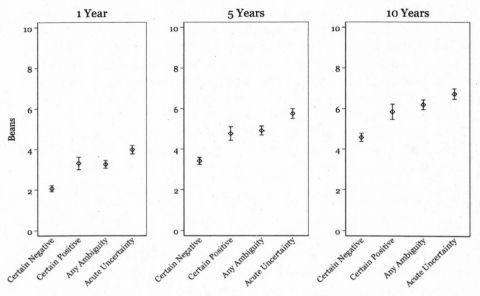

FIGURE 8.9 Women's perceived mortality on three time horizons by HIV status uncertainty, 2019
Source: TLT-3.

(life history theory, in particular) support this intuition that short lives are lived in a fundamentally different way, especially with regard to family formation and fertility. The basic model distinguishes between two speeds at which life history trajectories unfold: settings characterized by "harsh ecology" (i.e., high extrinsic mortality and food insecurity) tend to feature early reproduction, large numbers of children, and short birth intervals—each of which conveys additional mortality risk of its own. In contrast, the slow life history pathway tends to dominate in resource-abundant settings, where daily life is relatively safe and predictable; this trajectory is defined by delayed childbearing, few offspring, and strong attachments.[49]

Importantly, this theory does not emphasize the dispositions of individuals or cultures but the responsiveness of patterns of behavior *for all species* to local mortality conditions. In this model, both "real" and perceived mortality risks leave an indelible mark on human fertility, and the patterns are set long before young people become parents. Even though children may not perceive mortality rates in any articulable way, their lives become collectively patterned by the levels of attachment they experience as children. The psychosocial experiences of individuals are a direct consequence of the overall mortality regime, and in this way, the personal losses individuals experience and the demographic reality of mortality rates are two sides of the same coin.

Applying this insight to the early-life experiences of the TLT cohort specifically, life course theory emphasizes a subconscious "working model" of the
reliability of social relations that emerges between the ages of 5 and 7, at which
time the prevalence of maternal orphanhood stood at about 8 percent, pater-
nal orphanhood stood at about 10 percent, and sibling loss was even higher
(see fig. 8.5). Early-childhood stress through high mortality has measurable
consequences for marriage and fertility *in the population* even if those conditions improve (say, through available ART and new programs to support
maternal and child health) during adolescence and adulthood.[50]

Ordinary people tend to think about HIV and other health conditions in
terms of gross risks: the chance of an event happening per number of people
in the group. This is for good reason. It is intuitive, the math is simple, and
the vocabulary of probability and chance is nonexpert and widely used to
communicate information about health and risk to general audiences. Epidemiologists and demographers use net risks as standard practice. We consider,
for example, the probability of smokers who develop lung cancer in comparison to a parallel estimate of the proportion of nonsmokers who develop
that same condition. Our understandings of daily life amid an HIV epidemic
change considerably when we insist on the vocabulary of net risks and apply its logic to an experiential view of uncertainty. Adjusting the denominators and situating HIV within the broader mortality landscape approximates
more accurately how the epidemic is experienced from the inside.

A Postponed Wedding Demonstrates How Mortality
Accelerates the Life Course

Funerals are settings of thick sociality: they are events with high rates of interaction, often generating mischief and drama. But the consequences of frequent funerals extend beyond the burials themselves and beyond mortality
perceptions too. This example of the ramifications of mortality for marriage
begins at the salon and ends at the borehole.

> Early on Saturday morning Kondwani came in the salon to have her hair
> washed; she said she was preparing to go to attend the wedding of her young
> brother at her home village at Sosola. As her hair was being washed, Kond-
> wani received a call from her husband that her cousin has died and that the
> burial would be on that day—Saturday—at Sosola. When she hung up the
> phone, she asked Enid to stop washing her hair so that she could rush to
> the funeral.
>
> Enid said, "Of course. But what will happen with the wedding?"
>
> Kondwani said, "Well, we have to counsel them to stop the wedding and

do the burial ceremony. They cannot be celebrating while others are crying. The chief can't accept that."

"So what will happen with the *thobwa* and all the other food that they prepared?"

"That's the problem. All the wedding food will get eaten at the funeral."

"And when they want to do the wedding, you will have to start all the preparations all over again?"

"Yes. That will be after forty days, because from today till forty days that means people will be mourning the one who died. After those forty days, people can celebrate again. But before those forty days no one is supposed to celebrate."

Rushing straight from the hair salon to a funeral, Kondwani is among the many women who drop what they are doing to make the appropriate preparations and give the deceased a proper burial. In the example of this death, the costs of properly fulfilling bereavement obligations fall on the entire family but most heavily on the engaged couple. Having saved for their special day, they rented chairs, sewed wedding clothes, and prepared food for nearly three hundred guests. Because of the funeral, they will need to start saving again for their wedding. Couples save for many months to put on an event like this modest wedding; it is extremely unlikely that they will be able to secure the funds in a mere forty days.

This is just one example of how the mortality context has consequences that extend beyond the personal losses people experience—the bereavement, the funeral expenses, and the loss of income. Event planning and the ability to hold a ceremony as planned are constantly in jeopardy, with major resources being redirected to a different, more important ceremony. If mourning observations postpone celebrations—weddings, in particular—how can it be that a high-mortality context accelerates relationships and leaves marriages informal? Relationships are accelerated precisely because of examples like these. In a high-mortality context, couples see that it is foolish to wait, plan, save, and hold a real wedding. Marriage remains informal—despite best-laid plans and new government policies—because delays like these are prevalent and because delays so often become foreclosures.

If your heart broke a little for this couple, sit tight because their bad luck turns into bona fide tragedy. About four months later, Gertrude learns about the wedding that never was while fetching water early in the morning.

As we were at the borehole Deborah passed by; as usual, we all started gossiping. There are rumors that Deborah has aborted the pregnancy because her boyfriend was not taking care of her. They say she has now come back to the town to stay with her parents. Another woman said she felt bad for

Deborah's misfortune and that it was also sad that one of Deborah's sisters died just recently. The sister was fine. Totally healthy. Then she was dead. And her father kept his maize mill open instead of attending the funeral. At the funeral people gossiped that her father is the one who killed her. Another woman said that she had attended the funeral of that girl; a cousin was crying and making a scene: "Why have you killed her? What, do you plan to grind her in the maize mill?" The woman said that the girl who died was the one who was supposed to have a wedding ceremony in October. She had already done the engagement ceremony in June.

In a high-mortality context like Balaka, only fools are optimistic enough to delay their plans. Tomorrow is uncertain. Your relationship is uncertain. Even a wedding to be held in just hours is uncertain. This makes the work of coordinating futures, which is often invisible and taken for granted in many contexts, uniquely difficult.[51] Life course theory offers explanations for why high mortality—even if it is improving—accelerates the life course for young adults, especially in the domain of family formation. In Balaka, this period of the life course becomes so dense in terms of vital events that the uncertainties of HIV, relationships, childbearing, and death become inseparable, both practically (for the people living through it) and analytically (for social scientists seeking to understand the long arc of the HIV epidemic, after ART).

Despite the abundant estimation challenges, however, the analytic payoff of attending to the mortality landscape comprehensively may be substantial. Take, for example, the puzzle of Africa's "stalled" fertility transition, where despite relative decreases in mortality, high fertility has widely persisted across much of the continent in defiance of the classic demographic transition pattern. This anomaly becomes less puzzling when one recognizes that individual-level mortality perceptions are formed cumulatively rather than cross-sectionally, that persistently unpredictable life spans for adults may cultivate a now-or-never approach to many aspects of life, including childbearing, and that relatively small changes in individual lives can have population-wide consequences when amplified through social interactions and aggregated into rates.[52]

Mors certa, hora incerta

Unlike HIV, mortality has universal incidence and varies only in terms of when it strikes. *Mors certa, hora incerta.* Death is certain, its hour is uncertain. The mortality landscape is a broad, multidimensional concept that includes widely circulating stand-alone statistics, for example, crude death rate, life expectancy at birth, and infant and maternal mortality rates. In line with the goals of comprehensive demography (see chap. 1), these metrics need to be considered in real time and in life course time, lagged to account for the mortality levels adults experienced earlier, at developmentally crucial stages. The mortality landscape also captures the constellation of leading causes of death, funeral frequency, and mortality perceptions in the general population. This bundle of mortality-related conditions and their perceptions cannot be summarized with a single statistic. Nevertheless, the concept is crucial for understanding mortality as a population-level uncertainty with portentous relevance for the intimate aspects of everyday life—not just burials, but weddings and divorces too; not just mourning, but contraceptive use and childbearing; not just HIV, but the copresent threats of malaria and food insecurity.

In chapter 4, I demonstrated that a generalized HIV epidemic in the range of 6 to 10 percent saturates the population with uncertainty and that this uncertainty is consequential in the domains of fertility and health. In chapter 5, I showed that AIDS-related uncertainty is patterned but not resolvable through testing. Chapters 6 and 7 connected HIV to relationship uncertainty and showed the role of uncertainty for relationship formation, dissolution, and HIV transmission. In this chapter, I situated HIV within a broader set of things young Malawians worry about and deal with in their daily lives.

Despite prodigious improvements in infant survival, child survival, and survival for people living with HIV and AIDS, Balaka is still a high-mortality context. Malawi's crude death rate is among the highest in the world, and its life expectancy at birth is among the lowest. Life in a high-mortality context is not just a shorter version of life in a context of lower mortality. It is fundamentally different in subtle but important ways. For ordinary people, the experience of mortality is not read from the demographer's data but experienced through one's social network: attending funerals, witnessing illness and accidents, anticipating one's own eventual death. Two features of Balaka's mortality landscape, in particular, shape people's expectations of longevity, in contrast to low-mortality contexts: the sheer volume of funerals (a simple quantity, akin to a crude death rate) and the age distribution of mortality (understood from life-table parameters).

More than twenty years ago, the economist Mark Montgomery expressed surprise at the fact that mortality perceptions had received so little attention from demographers. Citing related work by Cynthia Lloyd and Serguey Ivanov, among others, Montgomery described a *transition effect,* by which mortality decline brings greater predictability to the external environment and enhances individual confidence and the sense of personal control. These developments, in turn, may encourage a longer-term view of family-building," with implications for marriage and fertility patterns.[53] Circling back to the Thomas theorem, it is not the empirical reality of improving material conditions that changes family life but individual- and population-level perceptions of lengthening life spans, infant survival, effective medical treatments within reach, fewer funerals, and a concentration of funerals for the old rather than the young. While all these trends are moving in a direction of stability from the demographer's point of view, for most Balaka residents the improvements are tentative and untrustworthy. From the lightning strikes in Karonga district to the burial of the triplets in Balaka and the food shortages that routinely force residents to choose between traveling to refill medications and eating lunch, Balaka remains a context of radical uncertainty, within which HIV—a principal actor on the global community's stage—plays, at most, a supporting actor's role.

9

Conclusion
Varieties of Uncertainty in Balaka

I close this book with a compilation of fieldnotes that focus on Gertrude's interactions with her neighbor Mai a Fatsani,[1] from when they first meet in June to an ominous final conversation in October. Because of their proximity, the two women interact regularly, almost daily, exchanging advice, jokes, and complaints. Consistent with earlier comments about the density and nature of boma life, Mai a Fatsani's hardships are publicly visible. She and her husband quarrel and make amends with a keen awareness that their neighbors notice everything, and Gertrude finds herself the primary audience of their squabbles. Gertrude notes fluctuations in her neighbor's health, her moods, how the couple is getting along, what is being eaten, what is lacking, and how the food is prepared. As Gertrude becomes more embedded in Balaka, her social networks begin to overlap, with members of the salon coterie and Stella's tumultuous family entering the orbit occasionally. Just as she did for Precious and numerous other friends in Balaka, Gertrude escorts a sick Mai a Fatsani to the hospital and observes for hours during an extremely long wait on a busy day. Mai a Fatsani's habits and struggles are infused with a variety of uncertainties; themes from my analyses of HIV uncertainty, relationship uncertainty, livelihood uncertainty, and existential uncertainty are woven together in a single season of this woman's life.

Mai a Fatsani

June 10

In the morning I started cleaning my house. My neighbor Mai a Fatsani was also sweeping, and she looked sick. I asked her if she was feeling well, and she said no, she had malaria and she didn't sleep well at night. (She is a bit old,

45 or 46.) I asked if she planned to go to the hospital, but she said, "No, I will be fine." She and her husband aren't from Balaka. They moved here for his work, and she followed the husband.

June 15

When I woke up in the morning I cleaned my house, and as I was sweeping I saw the landlord's son with the same woman as yesterday. The woman is married. She was coming out of his house again, and it was early in the morning.

I greeted Mai a Fatsani, and she said she was still not feeling well. Later on I saw her going to the nearby market; she came back with vegetables for lunch, but her husband had already left for work. He leaves very early because he is a teacher, and the school is a bit far. But he comes back around 2 p.m. He goes by bicycle.

June 16

After leaving the market, Tiyamike said she would escort me home. We passed by my house and found Mai a Fatsani cooking using a clay pot. Tiyamike laughed and asked her why she still likes using what people in the past were doing. Mai a Fatsani said cooking in the clay pot reminds her of her grandmother in the village. She said, "I can't stop doing what we were doing in the past. When cooking in the clay pot, everything smells good, and my husband likes it."

Tiyamike asked, "So do you advise that we should start cooking using clay pots? To keep the men happy?"

"No, your husband probably wouldn't like it. Here in town when you cook using a clay pot they think that you are poor and that you don't have modern pots to use. But it's not like that." She showed us another big clay pot that she uses to store water. She said, "I don't have a fridge, but my husband enjoys drinking cold water because it is very hot now."

Tiyamike said she would ask her grandmother to make one big clay pot for her so that she can enjoy cold water in October. "That's when it gets really hot." Then Tiyamike left to go meet someone.

June 20

When I reached the borehole I found a few people fetching water. Mai a Fatsani had arrived even before me, and everybody was just complaining about the water problem and electricity. Precious came to fetch some water, and another woman asked if she had had her baby, and she said yes. But it's a baby boy, while she wanted a baby girl, and all the clothes that she bought were for a baby girl.

The woman asked, "How many kilograms did the child weigh?"

Precious said, "2.8 kilograms, but the first child was born at 3.2."

One woman must have heard through gossip that Precious delivered on her way to the hospital. She asked, "So what happened for you to deliver on the way? This was not your first pregnancy. Did you not know that the labor pain had started?"

Precious said, "No, it was not my wish to give birth on the way. But when the labor pain started I thought that it was just some pains, because when I was pregnant with the first child, the pain would start and then stop, so I thought this was the same thing."

They all laughed. And the woman advised Precious not to be pregnant again until she is married. If she is failing to control herself, then she must use contraceptives, because she has too much responsibility for a single woman.

Precious said, "Yes, you are right."

Another woman came also to fetch water and complained that she doesn't have relish at home because her husband is a policeman and the government salaries are more than two weeks late again. Mai a Fatsani said that her husband is a teacher, and she has the same problem.

June 28

When I woke up in the morning I saw the son of my landlord digging a pit. I went nearby to ask what he was digging, and he said he was digging a pit latrine. Then I saw Mai a Fatsani slaughtering a chicken; she said it was the last of her livestock, and because she didn't have relish she decided to eat what she had.

July 22

When I woke up in the morning I went to fetch water at the tap, and I found Mai a Fatsani there, also drawing water. We greeted each other. I asked her why she didn't look happy. She said that one of her close relatives got very sick and died. I asked what happened to him. She said he started getting sick some time ago, but no one took him to the hospital because they thought that he was not very ill. Then he started being very thin like a child, and definitely it was due to low CD4 count because when they took him to the hospital the doctor started helping him. Then in the process he died, and now his relatives are crying a lot.

Then I said, "Sorry for that. Where will the burial happen?"

She said the burial will be in Mbera because although he was working at Toleza and married there, his home village is Mbera, so that's where he will be buried. I asked who made the decision for him to be buried at his village. She said we just decided that because his brothers were also buried there, and it is good for him to be buried near his relatives. I asked if he is going to be welcomed at his village. She said, "Yes, he will, because that's where he is from. And he paid the money to the chief when he got married. Had it been that he had bad behavior like stealing from neighbors or fines in the village, then it would be very difficult for the chief to accept that kind of a person."

August 21

When I reached home I found Mai a Fatsani quarreling with her husband; she was telling him to go for a walk after eating *nsima* because she didn't want to cook twice. Her husband refused to eat and said he would eat when he got back from his walk. Mai a Fatsani complained a lot. She shouted that it has been three weeks since he has been leaving her while cooking. Clearly, this means he has started seeing other women, because he doesn't eat again when he comes back home.

Her husband answered, "I am already old. I'm not proposing other women."

"If you are old, then stay home."

I laughed at them, respectfully, of course. And her husband refused to stay home. He left, and as he was leaving Mai a Fatsani shouted after him: "Go, but know that you will not find me here when you return."

When he had gone, Mai a Fatsani confided to me that she really thinks her husband has started seeing other women because since they got married he's never acted the way he's been acting recently.

"Why do you think he has changed?"

"Here in Balaka there are a lot of beautiful girls. I know he is admiring them."

August 25

In the morning I cleaned my house and prepared breakfast, cassava and some tea. I saw Mai a Fatsani just sitting on the veranda. I greeted her, and she said she was not fine. She had a headache, and I said sorry. I asked if she went to the hospital, and she said, "No, I am just tired. There's no need for me to go all the way to the hospital only to receive painkillers when I can just buy them."

August 31

When I returned from fetching water, I saw the husband just sitting on his veranda. He announced to me that he would be sitting on the veranda the whole day just to make his wife happy. "She always complains that I don't like staying home."

We laughed.

"Can I be chatting with women if I stay home the whole day? No. But if I stay home I hear a lot of problems."

I asked him, "Like what kind of problems?"

"Gertrude, women demand a lot. They tell you that there is no sugar, no salt, no relish, all at the same time. Then you give them 300, 400 kwacha, and somehow they manage to cover all the expenses. How do you suppose they do it?" Mai a Fatsani came out of the house and said, "Gertrude, don't listen to him. He is here at home because I told him that if he leaves me alone again I will pack my things and he will not find me."

Her husband laughed and said, "Tomorrow I will visit my friends again."

We all laughed.

September 1

Later in the morning Stella came to visit her parents, and no one paid attention to her, so she left in a snit. Mai a Fatsani came back from the market with vegetables. She didn't look happy, as usual, and her husband asked her what was wrong. She said she didn't want to eat vegetables only. She wanted fish. Her husband said, "Sorry I don't have money for that." She just entered the house, and she didn't cook. Instead she asked her son to cook.

September 22

In the morning I saw Mai a Fatsani going to the maize mill. She complained that her maize is about to finish. The problem is that they sold a lot of maize right after the harvest because they needed money, and they sold it at the cheapest price. So between that and the low salary her husband gets they don't know if they will make it to December.

September 30

In the morning when I woke up, I heard that Mai a Fatsani was down with malaria. She wanted to go to the hospital, but she didn't have any one to escort her because her husband was at work. I asked if I could escort her, and she was grateful.

The hospital was extremely busy, so Mai a Fatsani had to wait to be seen. I wandered to the section where they distribute ARVs, which was full of people—both men and women, boys and girls. A certain girl looked very, very sick; she was too sick to stay there and receive her medication, so she left. I saw one nurse weighing the patients and another nurse writing in the book, while the third nurse was doing counseling. He told the patients to be eating often, and apart from that they should make sure that in their diet they should eat vegetables; he said they should always remember the day of visit, because they always give the days to come back for refills, and if they know that they are going somewhere far they should make sure to walk around with a bottle of medication.

The nurse said, "A lot of you, when going to the funeral, for example, you leave the medicine at home because you are shy. You think other people might hear the medicine making noise in the bottle. Here's a tip: If you know that the medicine is making noise in the bottle, then put a lot of cotton wool inside to stop the noise. Or change from the bottle to plastic paper where it can't make noise. But make sure to take your medicine with you."

"If you know that you are traveling to South Africa [SA] or anywhere far, make sure you come with your stamped passport to show us that you are indeed traveling, and you will be given the ARV supply for six months. Then when you are in SA, keep taking your medicines. You can ask friends here to collect some for you, or you can go to the hospital there in SA. Just find out from your friends where they go if they're found HIV positive, or send a guardian to collect the medicine for you. Then make sure that at the next visit you go yourself, just for a checkup."

The nurse continued, "On the issue of vegetables, make sure you keep a garden of vegetables at home so that if you don't have money to buy you can eat from your own garden. And if you're too sick to walk from home to the hospital for a refill, send a guardian to collect the medicine for you." The people were going into the rooms one by one to get checked and receive their medicines.

Another nurse came out to give advice to the people who had just joined. "Let me give you the example of Miriam," she said. "Some people stop taking their medication when they are feeling better and starting to look nice. Other people have started admiring them, so they think they are OK. Others also stop coming to collect medicine because of something their church says. Or after being prayed over by the pastor, they throw the medicine away because they think are fine. But it is not like that. There was that girl called Miriam, she was on ARVs and she was coming to the hospital to collect the medicine. Then she started looking really good, and after being admired by people around town, she thought that she was fine and she stopped taking the ARVs. Of course, she started getting sick, and when she came to the hospital her CD4 count was low and she died because of the treatment that she was given.

"If you are sick, like if you have malaria, you might go to the hospital without taking the book you use to receive these ARVs with you. You get a new book there, and the nurse might give you normal treatment for malaria without knowing that you are HIV positive. This is like overdosing the patient. People with HIV can easily die while they have malaria, and you have to tell the nurses all the information so that you get the proper medication and the proper dosage."

The nurse was speaking angrily, like a Pentecostal preacher. "If you are able to eat nsima every day, how can you people fail to take your medicine every day?"

Then one woman (a patient) gave a comment: "Maybe some people are still shy to get their ARVs?"

"Well, if so, they are killing themselves."

One woman came with a small baby. She said she gave birth three weeks ago, and she was here for a checkup. The nurse helped her, and the woman said she doesn't care that she is HIV positive because she is still strong. She said she was tired of being checked by doctors often and also the child was not affected.

Another woman who was waiting to receive ARVs commented on the nurse's statement about belief in pastors and healers. She said, "People, beliefs cannot heal; just keep taking these medications for the rest of your life."

Then another man taking ARVs complained that he gives his wife money each day to buy some fruits to eat as a family, as they are both HIV positive. But his wife uses the money for gambling, and they eat poorly.

Only a few people remained, so I wandered back to the general section to see Mai a Fatsani. She was still waiting because there were a lot of patients. She said, "Let's leave. I'm tired of waiting. I'll just buy some painkillers on our way home."

When we reached the shop, Mai a Fatsani bought painkillers and said that she will never go back to the hospital again.

When we reached home, she slept. Stella came home and asked where Mai a Fatsani and I had gone.

I told her that we'd gone to the hospital. Stella gossiped saying, "ARVs with old people don't work properly. I've seen Mai a Fatsani going to collect medicines at Mponda hospital. She gets ill often because she is becoming weak. She needs to be eating a lot, to weaken the virus." Stella said, "Watch the old people on ARVs. That same thing is going to happen to us."

I started writing and slept.

October 1

In the morning, before sweeping, I went to see Mai a Fatsani to ask if she wanted me to escort her back to the hospital. She didn't want to go. "No, I will be fine. And my husband should return home tonight. Gertrude, just know that I have already paid to the chief of my village. If I die today, everything is set. They should be able to bury me properly."

HIV as Continuous Uncertainty

Although most people in Balaka eat well between June and September, some families are lacking, Mai a Fatsani and her husband among them. Government employees' salaries are not being paid on time, and the anticipation of hunger season looms large for this family. Through the neighbor's complaints and ailments, Gertrude documents the intersection of food insecurity, water shortages, HIV uncertainty, and relationship uncertainty—combined with aging, mortality, and the stress of burials on families. Gertrude sits for hours in a hospital waiting room, listening to nurses dispense advice, along with ARVs, to Balaka's HIV-positive residents.

The anthropologists Eileen Moyer and Anita Hardon refer to life with HIV both in North America and in sub-Saharan Africa as continuous uncertainty. They write, "Continuous uncertainty in relation to drug supplies, food availability, work opportunities, housing, social support systems, and family life prevent people from leading a normal life with HIV."[2] In a similar vein, the geographer Brian King refers to managed HIV in South Africa as "an uncertain lived experience."[3] Fluctuations in viral loads are a matter of constant concern; as the Balaka nurse pointed out, the nutritional needs of HIV-positive households are exacting, while nutrient-rich foods are scarce, and in a particularly cruel irony, stress and worry—about HIV, about medicine, about food, water, children, husbands, comorbidities, and burials—are said to cause a patient's CD4 count to drop, leading to weight loss and serious illness.[4] While ARVs work to prevent an HIV infection from turning into illness, the conditions under which first-line ARVs work well are specific and difficult for many in Balaka to achieve. Side effects can be unpleasant, policies are changing frequently, and the risk of drug resistance is real, especially as HIV-positive individuals age. "For many HIV-positive people," King writes, "the certainty that is generated by testing and ART either reinforce, or generate, other uncertainties," including food insecurity, relationship uncertainty, and burial anxiety.[5]

How might one go about maintaining strong nutrition, avoiding stress, and preventing comorbidities in a food-insecure context riddled with infectious diseases and relationship uncertainty? Mai a Fatsani is making a heroic effort. Stella remarks, quite ominously, that the fate of deteriorating in middle age, while eating nonpreferred food, taking ARVs, and trying to stretch a husband's paltry salary, is probably inevitable. In anticipating that "that same thing is going to happen to us," Stella conveys both a sobering assessment of HIV uncertainty—that it is more likely than not to become part of the struggles of aging and eventually cause death—and a remarkably accurate perception of mortality shifts over time. Few Balaka residents will die of HIV as young adults. Instead, with abundant supplies of ART and a universal treatment policy, HIV-positive individuals are aging with HIV.[6] Some will live long lives on ART, while others will develop drug resistance and die from HIV about a decade from now, after their own children are nearly grown.

Policy Failures and Possibilities

The brief glimpse of Precious's life after the delivery of her baby underscores fertility as a domain of profound uncertainty affecting women, in particular. Despite all the improvements in maternal health and child survival, Malawi remains a context of a 1 in 60 lifetime risk of maternal mortality.[7] The shopkeeper's daughter's death is just one of those (see chap. 2), and every young-adult woman living in Balaka knows someone who died in childbirth. Pregnancy and childbirth remain extremely uncertain events for every mother in Balaka.

Precious's third child is alive at the time of this writing (April 2022), but the early days of this baby's life were uncertain. The hospitalization recorded in chapter 6 was the first of dozens of trips to treat an underspecified respiratory condition, clinical stunting, and recurring dehydration during the child's first year. Absent further improvements to basic infrastructure and health care in Balaka, 50 of 1,000 children born this year will not live to their fifth birthday. As seen in the example of Alice's respondent, these losses can have cascading effects on other vital events, including divorce, remarriage, future childbearing, and longevity. And recent literature on maternal care emphasizes that African women who deliver outside facilities are often labeled as "backward" by community leaders, punished by health workers, and stigmatized by their peers.[8]

Precious's engagement with prenatal care and her delivery, diligent adherence to postnatal visit recommendations, and efforts to care for an ailing infant are an example of Malawi's almost miraculous reduction in infant and child mortality. But because she delivered prematurely en route to the hospital, Precious was ineligible for the 5,300 MK stipend from the RBF4MNH program. The stipend may have gone a long way to support this family. With support from Gertrude and one of the tailors, Precious managed to fight the fine imposed on women who deliver outside of the facility. Precious's empty-handedness despite the IOU written on her health card underscores the unintended consequences of well-meaning policies; they can cause confusion and exacerbate uncertainty, even if they were designed to accomplish something else. The RBF4MNH program is a case in point. Designed to reduce infant and maternal mortality in Balaka, the program managed to create a lot of confusion, introducing questions about who merits payment and why, what it takes to be a good patient, and who benefits from a program that makes perfect sense to those who designed it but seems arbitrary to recipients. Having generated no measurable improvements in key measures of maternal and child health (maternal mortality, infant mortality, or stunting), by tying a conditional cash transfer to a dangerous event and following through selectively on payments, the RBF4MNH program may have made childbearing in Balaka more rather than less uncertain.[9]

This observation raises a question about whether there is any role for policy in combating uncertainty at the societal level. I think so. One clear policy issue is a technological one: we desperately need better tests to detect HIV. The window period of 45 to 90 days for the widely available ELISA tests is too long to curb an epidemic of uncertainty that affects, at any given moment, *at least 40 percent of young adults*. Development of a cheap, rapid, antigen test to detect acute HIV-1 infections sooner should be a high priority. The basic technologies to provide real-time information on HIV status from a finger prick already exist. US-based clinicians regularly use them to screen the blood supply and to test for acute HIV-1 infections in emergency cases.[10] But they remain expensive and difficult to process in Malawi and across most of sub-Saharan Africa—the world region most affected by HIV. Forty years into the epidemic, it is time for these technologies to be made cheap, portable, and available in HIV-endemic contexts. Doing so will advance the important goal of early detection for HIV prevention at the macro level and will help clinicians provide definitive results to *all* HTC clients, not just those who test positive.[11] A better test could reduce (though not eliminate) the shadow of HIV uncertainty by providing people with real-time information about their HIV status.

The findings from TLT push an empirically based conversation about uncertainty into the clinical arena. Compared to people who know their HIV status, people who are uncertain about HIV have poorer self-rated health, they miss more days of school and work, and their expectations of survival are low. Discerning an uncertain person's "true" HIV status can, of course, remain the clinician's top priority. After all, this information is essential to the sound exercise of clinical judgment with respect to patient care. But the TLT study demonstrates a strong, negative relationship between uncertainty and health that exists independent of HIV status. So there could be clinical benefits to recognizing uncertain patients as uncertain and treating them— beyond testing them repeatedly—with the *condition of uncertainty* in mind. Whether the uncertainty is temporary or perpetual, it is likely wrapped up in issues outside the health care provider's domain: relationship uncertainty, livelihood uncertainty, and food insecurity may not be treatable in a clinical setting. Many clinicians now inventory violence in the household and protein intake as standard procedure. Uncertainty about HIV is a clinically relevant condition to integrate with such other pieces of information.

The framework of uncertainty can also be leveraged to support a new era of prevention efforts, as pre-exposure prophylaxis (PrEP) becomes available in Balaka and worldwide. PrEP cannot be used to treat an existing HIV infection; however, people who express concern about a partner's unknown status or uncertainty about their own future status may be especially good candidates for PrEP enrollment. As Malawi's national prevention strategy moves toward the target of enrolling sixteen thousand new clients on PrEP, the focus has been on "key populations," especially men who have sex with men and female sex workers.[12] However, as figure 1.2 shows, a large number of new infections occur to young women during their peak childbearing years. Qualitative research on the acceptability of PrEP for prevention suggests that most adolescent girls and young women know little about this option; however, on learning that PrEP pills can be taken daily to prevent infection on exposure to HIV, some are intrigued.[13] In yet another moment of technological transformation in treating and preventing HIV, good measures of HIV uncertainty

could be combined with life course insights about the most epidemiologically dangerous seasons of life to structure equitable delivery systems and aid
health care providers' efforts to prioritize those who stand to benefit most.[14]

More than anything, the finding that HIV takes second place to other
uncertainties underscores the crucial but Herculean task of providing safe
water, sufficient food, adequate shelter, and basic health care for all residents
of Balaka, of Malawi, and of the planet. Second-order concerns would include
employment (e.g., for Patrick, Linda, and Blessings) and educational access
(e.g., eliminating the stream of nonfee school expenses that constantly surprise Blessings).

Although a transformative HIV test and food and employment for all
are tall orders, an intervention as simple as consistently delivered paychecks
could go a long way toward reducing livelihood uncertainty in Balaka. I offered multiple examples of how livelihood uncertainty destabilizes daily life
and romantic relationships. Many Balaka residents live in conditions of abject
poverty, but livelihood uncertainty is not solely a problem for the poor. Mai
a Fatsani's husband is one of Malawi's educated, working professionals; he
is employed as a teacher. He, his wife, and others like them end up having
to do things like skip meals, kill their last chicken, and miss a beloved relative's funeral while waiting for their paychecks. This happens regularly, and
regardless of underlying health conditions, this is not okay. At a time when
technology allows for the sweet potato seller to receive transportation money
via Airtel from a man she has never met in just minutes, it seems absurd that
government agencies, businesses, and NGOs should lack the infrastructure
(or the resolve) to pay workers on time, all the time. When payments to sala-
ried workers are delayed and money stops circulating, the problems cascade:
goods stop circulating, food goes to waste, families get stressed, and workers
in the informal economy suffer acutely. The consequences of not knowing
when you might get paid are real. While some amount of livelihood uncertainty might always be part of the fabric of social life, salary delays are a resolvable problem.

In a context where the vast majority of deaths could be prevented by improvements to basic infrastructure, nutrition, and health care services, further reductions to mortality and an accompanying compression of death at
older ages are eminently possible. A taming of the mortality landscape should
reduce much of the existential uncertainty described in chapter 8. The transformation already under way could be advanced by pumping resources into
Professor Kalindekafe's research group on lightning strikes, by designing maternal health programs to support poor women rather than burdening them
with fines, and by increasing the clinical staff and decreasing wait times for

Mai a Fatsani and others who seek care at clinics in and around Balaka *while* continuing to ensure a steady supply of ART—both first- and second-line treatments—for those who need it.[15] Awareness of these changes may take some time to seep into the collective conscious, as mortality perceptions do not typically reflect the demographer's view instantaneously, and new varieties of uncertainty may crop up in its place. After all, uncertainty also pervades low-mortality contexts; it just takes different shapes.

The paradox of uncertainty is that it represents both problem and possibility for those experiencing it. In this book, I have documented many of the negative consequences of uncertainty—particularly in the domains of health and relationships. My own assessment, based on two decades of research and engagement in Balaka, is that uncertainty levels in this particular corner of the world exceed even the conventional understanding of radical uncertainty.[16] If they were asked directly, I reckon that the vast majority of TLT respondents would agree that they crave a more predictable tomorrow, season, year ahead. Although the negative consequences of uncertainty are extremely real, the productive, optimistic, and generative capacities of uncertainty are important to recognize. HIV-related uncertainty tends to be related to poor mental health, relationship dissolution, delayed treatment, and a host of other negative consequences. More generally, however, there are theoretical reasons to think about the possibilities of uncertainty and why people may be motivated to maintain rather than resolve it. In settings where certainty more often reveals a negative outcome than a positive one, the shadows of uncertainty sometimes offer a comfortable shade—a hiatus from a harsh landscape. In fact, many of the joys of life are impossible without uncertainty. The happy side of uncertainty includes hope, anticipation, and surprise.[17] So while it is true that a lot of social life is driven by the desire to curb uncertainty, humans also engage in myriad behaviors to allow for it and let it linger. Completely eliminating uncertainty from life would do just as much to impoverish it as it would to improve it.

Uncertainty Demography beyond Balaka

The philosopher Jürgen Habermas remarked in a recent interview, "There has never been a time when our knowledge about what we don't know was bigger."[18] Few would quibble with the assertion that we are living in uncertain times, and I expect uncertainty to be among the defining concepts of our century. In sociology, demography, and the social sciences broadly, now seems a good moment for uncertainty to assume its rightful place in the pantheon of social forces. The matter of how to study uncertainty—its sources, our strategies for coping with it, and its unique influence on daily life—is less clear. While I will applaud efforts to advance deeper theoretical developments of uncertainty and related concepts (certainty, risk, vulnerability, predictability, etc.), theoretical musings alone are unlikely to produce the kind of knowledge needed to address our most intractable problems, many of which are dilemmas of uncertainty. To address deadly epidemics, to anticipate the future of marriage and childbearing, to build structures to deal with massive migration flows in an era of climate crisis, we need more research that grapples empirically with the shadows of uncertainty tangible things (e.g., viruses, markets, temperatures, gossip) project upon people and upon social landscapes. Producing this kind of work requires serious investments from foundations, institutes, research groups, and individual scholars; it also requires rethinking some standard research practices and going about our work differently in the future.

In the words of the anthropological demographer Eugene Hammel, "The virtue of ethnographic approaches for the demographic enterprise is that the actors, who know the ground, are permitted to lead the way. The value of culture for social analysis is not so much that the informants speak to the investigator, but rather that they speak to one another and can be overheard."[19] Gertrude's ethnographic observations offered many clues to how uncertainty affects human behavior in Balaka, but it is by using the more conventional quantitative demographic data and techniques that I have attempted to measure uncertainty and demonstrate its effects. Uncertainty is a population-level phenomenon with population-level consequences. Arguments like this require population-level data, which need not be nationally representative to be rigorous. Deep engagement with specific communities and cohorts can be extremely valuable when the research design is anchored in deep knowledge of the context (geographic and life course) and guided by core principles of comprehensive demography: careful sampling, an emphasis on change and response (i.e., prioritizing insights from the longitudinal, moving picture over cross-sectional snapshots), and a commitment to interweaving field observations and survey items together over the duration of the project.[20]

Creative scholars may be able to productively identify uncertainty in the residue of existing data sources and found data. Big-data scholars using a large corpus of text may be able to "see" how uncertainty permeates daily conversation (including population chatter) by paying attention to the use of conditional rather than future-simple tenses. (Just imagine access to a corpus of personal diaries from randomly selected adolescents, sampled over time.) In particular contexts, long-run increases in non-numeric responses and nonresponses to questions about family formation may be reasonably read as evidence that the world is becoming too uncertain for young adults to be able to even imagine their future families. But reliance on found data and secondary sources has limits, and while these are valuable for a specified set of research purposes, I do not believe we can understand the force of global economic uncertainty in any real way by counting the number of mentions of the word *uncertainty* in quarterly Economist Intelligence Unit reports and tallying these by country. Materials for studying uncertainty seriously will not create themselves. We decide to create them (or not), and their value will depend on the insight, care, and rigor of the collective effort.

Reflecting on John Snow's infamous discovery of cholera on the pump handle, the statistician David Freedman remarked that the key ingredients for scientific advancement are logic and shoe leather, and it would be impossible for me to fully convey the amount of shoe leather more than seventy contributors to the TLT project collectively burned during our decade of work together.[21] Gertrude alone wrote 600 pages of fieldnotes in a six-month period. Over ten years, we spent more than US$5 million in NICHD support; we collected 25,000 surveys and pricked over 12,000 fingers for rapid HIV tests. At two hours per interview, that amounts to 50,000 hours of data collection before data entry, processing, or analysis even begins. Stated differently, the simple graphs of HIV prevalence by cohort (fig. 2.5) and HIV uncertainty over time (fig. 4.3)—on which my basic argument about HIV uncertainty rests—are underpinned (in hours) by what would amount to five solid years of research time and close to two million pieces of paper.

One consequence of disclosing things like mischievous responses about coital frequency and the obvious underestimates of sexual frequency (and overestimates of fidelity) in self-reports is admitting that the TLT survey data are imperfect. But our data are excellent, nonetheless. They are uniquely valuable for the study of several varieties of uncertainty that ebb and flow during young adulthood because they were designed to accomplish precisely that. The weaknesses of the TLT data are compensated for by other data sources: ethnographic material, high-quality nationally representative studies, and vital statistics compiled by fieldworkers and statisticians laboring in national capitals and international agencies around the world. To the extent that uncertainty demography becomes recognized as a worthy intellectual project for future investment, it will flourish when advanced by teams that locate uncertainty at the core of their questions and likewise draw on a wide variety of materials, disciplinary perspectives, and methodological approaches.

For scholars involved in survey research, the findings from TLT raise two concrete issues I believe we could productively address in the near term to improve the study of uncertainty. One concerns the general disposition

toward "don't know" responses in surveys, that is, how unknowns get physi-
cally encoded in our instruments and how we allow for (or willfully conceal)
their expression in the field. "Don't know" responses are a dreadful problem
in survey research; after going to great lengths to identify a representative
sample, we hate nothing more than having to drop cases due to nonresponse,
and because "don't know" answers are so costly to analysts, interviewer training procedures are designed to minimize them.[22] In this sense, ostensible
population-wide certainty about many issues may simply be an artifact of
contemporary data collection practices. Good interviewers probe, sometimes
insistently, to arrive at a "real" response to the questions researchers have
crafted, but the effort of probing (perhaps itself an indicator of uncertainty)
is rarely documented. If we are indeed living in an era of uncertainty, the
standard practice of discouraging "don't know" responses conceals the levels
of uncertainty people and populations experience and conveys a false sense of
precision about the things people think, expect, and know. Even worse, varying practices about whether and how to allow for and record "don't know" answers (within and across data sets) should give any thoughtful analyst pause.
I am not suggesting that every project adopt probabilistic phrasing and solicit answers using ten beans and a plate. But to the extent that well-designed
surveys based on strong samples are among the tools researchers will use to
study uncertainty in the social world, uncertainty demography will demand
more deliberate and coordinated conversations about how to handle statements and gestures of uncertainty in response to the questions we ask.

A second tractable issue concerns how scholars study sexual and romantic relationships.[23] Patuma's adventure in the bush is a story for the ages. Although the details of the bush buffalo, the four eggs in the jumbo, and hanging her husband's trousers up to dry tell a uniquely Balaka story, I recognized
it as a universal one. Gay or straight, married or dating, relayed as tragedy or
as comedy, we all know someone who has set aside their pride for a moment
or longer to find out the truth about their relationship. In global perspective, the social organization of romantic relationships is changing in unprec-
edented ways; even so, relationship uncertainty will remain an integral part
of the human experience, as the grist of the intimate sphere both assuages and
exacerbates uncertainty.

Patuma's story further highlights how poorly marriages and relationships
are measured in most surveys. In terms of data quality, researchers often fail
to capture brief relationships, and we regularly misclassify relationships that
are ambiguous, informal, secretive, and complex.[24] For researchers, this represents a serious problem if many relationships are ambiguous, informal, secretive, and complex, and it represents a different kind of serious problem if the

ambiguous, informal, secretive, and complex relationships are socially salient, as they were in Patuma's case, in Patrick's case, in Tiyamike's case, in Precious's case, and in Njemile's case. Beyond the information we attempt yet fail to capture, researchers rarely even think to inquire about stages of the relationship process—the many small steps involved with starting and ending a relationship.[25] That "marriage is a process" circulates widely in the anthropological literature on African families. Indeed, the variety of ceremonies and official steps are highly visible to foreign researchers. But marriage (i.e., relationships generally) is "a process" everywhere. From first encounters and exchanges of phone numbers to physical intimacy, beginning to share money, and introductions to the others' families and friends (as well as for relationship dissolution: sleeping at a friend's place, moving out, hiring a lawyer, beginning to date someone new), the process of forming (or stepping away from) a relationship is highly scripted; nonetheless, the myriad steps involved vary and inform, if not constitute, the sense of certainty that relationship conveys.

Something resembling uncertainty demography has been on the precipice of emerging for at least a decade. My analysis of HIV in an endemic context has made this variety of uncertainty legible in Balaka. Other applications for the questions weighing on the field today include aging with Alzheimer disease, retirement planning, and new infectious diseases. Throughout much of the world, the climate crisis is exacerbating wildfires and floods. For weather forecasters, product actuaries, and disaster preparedness experts, these are matters of risk assessment; as the science evolves, patterns may become more predictable and may even get converted into mere ambiguities. For individuals making decisions about their own lives and their family's well-being, uncertainty is the more appropriate concept. Just as Balaka residents navigate around HIV and the associated uncertainties, Californians navigate a landscape wherein both the wildfires themselves and the uncertainty about them pattern daily life. The prominent uncertain shadows in my own community include gun violence, flooding, inclement weather, and now, of course, COVID-19.

The key insight from two decades of research in Balaka is not simply that we might learn something interesting when we begin to take uncertainties into account; it is that scholars will fundamentally misunderstand the very thing they attempt to study when they do not. In estimating HIV as a condition that affects between 6 and 12 percent of young adults, HIV scholars have for decades overlooked the fact that the epidemic's shadow of uncertainty captures a population nearly four times as large, and they have failed to understand that the bright line for most behavioral outcomes is not serostatus but the experience of uncertainty. In the economic sphere, the example of employment uncertainty is instructive and well documented in the literature; comparing the fertility intentions of the unemployed and the employed conceals the fact that the forces of uncertainty often lead the precariously employed to more closely resemble the behavior of the unemployed than the securely employed. About newer uncertainty dilemmas facing our world today, less is clear at the population level. In medical sociology, the category "patients-in-waiting" has emerged to describe the unique situation of people trapped between a state of sickness and health due to uncertainty about disease.[26] That this state is consequential for patients (and parents) is irrefutable from the ethnographic data. How to understand this kind of uncertainty and its consequences at the population level—as a function of disease prevalence, disease visibility, evolving bodies of scientific knowledge, health-seeking behaviors, and diagnostic technologies—forces the inquiry into different directions. Likewise, what uncertainty demography brings to the topic of climate change and migration extends beyond the individual-level relationship between displacement and migration (or perceptions of vulnerability and probability of emigration). We may, instead, productively apply population-level thinking to link macrolevel uncertainties about land suitability to changing marriage patterns (altered, unintentionally, through migration) or use demographic tools to see the phenomenon more clearly, decomposing migrant populations into component parts: the proportion displaced by climate events, the proportion motivated by uncertainty about climate events, and the proportion migrating for totally unrelated reasons.

Most of this analysis has been specific to Balaka: its mortality landscape and burial rituals, its marriage regime, its HIV epidemic and other disease patterns. Balaka is, after all, a site of staggering uncertainty, with high rates of child mortality, relationship churning, lightning strikes, and food insecurity layered over a sustained HIV epidemic and more prosaic varieties of social change. At the same time, there is something universal about the role of uncertainty in daily life that is just as relevant to my own experiences in Chicago and to friends' experiences in Seoul, Milan, and Minas Gerais. Our individual lives are shaped by things we know we don't know, and so are the structural contexts we collectively inhabit. Building on the twin traditions of population thought and empirical investigations of population processes from diverse contexts, uncertainty demography is about making the unknown legible in individual lives and in populations. Engaged in a simultaneous effort of elaboration and enumeration, we take good measure of the shadows cast onto our landscapes and acknowledge uncertainty as an enduring aspect, a central feature, and a powerful force in everyday life.

Acknowledgments

This research uses data from Tsogolo La Thanzi, a research project designed by Jenny Trinitapoli and Sara Yeatman and funded by grants R01-HD058366 and R01-HD077873 from the National Institute of Child Health and Human Development. Data files are archived with and available through Data Sharing for Demographic Research, thanks to additional support from NICHD R03-HD095690. TLT-3 (fielded in 2019) was funded by a Max Planck Society grant awarded to Emily Smith-Greenaway and facilitated by the Max Planck Institute for Demographic Research. At the University of Chicago, the Department of Sociology provided a subvention through the Albion Small fund that allowed me to include tables and figures beyond the typical limits, and the African Studies Committee provided support to source key illustrations. Anna Beck at the University of Wisconsin cartography group made the maps in the front matter and chapter 1, Claudia Mastrogiaccomo constructed the Sankey chart in chapter 5, Kelvin Maigwa graciously allowed dear Nyanga to brighten chapter 5, and Grace Wagner assisted with the construction of demographic transition figures in chapter 8.

Foggy conversations about a new data collection venture began in 2007; since that time the Tsogolo La Thanzi project has evolved into a constellation of friendships and collaborations that spans continents, institutions, and now decades. The brightest star in that constellation is the more than decade-long friendship and collaboration with Sara Yeatman, from whom I am always learning new things. The unsung hero is Abdallah Chilungo, who is invisible in this manuscript yet has been central to every phase of TLT since the design period in 2008. More than anyone else I know, Abdul possesses a skill set of astonishing range that balances the intellectual and practical demands of data collection. From questionnaire design and supervising translations to designing innovative recruitment strategies and making sure salaries get paid on time, Abdul is the good heart of TLT. None of these data would exist without Sara and Abdul, and it has been my great joy to work side by side with brilliant people I also consider friends.

Over the years, many others contributed to aspects of study design, implementation, and dissemination of TLT data, especially Angela Chimwaza, Winford Masanjala, Susan Watkins, Hans-Peter Kohler, Victor Agadjanian, Gowokani Chijere-Chirwa, Rose Muheriwa, Pilira Msefula, Sydney Lungu, Eric Lungu, Hazel Namadingo, Isabella Khuleya, Janneke Verheijen, Adam Ashforth, Kathleen Broussard, Amy Conroy, Courtney Allen, Lauren Bachan, Stephanie Chamberlin, Nell Compernolle, Kate Dovel, Sarah Garver, Hannah Furnas, Ashley Larsen Gibby, Elizabeth Morningstar, Christie Sennott, Emily Smith-Greenaway, and Selena Zhong. At NICHD, Regina Bures, Rosalind King, and Susan Newcomer provided valuable guidance about grant management during the funding period.

Along with the Balaka District Executive Committee, Traditional Authorities Nsamala and Sawali warmly welcomed TLT to Balaka. Essential to helping us find a space in the community were District Commissioner Shadreck Manyetera and Town Assembly chief executive Hamisi Twabi. When it came to monitoring safety and installing essential utilities, Noel Banda and Isaac Lekison Kazuwa performed small miracles. The Balaka District Health Office supported our efforts to stay abreast of evolving testing and treatment protocols and technologies; they provided valuable supplies and connected us to a wonderful team of nurses and trainers who facilitated and supervised the integrated voluntary testing and counseling services within TLT. In particular, I thank Lyoid Piringu, Ruth Gondwe, John Chauma, Edson Banda, Martha Muyaso, and Ruth Kasiyamphanje for building a solid bridge between the research and clinical aspects of our study. Our friends at the Catholic Women's Association, especially Patricia Fatchi and Emma Dumbo, and at Fourways, especially Andrea Rodigari, Tamara Hudson, Patrick Fourways, and Joseph Kayira, made Balaka a home.

Nearly one hundred people contributed to the collection of TLT data before any analysis even began. In addition to thirty interviewers at any given point in time, our team was composed of data-entry clerks, project supervisors, an accountant, a gardener, cleaners, watchmen, translators, computer programmers, bicycle-taxi drivers, and a granny who attended to fussy babies so mothers could complete their interviews without interruptions. During the course of the study, every member of our research team went through transitions in the realm of family formation, and we interacted with many of the same institutions our respondents did. We made visits to receive ante-

ACKNOWLEDGMENTS 231

natal care and obtain contraception, following some of the nurses' recommendations and ignoring others. We had engagements, wedding ceremonies, marriage counseling, divorces. We participated in routine and voluntary HIV testing and received the results of those tests. We buried friends and family members as a consequence of AIDS, accidents, and other maladies. While collecting systematic data on the complexity of young adulthood in a setting of high HIV prevalence, our research team navigated these waters too. The knowledge generated by those collective experiences is an integral part of the account of uncertainty I have advanced in this book.

Each member of the interviewing, data, and facilities teams merits recognition for their contributions to TLT: Allie Mulama, Annette Kasambala, Bernard Kwenyengwe, Caroline Kandaya, Esnat Sanudi, Fransisca Zuza, Gift Chirwa, Grace Azizi, Ivy Missi, Jasintha Fatchi, Jenipher Matenje, John Kafuwa, Joyce Kayoka, Kenstone Mambo, Laureen Chingwengwe, Lilian Majawa, Linda Kabango, Linda Kalitela, Linely Chinyama, MacDaphton Bellos, Madalitso Potani, Maggie Tengatenga, Maisha Nyasulu, Mussa Mtayamo, Nelson Chitsonga, Nolia Phiri, Patrick Simbewe, Rehima Mitochi, Reuben Chitekwe, Robert Chibweya, Ronald Kamwendo, Rose Aliseni, Sam Kanyama Khwiya, Stafel M'bwerazino, Thokozani Dzingo, Treza Likomwa, Veronica Kuchipanga, Willey Zakudimba, Wilson Gondwe, Zacharia Nkhoma, Zynab Njerenga, Lawrence Kapasule, Adrian Chiwaula, Agnes Kalupsa, Anthony Kulemba, Austine Ayami, Chisomo Kalogwire, Dinala Chilembe, Edith Golowa, Gerald Imedi, Kiyare Matiki, Linely Nsamala, Ruth Kazembe, Siyeni Sitima, Tiwonge Mkandawire, Yahya Kamtunda, Elias Devison, Grace Nyson, Sellina Materechera, Stella Kasiyamphanje, Charity Mikundi, Kitty Gomonda, Billy Harrison, Hajira Manyamba, Andy Mguntha, Crissy Iphani Nyirenda, Moosa Laudon James, Wyson Dailes, Davie Chitimbe, Mirrium Nyirenda, Francis Kamungu, Caroline Kumbuyo, and Janet Nlashi.

To our departed friends Catherine Matewere, Tereza Matewere, Cedric Butao, Fanizo George, and Victor Nyoni: May you rest in eternal peace.

While working on this book, I benefited from many opportunities to present in-progress pieces of the analyses, and it would be impossible to overstate how this culture of serious and friendly feedback shaped my thinking about uncertainty demography and population chatter. Conversations with workshop participants at the University of Texas at Austin Population Research Center, the Harvard Center for Population and Development Studies, the University of Pennsylvania's Population Studies Center, the Max Planck Institute for Demographic Research, the African Population History Network at the London School of Hygiene and Tropical Medicine, the University of Chicago Sociology Department Colloquium Series (twice), Columbia University's INCITE group, the Third Coast Center for AIDS Research Monday Seminar, the Graduate Institute of International and Development Studies in Geneva, and the Dondena Center at Bocconi University (especially the Alpine Population Conference participants) helped me hone core ideas, cut distracting examples, and sharpen important details.

During an estimated 150 hours of writing with one another, the CISSR faculty writing group provided me with encouragement and the sound of clicking keyboards, which spurred my word count each Thursday. Marco Garrido, Emily Lynn Osborn, Jim Sparrow, Kimberly Hoang, Andrew Abbott, Eman Abdelhadi, Monika Nalepa, Paul Cheney, Paul Staniland, and Steve Pincus, I look forward to writing more in your kind presence. Many other scholars paused what they were doing to respond to queries along the lines of, "Will you take a quick look at this passage [or page or chapter] for me?" Since I am an intellectual extrovert, these kinds of queries were numerous, and I tried to spread them out. To Rose Aliseni, Rafael Batista, Christof Bradtner, Francis Dodoo, Darby English, Margaret Frye, Adom Getachew, Sarah Hayford, Caroline Kandaya, Jon Levy, Johanna Oh, Etienne Ollion, Michelle Poulin, Mariano Sana, Guy Stecklov, Ashton Verdery, Susan Watkins, and Alex Weinreb: Thank you for reading and responding generously, even though you didn't have time to spare.

During my sabbatical year at the Dondena Center at Bocconi University, Francesco Billari, Nicoletta Balbo, Marco Bonetti, and the DisCont team provided me with the perfect combination of solitude and scholarly interaction. The environment at Bocconi—the conversation and the coffee—was precisely what I needed to finish the manuscript. Once the first draft was complete, Abdul Chilungo, Gertrude Finyiza, Jessica Jerome, and jimi adams read every word and provided me with detailed feedback that helped me clarify fuzzy aspects of my thinking and improve the array of words on each page. Two anonymous reviewers make me grateful to be part of an intellectual community in which people critique so generously, even from behind the veil of anonymity where their ideas and effort will never be given due credit publicly.

In addition to being the constellation of my own intellectual life, TLT became an organizing force for my family, none of whom asked to have so much of their life structured by my research activities. The fieldwork demands that have supported my career have also shaped my marriage and my children's childhoods. Cassia and Luce got to participate in fieldwork rather than summer camp and missed more Fourth of July celebrations than they celebrated. Their very presence enhanced my credibility as a fertility scholar; they brought laughter and energy to the research center and helped in myriad ways—from alphabetizing recruitment cards to mopping floors and holding babies. Although it was never fully voluntary on their part, I do not take their cheerful participation in my work for granted. Gregory Collins put his own projects on hold to keep our family together during critical periods and tolerated long absences when that strategy seemed to make more sense. Our ongoing, decades-long conversation about balancing numbers and narrative and about the importance of getting the lighting right is woven into the fabric of this book, without attribution.

Elizabeth Branch Dyson embraced the project, offered incisive editorial judgments, and allowed me to craft this book using as many vignettes and figures as I needed—no more and no less. Emily Williams began working with me as a research assistant and quickly became a trusted reader and editor. Mollie McFee, Carrie Olivia Adams, and the editorial team at the University of Chicago Press treated every step of the publication process with professionalism. Sheila Berg elevated my prose with careful, kind, and instructive copyediting. Production editor Christine Schwab and indexer Bonny McLaughlin brought fresh eyes and stellar edits to the final polish.

Over the course of a decade, more than 3,500 Balaka residents shared their time and stories with TLT. Each one allowed us a glimpse—however sincerely or mischievously, eagerly or reluctantly—into their life. Only a few are featured in this book as individuals, beyond the aggregated data, and none of their real names will ever be disclosed. I nonetheless wish to acknowledge the contribution of each and reiterate here my deep appreciation.

Appendix

TABLE A.1 Mortality trends in Malawi, 1990–2020

	1990	1995	2000	2005	2010	2015	2020[a]
Total population	9,404,500	9,844,415	11,148,758	12,625,952	14,539,612	16,745,303	18,628,747
Crude death rate[b]	19.22	18.50	18.14	15.62	10.79	7.42	6.42
Total deaths	180,754	182,082	202,205	197,179	156,868	124,166	119,559
Life expectancy	46.10	45.85	45.09	47.84	55.56	61.95	64.26
Adult population[c]	5,191,284	5,414,428	6,009,181	6,767,510	7,793,232	9,193,171	10,904,100
Adult death rate[b,d]	299	406	533	633	558	423	412
Adult deaths from HIV	11,000	29,000	50,000	58,000	27,000	14,000	9,800
Population (ages 0–14)	4,212,558	4,429,487	5,137,348	5,856,043	6,739,256	7,550,122	8,224,350
HIV deaths (ages 0–14)	8,100	15,000	18,000	18,000	12,000	4,700	1,800
Infant mortality rate[b]	141	119	100	65	53	36	29
Under-5 mortality rate[b]	243	206	173	110	85	54	39

Source: United Nations Population Division.

[a] Some 2020 estimates are actually from 2019.

[b] Crude death rate, adult death rate, under-5 mortality, and infant mortality are all stated per 1,000 population.

[c] Age 15 and over.

[d] Data are averaged over five-year intervals beginning with the column year (i.e., estimates for 1985 span 1985–89; estimates for 2000 span 2000–2004; the table ends with single-year estimates for 2020).

Glossary of Chichewa and Technical Terms

ankhoswe (sing., nkhoswe)   Traditional marriage guardians.

Boma   Term for government administration blocks used across much of Southern and East Africa. Boma refers to a district headquarters (historically and today) and has become a meaningful geographic unit for the compilation of population data for Malawi.

chinkhoswe   Traditional marriage ceremony; related to ankhoswe above.

chitenje   Cloth wrapper women use as a long skirt to protect the clothes underneath (while cooking or walking) or to carry a baby or goods.

lobola   Bride-price paid in cash or kind. Lobola is uncommon in Balaka but practiced in a variety of forms throughout other parts of Southern and East Africa.

ndiwa   Chichewa term for relish, nourishing food with flavor (vegetables, meat, fish, beans) eaten in small quantities alongside nsima for calories.

90–90–90   A set of targets by UN member states, agreeing to ensure that 90 percent of all people living with HIV know their status, that 90 percent of those diagnosed receive sustained antiretroviral therapy, and that 90 percent of those receiving treatment achieve a state of viral suppression.

nsima   Maize-meal porridge; the staple food across Malawi.

Option B+   A policy implemented in Malawi in 2012 that made lifelong ART treatment available for all pregnant women. The policy was scaled to 20 other countries before 2016 and has subsequently been replaced by universal test and treat policies.

thobwa   Fermented maize-based drink often served at celebratory events such as weddings or funerals.

Notes

Chapter One

1. All names are pseudonyms except Caroline and Gertrude.
2. Trinitapoli, fieldnotes, August 7, 2019.
3. Caldwell 1995; Heimer 2012; adams and Light 2014.
4. Johnson-Hanks 2006; Johnson-Hanks et al. 2011.
5. "Boma" refers to a district headquarters (historically and today) and has become a meaningful geographic unit for the compilation of population data for Malawi.
6. Reniers 2003; Chimbiri 2006. Nearly half of first marriages in the south end in divorce within ten years.
7. MDHS 2004, 2010, 2016.
8. This explains in part why condom use remains low in stable partnerships. See Chimbiri 2007; Tavory and Swidler 2009.
9. Smith 1982, 443–44.
10. Petit 2013, xiii–xiv.
11. Schneider and Schneider 1996, 3.
12. Johnson-Hanks 2018; Bolu-Steve, Adegoke, and Kim-Ju 2020.
13. Hauser and Duncan 1959, 34.
14. Smith 1982, 443.
15. Mishra 2006; Timberg 2006.
16. Michelo, Sandøy, and Fylkesnes 2008; UNAIDS 2016.
17. Green et al. 2006; Trinitapoli and Weinreb 2012; Vandormael et al. 2019.
18. Vance 1952, 10.
19. Ryder 1964, 1965. See also Alwin and McCammon 2003; Abbott 2005.
20. Watkins 1991, 2004; Watkins, Swidler, and Biruk 2011.
21. Johnson-Hanks et al. 2011, 15.
22. Kreager 2009; Eloundou-Enyegue and Giroux 2012; Billari 2015; Frye 2017.
23. Thomas and Thomas 1938, 572.
24. The accuracy of the perceptions is a separate question, also important and consequential but for reasons that run in parallel to the point I'm making here.
25. Trinitapoli, fieldnotes, January 5, 2010.
26. Balaka is a matrilocal area, so the men come and go while the women stay in their villages.

27. Smith 1982, 442.

28. For this Geertzian distinction between models for and models of, usually invoked for understanding religious phenomena, see Geertz 1966.

29. Trinitapoli 2021.

30. Watkins 1990, 1991.

31. Watkins 1990, 256.

32. Randall 1996.

33. Watkins 1990.

34. Benton 2015; Dionne 2017.

Chapter Two

1. Yeatman 2009a, 2009b.

2. E.g., Trinitapoli 2006; adams and Trinitapoli 2009.; Trinitapoli and Weinreb 2012.

3. See Makofane et al. 2020 for an important critique of the term "generalized epidemic," which I use in the technical, not the normative, sense.

4. Crampin et al. 2012; Dube et al. 2012; Kahn et al. 2012; Sifuna et al. 2014.

5. Watkins et al. 2003; Kohler et al. 2014.

6. Matrilocality makes the task of actually following women over time during a time of concentrated transitions (especially marriages and migrations) slightly less Sisyphean.

7. Male partners were interviewed again in 2015, through the same recruitment procedures—tokens—but only current partners were interviewed during this round. Due to funding constraints, the 2019 round (TLT-3) focused only on women. See Yeatman et al. 2019 for more details about the study design.

8. Hooper 1990; Setel 2000; Iliffe 2005.

9. Heimer 2007; adams 2015.

10. Watkins 2004.

11. Muula 2008.

12. Munthali, Chimbiri, and Zulu 2004; Watkins 2004. See also Munthali et al. 2004.

13. Calculations are my own, using MDICP data.

14. Zulu and Chepngeno 2003; Smith and Watkins 2005; Green et al. 2006; Gregson et al. 2006; Muula 2008; Reniers 2008.

15. Muula 2002.

16. Joint United Nations Programme on HIV/AIDS and World Health Organization 2006.

17. Harries et al. 2016; Jahn et al. 2016.

18. Johnson et al. 2013; Nsanzimana et al. 2015; Wandeler, Johnson, and Egger 2016; Price et al. 2017; Watkins-Hayes 2019.

19. Daire 2007; Matovu and Makumbi 2007; Jereni and Muula 2008.

20. Rosenthal 2017.

21. By "low-cost," I mean about US$20–25 each month, which would be absolutely unattainable for most Malawians.

22. MDHS 2010, 2016.

23. More specifically, the eligibility criteria for ART was set by the WHO clinical staging system; patients in stages 3 (moderately symptomatic) or 4 (severely symptomatic) could initiate treatment.

24. Schouten et al. 2011.

25. Jahn et al. 2016.

26. Dovel et al. 2015; Dovel et al. 2016.

27. Kieffer et al. 2014; UNAIDS 2015.

28. Yeatman et al. 2013.

29. For further reading on the political backdrop, see Kalipeni 1992; Ihonvbere 1997; Mc-Cracken 1998; Mweso 2014.

30. Election investigations revealed the use of white out (called Tipp-ex in Malawi) to doctor result sheets during the 2018 election. Widespread protests throughout 2019 led to a recall election in 2019 and the installation of the current president, Lazarus Chakwera, in 2020.

31. Nishimura et al. 2009; Behrman 2015; Grant 2017.

32. Muchabaiwa, Mutambirwa, and Chilombo 2020.

33. Attending school with a dirty uniform is not prohibited, but it is considered shameful.

34. UNICEF 2014; Muriaas et al. 2019; Maiden 2021; "Malawi: 2nd Periodic Report on the African Charter on Human and People's Rights and the Maputo Protocol, 2015–2019" 2020.

35. Religious leaders are implicated too but not to the same extent as chiefs.

36. Balaka is not a lobola society; there is no bridewealth, so the financial barriers to marriage are quite low. The primary financial obstacles are the couple's ability to find or construct a house and bring appropriate (modest) gifts to a traditional ceremony with ankhoswe.

37. These violations carry the possibility of imprisonment too. The MDFRA, like all legislation in Malawi, has to balance protecting human rights, for example, women's rights in marriage and divorce, and not violating the "right to culture" (Mwambene 2007, 115). State legislation is not legally or practically equipped to overrule the customs and traditions of marriage in Malawi. But both the broad discouragement (norms) and official prohibition (laws) of polygamy color the earlier conversation between Alice and her respondent, in which both the respondent and her husband quickly dismiss polygamy as a solution to their fertility problem.

38. Brenner et al. 2018; De Allegri et al. 2019.

39. Verheijen 2017, 6.

40. Mojola et al. 2021.

41. Verheijen 2011, 2013.

42. *Mudzi* simply means "village" in Chichewa.

43. For a lucid discussion of what constitutes "quality" in qualitative demographic research, see Coast, Mondain, and Rossier 2009.

44. Emailing fieldnotes necessitated regular trips to town for internet access, and while in town Gertrude began to overhear chatter about TLT: Why are the TLT people back? How can I get a job there? How do they decide who they interview? What are they after, actually? The project's return after a three-year hiatus involved renovating an old rest house to function as our new research center; much of the chatter Gertrude captured in those early months (January and February) was specific to curiosity about the building and associated employment opportunities. But the chatter about our project was valuable in its own right at the planning stage in 2015 and later became central to research about the effects of data collection in longitudinal studies. See Oh, Yeatman, and Trinitapoli 2019.

45. Following local naming conventions, Gertrude always refers to her landlords by their relationship to Stella, their eldest daughter: Bambo a Stella (father to Stella) and Mai a Stella (mother to Stella).

46. "Scissor" means cesarian section.

47. Schroder, Carey, and Vanable 2003; Nnko et al. 2004; Das and Laumann 2010; Yeatman and Trinitapoli 2011.

48. Malawians subsist on a maize-meal porridge called *nsima*, which is eaten every day, in large quantities; *ndiwa* or *relish* refers to any kind of nutritious side dish (e.g., vegetables, legumes, fish, meat), eaten in much smaller amounts and only when it can be afforded.

49. Manda 2013; CEIC 2020.

50. Rindfuss 1991.

51. Given what is known about the accuracy of pregnancy and birth histories, these self-reports should be read as lower-bound estimates. See Mwale 2005; Haws et al. 2010; Szwarcwald et al. 2014; Helleringer et al. 2018.

52. The increase in prevalence across this age gradient of 15 to 25 is fairly monotonic; at each age, prevalence is a little higher. A detailed view showing prevalence by age, in single years rather than five-year cohorts, is available on the TLT website. The website contains replication files for most of the analyses presented in this book, as well as supplementary materials to support selected other claims.

53. Note that "this point" refers to the combination of age and period—not to one or the other. We have evidence of new infections in the younger cohort after 2015.

54. Based on searches of Medline via PubMed (1945–2021) and Web of Science conducted in July 2021.

55. Whyte 1998; Setel 2000; Preston-Whyte 2003; Benton 2015; Dionne 2017.

Chapter Three

1. King 2005; Manning 2020; Damaske 2021; Barnett, Brock, and Hansen 2021.

2. Stigler 1986.

3. Knight 1921; LeRoy and Singell 1987.

4. Keynes 1921; Dequech 2003, 2006.

5. Dequech 2000; Kay and King 2020.

6. Levy 2020, 17. A popular version of radical uncertainty likewise follows Keynes over Knight, distinguishing resolvable from radical uncertainty. According to David Kay and Mervyn King (2020), resolvable uncertainty can be addressed with new information—either through facts or through known probability distributions. Radical uncertainty, in contrast, cannot be easily resolved because of difficulty predicting the future, because of dependencies on another person or on entire structures that are themselves susceptible to change, and because the transformative role of relevant new technologies is impossible to anticipate.

7. I am excluding actuarial science and insurance markets from my definition of "the scholarship" here not because they aren't useful but because they are seldom cited or read by social scientists.

8. Johnson-Hanks et al. 2011; Abend 2018.

9. Schneider and Schneider 1996; Kertzer and Fricke 1997; Bernardi and Hutter 2007; Cooper and Pratten 2015.

10. Smith 1995, 317.

11. Stolzenberg and Margolis 2003, 860, 863.

12. Bongaarts 1978; Bongaarts, Frank, and Lesthaeghe 1984; Scheper-Hughes 1993; Montgomery and Cohen 1998.

13. Becker 1960; Becker and Barro 1988.

14. Caldwell 2004.

15. Caldwell 2004, 400–401.

16. Caldwell 2004, 401.

17. Swidler 1986, 2001.

18. Dyson 2005; Macamo 2017; Sasson and Weinreb 2017; Entwisle, Verdery, and Williams 2020; Muttarak 2021.

19. Billari and Kohler 2004; Mills, Blossfeld, and Klijzing 2005; Blossfeld, Buchholz, and Hofäcker 2006.

20. Kohler, Billari, and Ortega 2002.

21. Lesthaeghe 1989; Balbo and Barban 2014; Bernardi and Klaerner 2014.

22. Comolli 2017.

23. Adsera and Menendez 2011; Sobotka, Skirbekk, and Philipov 2011; Bloom 2014; Buh 2021; Ahir, Bloom, and Furceri 2022.

24. Schneider 2015, 1155.

25. Perelli-Harris 2006, 2008.

26. Zaba and Gregson 1998.

27. Marteleto et al. 2020; Rangel, Nobles, and Hamoudi 2020.

28. Aassve et al. 2020; Lindberg et al. 2020; Trinitapoli 2021.

29. Johnson-Hanks 2005, 364.

30. See, e.g., Musick et al. 2009; Rocca et al. 2010; Hayford and Agadjanian 2011; Ní Bhrolcháin and Beaujouan 2011; Trinitapoli and Yeatman 2011; Kodzi, Johnson, and Casterline 2012; Bachrach and Morgan 2013; Plummer and Wight 2013; Bernardi, Mynarska, and Rossier 2015.

31. Mills, Blossfeld, and Klijzing 2005; Johnson-Hanks 2014; Brown and Patrick 2018, 25.

32. Sandberg 2006.

33. Weitzman et al. 2021.

34. Smith-Greenaway, Yeatman, and Chilungo 2022.

35. Kohler and Kohler 2002; Perelli-Harris 2006; Bernardi, Klärner, and Lippe 2008; Raymo and Shibata 2017; Aassve, Moglie, and Mencarini 2021.

36. Bolano and Vignoli 2021.

37. Mische 2009; Beckert 2016.

38. Huinink and Kohli 2014; Bernardi, Huinink, and Settersten 2019; Vignoli et al. 2020.

39. Crosnoe and Cavanaugh forthcoming.

40. Coale 1973.

41. Van de Walle 1992.

42. Van de Walle 1992, 491–92.

43. Frye and Bachan 2017.

44. Morgan 1981, 1982.

45. Schaeffer and Thomson 1992.

46. Ní Bhrolcháin and Beaujouan 2011, 2019.

47. Bell and Fissell 2021.

48. Kennedy 2012; Kennedy et al. 2022.

49. Duden 1991; Rublack 1996; Bell and Fissell 2021.

50. Ghalioungui, Khalil, and Ammar 1963.

51. Bledsoe, Banja, and Hill 1998; Mukherjee et al. 2013; Finocchario-Kessler et al. 2018; Li et al. 2018.

52. Brown and Patrick 2018; Brown 2020.

53. Burton and Tucker 2009, 135.

54. Wood 2001, 2003.

55. Burton and Tucker 2009, 140.

56. Kalwij and Kutlu Koc 2021.

57. Hurd and McGarry 1995, 2002; Delavande and Rohwedder 2011; Elder 2013.

58. Hamermesh 1985; Fischhoff et al. 2000; Manski 2004; Wu, Stevens, and Thorp 2013.

59. Kahneman 1974; Montgomery 2000; Tversky and Kahneman 2011; Sandberg et al. 2012; Ludwig and Zimper 2013; Apicella and De Giorgi 2022.

60. Keyfitz 1971, 1980.

61. Fries 1980.

62. Fries 1980, 135.

63. Wilmoth and Horiuchi 1999.

64. Goldstein 2015; Billari 2022.

65. For the sake of clear reasoning differentiating certain from uncertain times when the historical record is insufficiently clear, I bracket from this discussion large-scale mortality events, including war, genocide, and natural disaster. However, an excellent literature is also highly relevant to the topic; see, e.g., Frankenberg et al. 2011; Heuveline 2015; Nobles, Frankenberg, and Thomas 2015; Alburez-Gutierrez 2019; Kraehnert et al. 2019.

66. Pesando et al. 2021. See also: Elder 1998; Zimmermann and Konietzka 2018; Beaujouan 2020; Sironi and Billari 2020; Bernard and Kalemba 2022; Tocchioni, Caltabiano, and Meggiolaro 2022.

67. For clarity on the stakes of bridging the micro/macro divide and the need to balance statistical detail with theoretical insight when using aggregation methods, see Eloundou-Enyegue and Giroux 2012.

68. Dewey 1929; Shackle, Carter, and Ford 1972; Swidler 1986; Weber 2001.

Chapter Four

1. UNAIDS 2007; Brookmeyer 2010; Makofane et al. 2020.

2. It is common for Malawian parents to be referred to by the name of their eldest child.

3. Malawian women seldom express anger outright, and speaking ill of the dead is forbidden, so the word *bad* here is strong in a way that may not be understood when I stay faithful to Blessings's actual words.

4. Queen Elizabeth is the best hospital in Malawi. See Wendland 2010 for a description.

5. Timæus and Moultrie 2008.

6. Depo-Provera, i.e., medroxyprogesterone acetate.

7. The language sounds clunky because this is the literal back-translation from Chichewa to English.

8. Fernald 1978; Mkondiwa 2019, 2020.

9. Hayford, Agadjanian, and Luz 2012.

10. Anglewicz and Kohler 2009; Trinitapoli and Yeatman 2011.

11. The approach follows the spirit of decades-old advice from Nora Cate Schaeffer and Elizabeth Thomson about how to productively embrace expressions of uncertainty in survey research. Shaeffer and Thomson 1992.

12. Trinitapoli and Yeatman 2011.

13. Manski 2004.

14. Underlying every figure is a portion of the TLT data that covers (usually) between and 1,000 and 3,000 respondents—always representative of the population as a whole unless otherwise noted, for example, "married women only," "among the sexually active," or "among those

who tested positive." Readers interested in the more technical aspects of these analyses can consult the online supplementary material, which includes replication files and details about every aspect of measurement. Here I present the results (always estimated in several different ways to confirm robustness) in their simplest possible form, usually graphically.

15. Wändi Bruine de Bruin, Baruch Fischhoff, and colleagues refer to fifty-fifty answers as expressions of epistemic uncertainty and warn scholars not to confuse these answers with a true probabilistic response. Their caution supports the present approach of characterizing fifty-fifty responses as expressions of acute uncertainty about HIV. Fischhoff and Bruine De Bruin 1999; Bruine de Bruin et al. 2000.

16. Incidence is 6 per 1,000 person-waves among our sample of women ages 15–25 in 2009. The incidence rate for men of the same age could not be calculated due to the small number of cases.

17. Watkins 2004; Anglewicz and Kohler 2009; Kerwin and Ordaz Reynoso 2021.

18. For these calculations, I limited the definition of "insulated" to respondents who participated in at least four waves of the study. Measured at the threshold of participation in seven waves (allowing one missed wave), I identified 13 insulated women and 10 men in the full study. The insulated respondents are a diverse group in terms of their education level, socioeconomic status, religion, and occupation. What they share is that an unusually high number of them are never-married, and none of them has ever been divorced.

19. Trinitapoli and Yeatman 2011.

20. See Yeatman, Trinitapoli, and Garver 2020.

21. Hayford, Agadjanian, and Luz 2012.

22. Wilson and Daly 1997; Kohler and Kohler 2002; Sobotka, Skirbekk, and Philipov 2011; Mace 2014; Nobles, Frankenberg, and Thomas 2015.

23. I'll note that very little of this literature is key worded with the term "uncertainty," making the compilation of such findings a challenge. A more unified conversation about uncertainty in its many dimensions would be productive for future researchers.

24. Despite the considerable debate about the wisdom of single-item measures vs. validated scales, these four outcomes are widely used in the literature on health and well-being worldwide. See the following examples from Malawi and elsewhere: Idler and Benyamini 1997; Chima, Goodman, and Mills 2003; Kahneman, Diener, and Schwarz 2003; Williams et al. 2008; Baranov, Bennett, and Kohler 2015; Smith-Greenaway 2015; Kilburn et al. 2018; Yeatman and Smith-Greenaway 2018.

25. Remember also that if we had been relying exclusively on the known HIV status, as most studies do, we would have lost between one-third and one-half of the sample while generating these estimates.

26. Kumwenda et al. 2006; Lopman et al. 2008; Moodley et al. 2009; Santelli et al. 2015.

27. Birdthistle et al. 2019; Karim and Baxter 2019.

Chapter Five

1. Most immediately, this means keeping those who just learned about infection from despair and giving seronegative individuals additional tools with which to protect themselves and continue to avoid infection.

2. UNAIDS 2014.

3. Based on searches conducted on June 15, 2021, using PubMed and Web of Science.

4. Analyses were repeated in 2019 and produced nearly identical results.

5. Yeatman et al. 2015.

6. Branson 2010; Taylor et al. 2015; Chen et al. 2021.

7. In addition to describing the limited clinic capacities in Kenya, Tanzania, and Uganda during this period, Ed Hooper describes his own experience waiting for the results of a third test taken within one calendar year. "I felt decidedly nervous as I waited more than a fortnight for the result to come through," he writes. Hooper 1990, 109.

8. Trinitapoli and Weinreb 2012, 118.

9. By 2015, 83 percent of women and 70 percent of men had ever been tested, with a full 44 percent of women and 42 percent of men having been tested in the past year, but these estimates are less germane to our task here, which is to understand the testing landscape at the time TLT began. See Kim et al. 2016; MDHS 2016.

10. I say "relatively easy" because one hears many stories of lacking supplies such as gloves, pipettes, or the solutions needed to develop the test. Valuable medical supplies can be stolen or simply delayed in transit. Despite these challenges, testing was transformed from expert work done in faraway laboratories to a routine procedure available in local clinics.

11. Trinitapoli and Weinreb 2012.

12. Thornton 2008; Obare et al. 2009.

13. The 5 Cs were established in 2012 in the wake of much concern about coerced testing and other irregularities. They are Consent, Confidentiality, Counseling, Correct test results, and Connection/linkage to prevention, care, and treatment. The 5 Cs were preceded by an earlier constellation of three. See Angotti et al. 2009; WHO 2015.

14. Magwira 2016.

15. Providing free, confidential testing to all respondents at the end of the study was something we wanted to do for ethical reasons, and it was also analytically useful for calculating HIV prevalence for the entire sample.

16. These models adjust for the fact that among those we offered to test, some refused and for the fact that among those we did not test at TLT until wave 8, some sought testing on their own outside the study.

17. Ancillary analyses confirm similar associations for men and women, not shown.

18. As with earlier discussions of uncertainty, these relationships can be tested at every possible threshold along a scale and modeled in myriad linear and nonlinear ways; the possibilities are almost endless. The analyses I present here are not exhaustive but represent a selection of substantively important relationships that are robust to multiple specifications.

19. The underlying model includes controls for marital status, education, socioeconomic status, parity, religious affiliation, and religious switching. Results from a model that expanded the threshold of uncertainty to 3–7 beans are substantively consistent with the acute uncertainty model in figure 5.4.

20. Beegle, Poulin, and Shapira 2015, 666.

21. Beegle, Poulin, and Shapira 2015, 675.

22. Abdul Latif Jameel Poverty Action Lab, n.d., para. 12. See also Thornton 2008; Delavande and Kohler 2012.

23. Landis, Earp, and Koch 1992; Matovu et al. 2005; Gray et al. 2013.

24. Analysis of men's pre-post-test responses are nearly identical, with 77 percent of men who received a negative result expressing certainty about their status.

25. Muula 2008; Balbo and Barban 2014.

26. Having surprised many interlocutors with these results, I decided to repeat the pre-post-

test analysis in the 2019 survey round, just to be sure. After the test, 90 percent of those who test positive are certain of their status, while just 81 percent of those who received a negative result were certain. The predictors of certainty in 2019 were not identical to the 2015 results presented here, but they are extremely similar in terms of the demographic and attitudinal patterns.

27. Being home in the afternoon stands in contrast to the full days women often spend accessing basic health care in local clinics. See Yeatman, Chamberlin, and Dovel 2018.

28. Work by Amy Conroy (2013) emphasizes the presence of doubt rather than leveraging accusatory language to indicate mistrust. For similar arguments, see also Wilson 2013.

29. This point is elaborated in chapters 6 and 7.

Chapter Six

1. Njemile felt strongly about not disclosing the name of the town they traveled to, hence "Faraway" town in "Faraway" district. It would take about 3 hours to get there by car.

2. I estimated concurrent partnerships for the randomly selected sample of men ages 15–25 in 2009, but very few of them were married at this time, so the estimates are unstable.

3. According to the men Gertrude met at the tailoring shop, men's reports of coital frequency may be exaggerated, but that seems to be an optimistic recounting of their prowess in their primary relationships. However, it is not clear that even the most braggadocious men disclosed their informal partnerships to us. Most literature on self-reports of sexual behavior suggests that women, in particular, underreport in surveys almost everything having to do with their sex lives.

4. I omitted "can't know" responses from the results I present here, but about 3 percent of women gave this answer at each wave. If I were to include it in the estimate, I would group it with expressions of doubt about a relationship rather than confidence in it.

5. Technically speaking, this violates one of the principles of demographic estimation, because one needs to have a partner in order to have suspicions about that partner. The inclusion of unpartnered respondents inflates the denominator and therefore produces low-bound estimates that index trust levels in the population.

6. Treating the receipt of a heads-up from community members as an "event-ish" phenomenon ventures uncomfortably far from the kinds of topics survival models were designed to address. The point is not to identify predictors of who might experience this event but to appreciate, descriptively, what these models show us about the environment overall.

7. Results-Based Financing for Maternal and Neonatal Health (RBF4MNH).

8. Hunter 2016a, 2016b.

9. This is consistent with Jennifer Johnson-Hanks's insights about young Cameroonian women's expectations and with Daniel Jordan Smith's description of masculinity in Nigeria. Both argue that discretion in men's sexual activities outside marriage is the true standard by which faithfulness is measured. See Johnson-Hanks 2004; Smith 2017, 2020.

10. According to self-reports of occupational status, just three women in the TLT study identify as sex workers. The epidemiological literature strongly supports claims that transmission probabilities per coitus are low and that most transmission of HIV takes place in ongoing relationships. See, e.g., Gray et al. 2001; Wawer et al. 2005; Patel et al. 2014.

11. This cross-sectional evidence of negative selection out of first marriage and positive selection into second marriage is consistent with other research on marital selection, including Reniers 2008; Anglewicz and Reniers 2014; Angelucci and Bennett 2021.

12. Consistent with these patterns from the TLT data, Bracher, Santow, and Watkins (2003) estimated that 2 percent of Malawian brides are living with HIV at the time of their first marriage.

13. Although the estimates of divorce and remarriage across sub-Saharan Africa are plentiful, only a handful of other studies in the region focus on the reasons for divorce, as articulated by divorcees or cataloged in the courts. Some examples of the careful work on this topic, historical and contemporary, are Solivetti 1994; Toefy 2002; Adeniran 2015; and Osafo et al. 2021.

14. Marston et al. 2009; Trinitapoli 2015.

15. Similarly, just 9 of the 80 who were divorced in 2012 had not remarried by 2019.

16. Auvert et al. 2001; Clark 2004; Magadi 2011; Trinitapoli and Weinreb 2012; Greenwood et al. 2017.

17. In other words, women tell new love interests that their previous relationships are over, when in reality those relationships are ongoing, though possibly complicated, fragile, or uncertain.

18. Majiga 2 is a popular trading area outside the main market. It's a fun place to walk around in the evening, with tons of foot traffic and vendors selling their goods by candlelight.

19. Magruder 2011, 1402.

20. For notable exceptions, see Wyrod 2016; Pike, Mojola, and Kabiru 2018; Smith 2020; Pike 2021.

21. Poulin 2007. See also Moore et al. 2007 on the meaning of money in relationships; and Madise et al. 2007 on the relationship between poverty and risky sexual behavior.

22. Mojola 2015; Wyrod 2016; Smith 2017; Pike 2021.

23. I also document a negative relationship between suspicion of another partner and zero-beans responses to our question about current likelihood of HIV infection in the subsequent wave but do not depict that relationship in the conceptual diagram, because it can be reasonably inferred as the converse of the relationships shown.

24. Tawfik 2003; Tawfik and Watkins 2007.

25. Yeatman and Trinitapoli 2013.

26. Beckert 1996.

27. For other examples of research that pushes demography in a similar direction, see Johnson-Hanks 2006; Hobcraft 2007; Petit 2013.

Chapter Seven

1. Recall the reminders from Watkins and Ryder not to forget about the granny in the back bedroom, for she too has something to do with a couple's fertility preferences and behaviors. Ryder 1973; Watkins 1993.

2. Wilson 2013. See also Hayes 2016.

3. Marital insecurity is just one variety of relationship uncertainty, not the only kind.

4. Mair 1951.

5. Grant and Soler-Hampejsek 2014.

6. Mtika and Doctor 2002, 88. See also Mitchell 1956; Chimango 1977.

7. Hirsch and Wardlow 2006; Spronk 2009.

8. Twenty-four bags of maize is a huge yield, and the samosas are delicious.

9. Reniers 2003.

10. Wasserman 2005; Mutula 2008; Bruijn and Dijk 2012; Mutsvairo and Ragnedda 2019; Ragnedda and Gladkova 2020.

11. We found that women who owned mobile phones wanted smaller families and had fewer

children than women without phones. The relationship seems to be driven by a longer interval between births rather than by delays in marriage or first birth. See Billari, Rotondi, and Trinitapoli 2020.

12. Turkle 2009; Rainie 2017; Silver et al. 2019.

13. Furnas 2017.

14. Archambault 2013; Cole 2014.

15. Archambault 2017, p. 9.

16. Breckenridge 2000; Cole and Thomas 2009; Parikh 2004, 2015.

17. Archambault 2017.

18. Trinitapoli 2015; Achebe 2018.

19. Magruder 2011.

20. Bertrand-Dansereau and Clark 2016, 71–72.

21. Archambault 2013; Ranganathan et al. 2018.

22. This strategy of soliciting information from small children in a compound is a common practice, also discussed by Archambault 2013 and Ashforth 2018.

23. For more on the conundrum between love and money, see Cole and Thomas 2009; Hunter 2009.

24. It matters here that Stella is married, while Tiyamike is single.

25. Haitsma 2003; Nnko et al. 2004; Johnson-Hanks Forthcoming.

26. The best friend method was one of the first publications from the TLT project. More details about the method can be found in Yeatman and Trinitapoli 2011. More recently, the approach has been extended and improved by Helleringer et al. 2019.

27. Swidler 1986.

28. This is a revision and extension of the relationship uncertainty analyses discussed in chapter 6 (the hazard of knowing or suspecting your partner has other partners; fig. 6.2) and some elements of the conceptual model depicted in figure 6.6.

29. The results for men are not shown here. In the 2015 and 2019 survey rounds, cross-sectional relationships between trust and phone ownership are also strong and negative. Tiyamike's story and the comments from Stella about her mother's phone illustrate that phone *ownership* is not the only way to think about phones as mediators in the romantic sphere; there is a lot of borrowing and passing of messages through neighbors and mothers. However, the general point stands.

30. Recall figures 6.4 and 6.5, which show a shifting pattern of HIV prevalence for men and women through the process of divorce and remarriage.

31. Trinitapoli, fieldnotes, August 1, 2016.

32. Benton 2015; Kaler, Angotti, and Ramaiya 2016; Frye and Chae 2017; The themes of "looking good" and "looking well" as a topic of gossip and evaluation with respect to HIV status and treatment have been noted in research from a variety of contexts and research traditions.

Chapter Eight

1. Nation Online 2021.

2. See also stories about the death of Mrs. Esme Muluzi-Malisita, daughter of former president Bakili Muluzi, by lightning strike in 2016. Nyasa Times 2016, 2021.

3. Kalindekafe et al. 2018. The reasons for this are not completely clear but stem from at least four factors: (1) overall frequency of lightning strikes due to geography; (2) population density, which leads to high probability of death upon a lightning strike; (3) poor infrastructure such

as fragile homes and lack of lightning rods; and (4) (potential) reporting differences, though in searching I have found no reason to think that Malawian record keepers have any incentive to record lightning-strike fatalities more diligently than their counterparts in neighboring countries.

4. Mulder et al. 2012; Holle 2016; Cooper and Holle 2019.

5. Lexis 1879; Stigler 1986; Véron and Rohrbasser 2003; Rau et al. 2018.

6. Kannisto 2000; Colchero et al. 2016; Riffe, Schöley, and Villavicencio 2017.

7. Zureick 2010, 1.

8. Notestein 1945; Davis 1963; Kreager 2015.

9. Swidler 1986.

10. Lee 1987; Livi-Bacci 2015.

11. For an important discussion of social change and maternal mortality, see Wendland 2022.

12. See figure 2.2 in particular.

13. Palamuleni 1993; Walters 2021.

14. See appendix table A.1 for a more detailed summary.

15. United Nations, Department of Economic and Social Affairs, and Population Division 2019. Calculated for nations with populations over 90,000.

16. National Statistical Office 1987, 2018.

17. And with help from open-source software shared by Tim Riffe and Carl Schmertmann.

18. Montgomery 2000.

19. Manda 1987, 31.

20. Kilonzo and Hogan 1999; Kiš 2007; Klaits 2010; Jindra and Noret 2011.

21. From our original sample, just 30 respondents died during the course of the study, so we are "underpowered" as a mortality study. To be clear, this is not a mistake; TLT was never designed to generate mortality estimates. It is mortality perceptions, not mortality, that interest me here.

22. Newspaper stories from 2019 reporting the deaths of two men and one woman support this.

23. By "community" here, I mean face-to-face discussions among family, friends, and neighbors at and around the funeral and in other social spaces such as national newspapers, text messages, Facebook, and Whatsapp.

24. Geschiere 2013.

25. Ashforth and Watkins 2015.

26. Reniers 2008; Smith and Mbakwem 2010; Johnson et al. 2013; Trinitapoli 2015; Kim et al. 2020.

27. Flammant 2020.

28. Sangala 2018; Benjamin 2021.

29. Trinitapoli and Weinreb 2012.

30. Dionne, Gerland, and Watkins 2013; Dionne 2017.

31. Hirsch 2015, s27.

32. Oster operationalized risky behavior as more than one sexual partner in the past year, using self-reports. Her interpretations surpass the capacity of her data, and many scholars of HIV (including me) disagree with the conclusion of limited behavioral response.

33. Brezina, Tekin, and Topalli 2009; Davis and Niebes-Davis 2010.

34. Haynie, Soller, and Williams 2014.

35. Macamo 2017, 221.

36. Blacker and Zaba 1997, 50; emphasis added. Blacker and Zaba were charting new methodological territory, generating the first-ever estimates of lifetime mortality risks from HIV.

37. Madise, Matthews, and Margetts 1999; Martorell 1999; Alderman, Hoddinott, and Kinsey 2006; Hannum and Hu 2017; Ekholuenetale et al. 2020.

38. These questions about food insecurity and malaria since the last interview were introduced in wave 2, so these estimates are based on six intervals between waves rather than on eight discrete observations.

39. In all likelihood, these estimates of malarial episodes are overstated, as they are based on self-reported bouts of malaria (not clinically confirmed cases). Given the underspecified nature of the symptoms and the fact that malaria, in this context, can be a catch-all, lay diagnosis, our "malaria" measure may be better interpreted as "other illness." Regardless of whether the risk is malaria alone or some combination of factors, the general point about net risks (vis-à-vis HIV) stands. For a more in-depth elaboration about confusion between early HIV infection and malaria, see Yeatman et al. 2015.

40. Stated very plainly by one Durban sex worker interviewed by Helen Preston-Whyte: "It is better to die in fifteen years' time of AIDS than to die in five days' time of hunger." Preston-Whyte et al. 2000, 165. See also van de Waal and Whiteside 2003.

41. Muula 2008.

42. Montgomery 2000; Watkins 2004; Root 2010; Wilson 2013.

43. Trinitapoli and Weinreb 2012; Dionne 2017.

44. Benton 2015.

45. In other words, motor vehicles are a new problem and have had a more serious impact on this cohort than earlier ones. IHME 2015.

46. For robustness, analyses comparing the proportion of respondents who placed at least one bean when asked about that cause (a notion of any vulnerability) produced substantively identical results.

47. Delavande and Rohwedder 2011; Elder 2013; Kim and Kim 2017.

48. ; Davis and Niebes-Davis 2010; Scott-Sheldon et al. 2010; Bucher-Koenen and Kluth 2013; Nicholls and Zimper 2015.

49. Chisholm et al. 1993; Chisholm et al. 2005; Mace 2014.

50. Chisholm et al. 1993.

51. Tavory and Eliasoph 2013.

52. Watkins and Danzi 1995; Bongaarts and Feeney 1998; Casterline 2001; Cleland, Ndugwa, and Zulu 2011; Hayford, Agadjanian, and Luz 2012; Van Bavel and Reher 2013; Smith-Greenaway and Trinitapoli 2020.

53. Montgomery 2000, 796; emphasis added.

Chapter Nine

1. *Mai a Fatsani* means "mother to Fatsani." As with "father of Stella," Gertrude uses this honorific to show respect, since the two are not age-mates.

2. Moyer and Hardon 2014, 267.

3. King 2021, 145.

4. Weinstein and Li 2016; Zhou 2016; Effendy et al. 2019; Backe et al. 2021; King 2021, The link between stress and disease progression is well documented in both the clinical and social science literatures.

5. King 2021, 151.

6. Mojola et al. 2015; Vollmer et al. 2017; Rishworth and King 2022.

7. The lifetime risk of 1 in 60 women age 15 dying from causes related to childbirth is based on 349 deaths per 100,000 live births in 2017, using Wilmoth's method ℓ3. See Wilmoth 2009.

8. Cogburn 2020; Sochas 2021.

9. Pot, Kok, and Finyiza 2018.

10. Escudero et al. 2021; Haukoos et al. 2021.

11. Yeatman et al. 2013.

12. Zimba et al. 2019; National AIDS Commission 2020; Mpunga et al. 2021.

13. Maseko et al. 2020.

14. Philbin et al. 2022.

15. Manthalu et al. 2016; Magadi 2021; Ochieng et al. 2022.

16. Kay and King 2020; Levy 2020.

17. Kahneman, Diener, and Schwarz 2003; Maru et al. 2022.

18. I appreciate Roland Rau for pointing me to the interview and providing the English translation. Habermas, quoted in Schwering 2020, para 3.

19. Hammel 1990, 475.

20. Sieber 1973; Greenhalgh 1997, 2012; Casley and Lury 1987; Charbit and Petit 2011.

21. Freedman 1991, 298.

22. It is true that missing data are now often handled through multiple imputation techniques, but these are contested, imperfect, and forever changing. Careful analysts still worry a great deal about the implications of missing values—and even the most sophisticated imputation strategies—for their results.

23. An email exchange with Philip Anglewicz shed new light on the value of analyzing marriage steps and thinking about relationships as sources of uncertainty rather than as statuses.

24. Kennedy and Bumpass 2008; Chae 2016.

25. Frye and Trinitapoli 2015.

26. Timmermans and Buchbinder 2010. See also Aronowitz 2015; Aronowitz and Greene 2019.

References

Aassve, Arnstein, Marco Le Moglie, and Letizia Mencarini. 2021. "Trust and Fertility in Uncertain Times." *Population Studies* 75 (1): 19–36.

Aassve, Arnstein, et al. 2020. "The COVID-19 Pandemic and Human Fertility." *Science* 369 (6502): 370–71.

Abbott, Andrew Delano. 2005. "The Historicality of Individuals." *Social Science History* 29 (1): 1–13.

Abdul Latif Jameel Poverty Action Lab. n.d. "The Demand for and Impact of Learning HIV Status in Malawi." http://www.povertyactionlab.org/evaluation/demand-and-impact-learning -hiv-status-malawi.

Abend, Gabriel. 2018. "The Limits of Decision and Choice." *Theory and Society* 47 (6): 805–41.

Achebe, Nwando. 2018. "Love, Courtship, and Marriage in Africa." In *A Companion to African History*, edited by William H. Worger, Charles Ambler, and Nwando Achebe. 119–42. New York: John Wiley & Sons.

adams, jimi. 2015. "AIDS in Africa." *Contemporary Sociology* 44 (5): 591–603.

adams, jimi, and Ryan Light. 2014. "Mapping Interdisciplinary Fields: Efficiencies, Gaps and Redundancies in HIV/AIDS Research." *PLoS ONE* 9 (12): e115092.

adams, jimi, and Jenny Trinitapoli. 2009. "The Malawi Religion Project: Data Collection and Selected Analyses." *Demographic Research* 21 (10): 255–88.

Adeniran, Adetayo Olaniyi. 2015. "Analytical Study of the Causal Factors of Divorce in African Homes." *Research on Humanities and Social Sciences* 5 (14): 18–29.

Adsera, Alicia, and Alicia Menendez. 2011. "Fertility Changes in Latin America in Periods of Economic Uncertainty." *Population Studies* 65 (1): 37–56.

Ahir, Hites, Nicholas Bloom, and Davide Furceri. 2022. *The World Uncertainty Index.* NBER Working Paper 29763. Cambridge, MA: National Bureau of Economic Research.

Aiderman, Harold, John Hoddinott, and Bill Kinsey. 2006. "Long Term Consequences of Early Childhood Malnutrition." *Oxford Economic Papers* 58 (3): 450–74.

Alburez-Gutierrez, Diego. 2019. "Blood Is Thicker than Bloodshed: A Genealogical Approach to Reconstruct Populations after Armed Conflicts." *Demographic Research* 40 (23): 627–56.

Alwin, Duane F., and Ryan J. McCammon. 2003. "Generations, Cohorts, and Social Change." In *Handbook of the Life Course*, edited by Jeylan T. Mortimer and Michael J. Shanahan, 23–49. Boston, MA: Springer.

Angelucci, Manuela, and Daniel Bennett. 2021. "Adverse Selection in the Marriage Market: HIV Testing and Marriage in Rural Malawi." *Review of Economic Studies* 88 (5): 2119–48.

Anglewicz, Philip, and Hans-Peter Kohler. 2009. "Overestimating HIV Infection: The Construction and Accuracy of Subjective Probabilities of HIV Infection in Rural Malawi." *Demographic Research* 20 (6): 65–96.

Anglewicz, Philip, and Georges Reniers. 2014. "HIV Status, Gender, and Marriage Dynamics among Adults in Rural Malawi." *Studies in Family Planning* 45 (4): 415–28.

Angotti, Nicole, et al. 2009. "Increasing the Acceptability of HIV Counseling and Testing with Three C's: Convenience, Confidentiality and Credibility." *Social Science & Medicine* 68 (12): 2263–70.

Apicella, Giovanna, and Enrico G. De Giorgi. 2022. *A Behavioural Gap in Survival Beliefs*. SSRN Scholarly Paper ID 3821595. Rochester, NY: Social Science Research Network.

Archambault, Julie Soleil. 2013. "Cruising through Uncertainty: Cell Phones and the Politics of Display and Disguise in Inhambane, Mozambique." *American Ethnologist* 40 (1): 88–101.

———. 2017. *Mobile Secrets: Youth, Intimacy, and the Politics of Pretense in Mozambique*. Chicago: University of Chicago Press.

Aronowitz, Robert. 2015. *Risky Medicine: Our Quest to Cure Fear and Uncertainty*. Chicago: University of Chicago Press.

Aronowitz, Robert, and Jeremy A. Greene. 2019. "Contingent Knowledge and Looping Effects—A 66-Year-Old Man with PSA-Detected Prostate Cancer and Regrets." *New England Journal of Medicine* 381 (12): 1093–96.

Ashforth, Adam. 2018. *The Trials of Mrs. K.: Seeking Justice in a World with Witches*. Chicago: University of Chicago Press.

Ashforth, Adam, and Susan Cotts Watkins. 2015. "Narratives of Death in Rural Malawi in the Time of AIDS." *Africa* 85 (2): 245–68.

Auvert, Bertran, et al. 2001. "Ecological and Individual Level Analysis of Risk Factors for HIV Infection in Four Urban Populations of Sub-Saharan Africa with Different Levels of HIV Infection." *AIDS* 15 (S4): S15–S30.

Bachrach, Christine A., and S. Philip Morgan. 2013. "A Cognitive-Social Model of Fertility Intentions." *Population and Development Review* 39 (3): 459–85.

Backe, Emma Louise, et al. 2021. "'Thinking Too Much': A Systematic Review of the Idiom of Distress in Sub-Saharan Africa." *Culture, Medicine, and Psychiatry* 45 (4): 655–82.

Balbo, Nicoletta, and Nicola Barban. 2014. "Does Fertility Behavior Spread among Friends?" *American Sociological Review* 79 (3): 412–31.

Baranov, Victoria, Daniel Bennett, and Hans-Peter Kohler. 2015. "The Indirect Impact of Antiretroviral Therapy: Mortality Risk, Mental Health, and HIV-Negative Labor Supply." *Journal of Health Economics* 44: 195–211.

Barnett, Michael, William Brock, and Lars P. Hansen. 2021. *Climate Change Uncertainty Spillover in the Macroeconomy*. NBER Working Paper 29064. Cambridge, MA: National Bureau of Economic Research.

Beaujouan, Eva. 2020. "Latest-Late Fertility? Decline and Resurgence of Late Parenthood Across the Low-Fertility Countries." *Population and Development Review* 46 (2): 219–47.

Becker, Gary S. 1960. "An Economic Analysis of Fertility." In *Demographic and Economic Change in Developed Countries*, edited by George B. Roberts, Chair, Universities–National Bureau Committee for Economic Research, 209–31. New York: Columbia University Press.

Becker, Gary S., and Robert J. Barro. 1988. "A Reformulation of the Economic Theory of Fertility." *Quarterly Journal of Economics* 103 (1): 1–25.

Beckert, Jens. 1996. "What Is Sociological about Economic Sociology? Uncertainty and the Embeddedness of Economic Action." *Theory and Society* 25 (6): 803–40.

———. 2016. *Imagined Futures: Fictional Expectations and Capitalist Dynamics.* Cambridge, MA: Harvard University Press.

Beegle, Kathleen, Michelle Poulin, and Gil Shapira. 2015. "HIV Testing, Behavior Change, and the Transition to Adulthood in Malawi." *Economic Development and Cultural Change* 63 (4): 665–84.

Behrman, Julia Andrea. 2015. "Does Schooling Affect Women's Desired Fertility? Evidence from Malawi, Uganda, and Ethiopia." *Demography* 52 (3): 787–809.

Bell, Suzanne O., and Mary E. Fissell. 2021. "A Little Bit Pregnant? Productive Ambiguity and Fertility Research." *Population and Development Review* 47 (2): 505–26.

Benjamin, Foster. 2021. "Police Engage Chiefs on Cemetery Fracas." *The Nation Online*, February 17. https://www.mwnation.com/police-engage-chiefs-on-cemetery-fracas/.

Benton, Adia. 2015. *HIV Exceptionalism: Development through Disease in Sierra Leone.* Minneapolis: University of Minnesota Press.

Bernard, Aude, and Sunganani Kalemba. 2022. "Internal Migration and the De-standardization of the Life Course: A Sequence Analysis of Reasons for Migrating." *Demographic Research* 46 (12): 337–54.

Bernardi, Laura, Johannes Huinink, and Richard A. Settersten. 2019. "The Life Course Cube: A Tool for Studying Lives." *Advances in Life Course Research* 41: e100258. https://www.sciencedirect.com/science/article/pii/S1040260818301850.

Bernardi, Laura, and Inge Hutter. 2007. "The Anthropological Demography of Europe." *Demographic Research* 17: 541–66.

Bernardi, Laura, and Andreas Klaerner. 2014. "Social Networks and Fertility." *Demographic Research* 30: 641–70.

Bernardi, Laura, Andreas Klärner, and Holger von der Lippe. 2008. "Job Insecurity and the Timing of Parenthood: A Comparison between Eastern and Western Germany." *European Journal of Population / Revue européenne de Démographie* 24 (3): 287–313.

Bernardi, Laura, Monika Mynarska, and Clémentine Rossier. 2015. "Uncertain, Changing and Situated Fertility Intentions." In *Reproductive Decision-Making in a Macro-Micro Perspective*, edited by Dimiter Philipov, Aart C. Liefbroer, and Jane Klobas, 113–39. Dordrecht: Springer Netherlands.

Bertrand-Dansereau, Anais, and Shelley Clark. 2016. "Pragmatic Tradition or Romantic Aspiration? The Causes of Impulsive Marriage and Early Divorce among Women in Rural Malawi." *Demographic Research* 35 (3): 47–80.

Billari, Francesco C. 2015. "Integrating Macro- and Micro-Level Approaches in the Explanation of Population Change." *Population Studies* 69 (Suppl.): S11–S20.

———. 2022. "Demography: Fast and Slow." *Population and Development Review* 48 (1): 9–30.

Billari, Francesco C., and Hans-Peter Kohler. 2004. "Patterns of Low and Lowest-Low Fertility in Europe." *Population Studies: A Journal of Demography* 58 (2): 161–76.

Billari, Francesco, Valentina Rotondi, and Jenny Trinitapoli. 2020. "Mobile Phones, Digital Inequality, and Fertility: Longitudinal Evidence from Malawi." *Demographic Research* 42 (37): 1057–96.

Birdthistle, Isolde, et al. 2019. "Recent Levels and Trends in HIV Incidence Rates among Adolescent Girls and Young Women in Ten High-Prevalence African Countries: A Systematic Review and Meta-Analysis." *The Lancet Global Health* 7 (11): e1521–e1540.

Blacker, John, and Basia Zaba. 1997. "HIV Prevalence and Lifetime Risk of Dying of AIDS." *Health Transition Review* 7 (S2): 45–62.

Bledsoe, Caroline, Fatoumatta Banja, and Allan G. Hill. 1998. "Reproductive Mishaps and Western Contraception: An African Challenge to Fertility Theory." *Population and Development Review* 24 (1): 15–57.

Bloom, Nicholas. 2014. "Fluctuations in Uncertainty." *Journal of Economic Perspectives* 28 (2): 153–76.

Blossfeld, Hans-Peter, Sandra Buchholz, and Dirk Hofäcker. 2006. *Globalization, Uncertainty and Late Careers in Society.* London: Routledge.

Bolano, Danilo, and Daniele Vignoli. 2021. "Union Formation under Conditions of Uncertainty: The Objective and Subjective Sides of Employment Uncertainty." *Demographic Research* 45 (5): 141–86.

Bolu-Steve, F. N., A. A. Adegoke, and G. M. Kim-Ju. 2020. "Cultural Beliefs and Infant Mortality in Nigeria." *Education Research International* 2020 (e6900629): 1–10.

Bongaarts, John. 1978. "A Framework for Analyzing the Proximate Determinants of Fertility." *Population and Development Review* 4 (1): 105–32.

Bongaarts, John, and G. Feeney. 1998. "On the Quantum and Tempo of Fertility." *Population and Development Review* 24 (2): 271–91.

Bongaarts, John, Odile Frank, and Ron Lesthaeghe. 1984. "The Proximate Determinants of Fertility in Sub-Saharan Africa." *Population and Development Review* 10 (3): 511–37.

Bracher, Michael, Gigi Santow, and Susan Cotts Watkins. 2003. "'Moving' and Marrying: Modeling HIV Infection among Newlyweds in Malawi." *Demographic Research* S1 (7): 207–46.

Branson, Bernard M. 2010. "The Future of HIV Testing." *JAIDS: Journal of Acquired Immune Deficiency Syndromes* 55 (S2): S102–S105.

Breckenridge, Keith. 2000. "Love Letters and Amanuenses: Beginning the Cultural History of the Working Class Private Sphere in Southern Africa, 1900–1933." *Journal of Southern African Studies* 26 (2): 337–48.

Brenner, Stephan, et al. 2018. "Impact of Results-Based Financing on Effective Obstetric Care Coverage: Evidence from a Quasi-Experimental Study in Malawi." *BMC Health Services Research* 18 (1): 791.

Brezina, Timothy, Erdal Tekin, and Volkan Topalli. 2009. "'Might Not Be a Tomorrow': A Multimethods Approach to Anticipated Early Death and Youth Crime." *Criminology* 47 (4): 1091–1129.

Brookmeyer, Ron. 2010. "Measuring the HIV/AIDS Epidemic: Approaches and Challenges." *Epidemiologic Reviews* 32 (1): 26–37.

Brown, Eliza. 2020. "Projected Diagnosis, Anticipatory Medicine, and Uncertainty: How Medical Providers 'Rule Out' Potential Pregnancy in Contraceptive Counseling." *Social Science & Medicine* 258: 113–18.

Brown, Eliza, and Mary Patrick. 2018. "Time, Anticipation, and the Life Course: Egg Freezing as Temporarily Disentangling Romance and Reproduction." *American Sociological Review* 83 (5): 959–82.

Bruijn, Mirjam de, and Rijk van Dijk, eds. 2012. *The Social Life of Connectivity in Africa*. New York: Palgrave Macmillan.

Bruine de Bruin, Wändi, et al. 2000. "Verbal and Numerical Expressions of Probability: 'It's a Fifty-Fifty Chance.'" *Organizational Behavior and Human Decision Processes* 81 (1): 115–31.

Bucher-Koenen, Tabea, and Sebastian Kluth. 2013. *Subjective Life Expectancy and Private Pensions*. Tech. Rep. 201214. MEA Discussion Paper Series. Munich Center for the Economics of Aging (MEA) at the Max Planck Institute for Social Law and Social Policy.

Buh, Brian. 2021. "Measuring the Effect of Employment Uncertainty on Fertility in Europe (a Literature Review)." *Institut für Demographie—VID* 1: 1–24.

Burton, Linda M., and M. Belinda Tucker. 2009. "Romantic Unions in an Era of Uncertainty: A Post-Moynihan Perspective on African American Women and Marriage." *ANNALS of the American Academy of Political and Social Science* 621 (1): 132–48.

Caldwell, John C. 1995. "Understanding the AIDS Epidemic and Reacting Sensibly to It." *Social Science & Medicine* 41 (3): 299–302.

———. 2004. "Social Upheaval and Fertility Decline." *Journal of Family History* 29 (4): 382–406.

Casley, Dennis J., and Denis A. Lury. 1987. *Data Collection in Developing Countries*. 2nd ed. Oxford: Oxford University Press.

Casterline, John B., ed. 2001. *Diffusion Processes and Fertility Transition: Selected Perspectives*. Washington, DC: National Academies Press.

CEIC Data. 2020. "Malawi Motor Vehicles Sales Growth, 2006–2012—CEIC Data." https://www.ceicdata.com/en/indicator/malawi/motor-vehicles-sales-growth.

Chae, Sophia. 2016. "Forgotten Marriages? Measuring the Reliability of Marriage Histories." *Demographic Research* 34 (19): 525–62.

Charbit, Yves, and Véronique Petit. 2011. "Toward a Comprehensive Demography: Rethinking the Research Agenda on Change and Response." *Population and Development Review* 37 (2): 219–39.

Chen, Jane S., et al. 2021. "A Randomized Controlled Trial Evaluating Combination Detection of HIV in Malawian Sexually Transmitted Infections Clinics." *Journal of the International AIDS Society* 24 (4): e25701.

Chima, Reginald Ikechukwu, Catherine A. Goodman, and Anne Mills. 2003. "The Economic Impact of Malaria in Africa: A Critical Review of the Evidence." *Health Policy* 63 (1): 17–36.

Chimango, L. J. 1977. "Woman without Ankhoswe in Malawi." *African Law Studies* 15: 54–61.

Chimbiri, Agnes. 2006. "Development, Family Change, and Community Empowerment in Malawi." In *African Families at the Turn of the 21st Century*, edited by Yaw Oheneba-Sakyi and Baffour K. Takyi, 227–48. Santa Barbara, CA: Greenwood Publishing Group.

———. 2007. "The Condom Is an Intruder in Marriage: Evidence from Rural Malawi." *Social Science & Medicine* 64 (5): 1102–15.

Chisholm, James S., et al. 1993. "Death, Hope, and Sex: Life-History Theory and the Development of Reproductive Strategies (with Comments and Reply)." *Current Anthropology* 34 (1): 1–24.

Chisholm, James S., et al. 2005. "Early Stress Predicts Age at Menarche and First Birth, Adult Attachment, and Expected Lifespan." *Human Nature* 16 (3): 233–65.

Clark, Shelley. 2004. "Early Marriage and HIV Risks in Sub-Saharan Africa." *Studies in Family Planning* (3): 149–60.

Cleland, John G., Robert P. Ndugwa, and Eliya M. Zulu. 2011. "Family Planning in Sub-Saharan Africa: Progress or Stagnation?" *Bulletin of the World Health Organization* 89: 137–43.

Coale, Ansley J. 1973. "The Demographic Transition Reconsidered." In *Proceedings of the International Population Conference, Liege*, 53–57. Liege: International Union for the Scientific Study of Population.

Coast, Ernestina, Nathalie Mondain, and Clémentine Rossier. 2009. "Qualitative Research in Demography: Quality, Presentation and Assessment." Paper presented at the XXVI IUSSP International Population Conference, Marrakech, Morocco, September 27. http://eprints.lse .ac.uk/36788/

Cogburn, Megan D. 2020. "Homebirth Fines and Health Cards in Rural Tanzania: On the Push for Numbers in Maternal Health." *Social Science & Medicine* 254: e112508.

Colchero, Fernando, et al. 2016. "The Emergence of Longevous Populations." *Proceedings of the National Academy of Sciences* 113 (48): e7681–90.

Cole, Jennifer. 2014. "The Téléphone Malgache: Transnational Gossip and Social Transformation among Malagasy Marriage Migrants in France." *American Ethnologist* 41 (2): 276–89.

Cole, Jennifer, and Lynn M. Thomas, eds. 2009. *Love in Africa*. Chicago: University of Chicago Press.

Comolli, Chiara Ludovica. 2017. "The Fertility Response to the Great Recession in Europe and the United States: Structural Economic Conditions and Perceived Economic Uncertainty." *Demographic Research* 35 (51): 1549–1600.

Conroy, Amy A. 2014. "'It Means There Is Doubt in the House': Perceptions and Experiences of HIV Testing in Rural Malawi." *Culture, Health & Sexuality* 16 (4): 397–411.

Cooper, Elizabeth, and David Pratten. 2015. "Ethnographies of Uncertainty in Africa: An Introduction." In *Ethnographies of Uncertainty in Africa*, edited by Elizabeth Cooper and David Pratten, 1–16. London: Palgrave Macmillan.

Cooper, Mary Ann, and Ronald L. Holle. 2019. "Current Global Estimates of Lightning Fatalities and Injuries." In *Reducing Lightning Injuries Worldwide*, edited by Mary Ann Cooper and Ronald L. Holle, 65–73. Cham, Switzerland: Springer International.

Crampin, Amelia C., et al. 2012. "Profile: The Karonga Health and Demographic Surveillance System." *International Journal of Epidemiology* 41 (3): 676–85.

Crosnoe, Robert, and Shannon Cavanaugh. Forthcoming. *The Journey to Adulthood in Uncertain Times*. New York: Russell Sage Foundation.

Daire, Judith. 2007. "Advocating for the Improvement of Adolescent VCT Services in Malawi." *Malawi Medical Journal* 19 (3): 118–21.

Damaske, Sarah. 2021. *The Tolls of Uncertainty: How Privilege and the Guilt Gap Shape Unemployment in America*. Princeton, NJ: Princeton University Press.

Das, Aniruddha, and Edward O. Laumann. 2010. "How to Get Valid Answers from Survey Questions: What We Learned from Asking about Sexual Behavior and the Measurement of Sexuality." In *The Sage Handbook of Measurement*, 9–26. Thousand Oaks, CA: Sage.

Davis, Kingsley. 1963. "The Theory of Change and Response in Modern Demographic History." *Population Index* 29 (4): 345–66.

Davis, Matthew J., and Allison J. Niebes-Davis. 2010. "Ethnic Differences and Influence of Perceived Future Certainty on Adolescent and Young Adult Sexual Knowledge and Attitudes." *Health, Risk & Society* 12 (2): 149–67.

De Allegri, Manuela, et al. 2019. "Effect of Results-Based Financing on Facility-Based Maternal Mortality at Birth: An Interrupted Time-Series Analysis with Independent Controls in Malawi." *BMJ Global Health* 4 (3): 1–7.

Delavande, Adeline, and Hans-Peter Kohler. 2012. "The Impact of HIV Testing on Subjective Expectations and Risky Behavior in Malawi." *Demography* 49 (3): 1011–36.

Delavande, Adeline, and Susann Rohwedder. 2011. "Differential Survival in Europe and the United States: Estimates Based on Subjective Probabilities of Survival." *Demography* 48 (4): 1377–1400.

Dequech, David. 2000. "Fundamental Uncertainty and Ambiguity." *Eastern Economic Journal* 26 (1): 41–60.

———. 2003. "Uncertainty and Economic Sociology." *American Journal of Economics and Sociology* 62 (3): 509–32.

———. 2006. "The New Institutional Economics and the Theory of Behaviour under Uncertainty." *Journal of Economic Behavior & Organization* 59 (1): 109–31.

Dewey, John. 1929. *The Quest for Certainty: A Study of the Relation of Knowledge and Action.* New York: Minton, Balch & Co.

Dionne, Kim Yi. 2017. *Doomed Interventions: The Failure of Global Responses to AIDS in Africa.* Cambridge: Cambridge University Press.

Dionne, Kim Yi, Patrick Gerland, and Susan Cotts Watkins. 2013. "AIDS Exceptionalism: Another Constituency Heard From." *AIDS and Behavior* 17 (3): 825–31.

Dovel, Kathryn, et al. 2015. "Men's Heightened Risk of AIDS-Related Death: The Legacy of Gendered HIV Testing and Treatment Strategies." *AIDS* 29 (10): 1123–25.

Dovel, Kathryn, et al. 2016. "Trends in ART Initiation among Men and Non-Pregnant/Non-Breastfeeding Women before and after Option B+ in Southern Malawi." *PLoS ONE* 11 (12): e0165025.

Dube, Albert L. N., et al. 2012. "Fertility Intentions and Use of Contraception among Monogamous Couples in Northern Malawi in the Context of HIV Testing: A Cross-Sectional Analysis." *PLoS ONE* 7 (12): e51861.

Duden, Barbara. 1991. *The Woman Beneath the Skin: A Doctor's Patients in Eighteenth-Century Germany.* Cambridge, MA: Harvard University Press.

Dyson, Tim. 2005. "On Development, Demography and Climate Change: The End of the World as We Know it?" *Population and Environment* 27 (2): 117–49.

Effendy, Elmeida, et al. 2019. "The Association between CD-4 Level, Stress and Depression Symptoms among People Living with HIV/AIDS." *Open Access Macedonian Journal of Medical Sciences* 7 (20): 3459–63.

Ekholuenetale, Michael, et al. 2020. "Impact of Stunting on Early Childhood Cognitive Development in Benin: Evidence from Demographic and Health Survey." *Egyptian Pediatric Association Gazette* 68 (1): e31.

Elder, Glen H. 1998. "The Life Course as Developmental Theory." *Child Development* 69 (1): 1–12.

Elder, Todd E. 2013. "The Predictive Validity of Subjective Mortality Expectations: Evidence from the Health and Retirement Study." *Demography* 50 (2): 569–89.

Eloundou-Enyegue, Parfait M., and Sarah C. Giroux. 2012. "Fertility Transitions and Schooling: From Micro- to Macro-Level Associations." *Demography* 49 (4): 1407–32.

Entwisle, Barbara, Ashton Verdery, and Nathalie Williams. 2020. "Climate Change and Migration: New Insights from a Dynamic Model of Out-Migration and Return Migration." *American Journal of Sociology* 125 (6): 1469–1512.

Escudero, Daniel J., et al. 2021. "How to Best Conduct Universal HIV Screening in Emergency Departments Is Far from Settled." *Journal of the American College of Emergency Physicians Open* 2 (1): e12352.

Fernald, Russell D. 1978. "A Comparison of Four Variations of Mancala Found in Central Africa." *Anthropos* 73 (1–2): 205–14.

Finocchario-Kessler, Sarah, et al. 2018. "High Report of Miscarriage among Women Living with HIV Who Want to Conceive in Uganda." *BMC Research Notes* 11 (1): 753.

Fischhoff, Baruch, and Wändi Bruine De Bruin. 1999. "Fifty-Fifty = 50%?" *Journal of Behavioral Decision Making* 12 (2): 149–63.

Fischhoff, Baruch, et al. 2000. "Teen Expectations for Significant Life Events." *Public Opinion Quarterly* 64 (2): 189–205.

Flammant, Cécile. 2020. "An Ongoing Decline in Early Orphanhood in France." *Population Societies* 580 (8): 1–4.

Frankenberg, Elizabeth, et al. 2011. "Mortality, the Family and the Indian Ocean Tsunami." *Economic Journal* 121 (554): F162–F182.

Freedman, David A. 1991. "Statistical Models and Shoe Leather." *Sociological Methodology* 21: 291–313.

Fries, James F. 1980. "Aging, Natural Death, and the Compression of Morbidity." *New England Journal of Medicine* 303 (3): 130–35.

Frye, Margaret. 2017. "Cultural Meanings and the Aggregation of Actions: The Case of Sex and Schooling in Malawi." *American Sociological Review* 82 (5): 945–76.

Frye, Margaret, and Lauren Bachan. 2017. "The Demography of Words: The Global Decline in Non-Numeric Fertility Preferences, 1993–2011." *Population Studies* 71 (2): 187–209.

Frye, Margaret, and Sophia Chae. 2017. "Physical Attractiveness and Women's HIV Risk in Rural Malawi." *Demographic Research* 37 (10): 251–94.

Frye, Margaret, and Jenny Trinitapoli. 2015. "Ideals as Anchors for Relationship Experiences." *American Sociological Review* 80 (3): 496–525.

Furnas, Hannah E. 2017. "Technology Use and Social Connection: Mobile Phone Ownership, Device Sharing, and Social Ties in Malawi." PhD dissertation, Pennsylvania State University.

Geertz, Clifford. 1966. "Religion as a Cultural System." In *Anthropological Approaches to the Study of Religion*, edited by Michael Banton, 1–46. New York: Routledge.

Geschiere, Peter. 2013. *Witchcraft, Intimacy, and Trust: Africa in Comparison*. Chicago: University of Chicago Press.

Ghalioungui, P., SH. Khalil, and A. R. Ammar. 1963. "On an Ancient Egyptian Method of Diagnosing Pregnancy and Determining Foetal Sex." *Medical History* 7 (3): 241–46.

Goldstein, Joshua R. 2015. "Turnover and Dependency Are Minimized When Population Growth Is Negative." Paper presented at the Annual Meeting of the Population Association of America, San Diego, CA, April 17. https://paa2015.princeton.edu/papers/153484.

Grant, Monica J. 2017. "De Facto Privatization and Inequalities in Educational Opportunity in the Transition to Secondary School in Rural Malawi." *Social Forces* 96 (1): 65–90.

Grant, Monica J., and Erica Soler-Hampejsek. 2014. "HIV Risk Perceptions, the Transition to Marriage, and Divorce in Southern Malawi." *Studies in Family Planning* 45 (3): 315–37.

Gray, Richard T., et al. 2013. "Increased HIV Testing Will Modestly Reduce HIV Incidence among Gay Men in NSW and Would Be Acceptable if HIV Testing Becomes Convenient." *PLoS ONE* 8 (2): e55449.

Gray, Ronald H., et al. 2001. "Probability of HIV-1 Transmission per Coital Act in Monogamous, Heterosexual, HIV-1 Discordant Couples in Rakai, Uganda." *The Lancet* 357 (9263): 1149–53.

Green, Edward, et al. 2006. "Uganda's HIV Prevention Success: The Role of Sexual Behavior Change and the National Response." *AIDS and Behavior* 10 (4): 335–46.

Greenhalgh, Susan. 1997. "Methods and Meanings: Reflections on Disciplinary Difference." *Population and Development Review* 23 (4): 819–24.

———. 2012. "On the Crafting of Population Knowledge." *Population and Development Review* 38 (1): 121–31.

Greenwood, Jeremy, et al. 2017. "The Role of Marriage in Fighting HIV: A Quantitative Illustration for Malawi." *American Economic Review* 107 (5): 158–62.

Gregson, Simon, et al. 2006. "HIV Decline Associated with Behavior Change in Eastern Zimbabwe." *Science* 311 (5761): 664–66.

Haitsma, Martha Van. 2003. "The Chicago Health and Social Life Survey Design." In *The Sexual Organization of the City*, edited by Edward O. Laumann et al., 39–65. Chicago: University of Chicago Press.

Hamermesh, Daniel S. 1985. "Expectations, Life Expectancy, and Economic Behavior." *Quarterly Journal of Economics* 100 (2): 389–408.

Hammel, Eugene A. 1990. "A Theory of Culture for Demography." *Population and Development Review* 16 (3): 455–85.

Hannum, Emily, and Li-Chung Hu. 2017. "Chronic Undernutrition, Short-Term Hunger, and Student Functioning in Rural Northwest China." *International Journal of Educational Development* 54: 26–38.

Harries, Anthony D., et al. 2016. "Act Local, Think Global: How the Malawi Experience of Scaling Up Antiretroviral Treatment Has Informed Global Policy." *BMC Public Health* 16 (1): 938.

Haukoos, Jason S., et al. 2021. "Comparison of HIV Screening Strategies in the Emergency Department: A Randomized Clinical Trial." *JAMA Network Open* 4 (7): e2117763.

Hauser, Philip M., and Otis Dudley Duncan. 1959. *The Study of Population: An Inventory and Appraisal*. Chicago: University of Chicago Press.

Haws, Rachel A., et al. 2010. "'These Are Not Good Things for Other People to Know': How Rural Tanzanian Women's Experiences of Pregnancy Loss and Early Neonatal Death May Impact Survey Data Quality." *Social Science & Medicine* 71 (10): 1764–72.

Hayes, Nicole C. 2016. "'Marriage Is Perseverance': Structural Violence, Culture, and AIDS in Malawi." *Anthropologien* 58 (1): 95–105.

Hayford, Sarah R., and Victor Agadjanian. 2011. "Uncertain Future, Non-Numeric Preferences, and the Fertility Transition: A Case Study of Rural Mozambique." *Etude de la population africaine / African Population Studies* 25 (2): 419–39.

Hayford, Sarah R., Victor Agadjanian, and Luciana Luz. 2012. "Now or Never: Perceived HIV Status and Fertility Intentions in Rural Mozambique." *Studies in Family Planning* 43 (3): 191–99.

Haynie, Dana L., Brian Soller, and Kristi Williams. 2014. "Anticipating Early Fatality: Friends', Schoolmates' and Individual Perceptions of Fatality on Adolescent Risk Behaviors." *Journal of Youth and Adolescence* 43 (2): 175–92.

Heimer, Carol A. 2007. "Old Inequalities, New Disease: HIV/AIDS in Sub-Saharan Africa." *Annual Review of Sociology* 33 (1): 551–77.

———. 2012. "Inert Facts and the Illusion of Knowledge: Strategic Uses of Ignorance in HIV Clinics." *Economy and Society* 41 (1): 17–41.

Helleringer, Stéphane, et al. 2018. "Using Community-Based Reporting of Vital Events to Monitor Child Mortality: Lessons from Rural Ghana." *PLoS ONE* 13 (1): e0192034.

Helleringer, Stéphane, et al. 2019. "Evaluating sampling biases from third-party reporting as a method for improving survey measures of sensitive behaviors." *Social Networks* 59:134–140.

Heuveline, Patrick. 2015. "The Boundaries of Genocide: Quantifying the Uncertainty of the Death Toll during the Pol Pot Regime (1975–1979)." *Population Studies* 69 (2): 201–18.

Hirsch, Jennifer S. 2015. "Desire across Borders: Markets, Migration, and Marital HIV Risk in Rural Mexico." *Culture, Health & Sexuality* 17 (S1): S20–S33.

Hirsch, Jennifer S., and Holly Wardlow, eds. 2006. *Modern Loves: The Anthropology of Romantic Courtship and Companionate Marriage.* Ann Arbor: University of Michigan Press.

Hobcraft, John. 2007. "Towards a Scientific Understanding of Demographic Behaviour." *Population-e* 62 (1): 47–51.

Holle, Ronald L. 2016. "The Number of Documented Global Lightning Fatalities." Paper presented at the 24th International Lightning Detection Conference and 6th Annual Lightning and Meteorology Conference, San Diego, CA, April 18–21. https://www.vaisala.com/sites/default/files/documents/Ron%20Holle.%20Number%20of%20Documented%20Global%20Lightning%20Fatalities.pdf.

Hooper, Ed. 1990. *Slim: A Reporter's Own Story of AIDS in East Africa.* London: Bodley Head.

Huinink, Johannes, and Martin Kohli. 2014. "A Life-Course Approach to Fertility." *Demographic Research* 30: 1293–1326.

Hunter, Mark. 2009. "Providing Love: Sex and Exchange in Twentieth-Century South Africa." In *Love in Africa*, edited by Jennifer Cole and Lynn M. Thomas, 135–56. Chicago: University of Chicago Press.

———. 2016a. "Introduction: New Insights on Marriage and Africa." *Africa Today* 62 (3): vii–xv.

———. 2016b. "Is It Enough to Talk of Marriage as a Process? Legitimate Co-Habitation in Umlazi, South Africa." *Anthropology Southern Africa* 39 (4): 281–96.

Hurd, Michael D., and Kathleen McGarry. 1995. "Evaluation of the Subjective Probabilities of Survival in the Health and Retirement Study." *Journal of Human Resources* 30: S268.

———. 2002. "The Predictive Validity of Subjective Probabilities of Survival." *Economic Journal* 112 (482): 966–85.

Idler, Ellen L., and Yael Benyamini. 1997. "Self-Rated Health and Mortality: A Review of Twenty-Seven Community Studies." *Journal of Health and Social Behavior* 38 (1): 21–37.

Ihonvbere, Julius O. 1997. "From Despotism to Democracy: The Rise of Multiparty Politics in Malawi." *Third World Quarterly* 18 (2): 225–47.

Iliffe, John. 2005. *The African AIDS Epidemic: A History.* Athens: Ohio University Press.

Institute for Health Metrics and Evaluation (IHME). 2015. *Malawi.* http://www.healthdata.org/malawi.

Jahn, Andraes, et al. 2016. "WHO—Scaling-up Antiretroviral Therapy in Malawi." *Bulletin of the World Health Organization* 94 (10): 772–76.

Jereni, Bwanali H., and Adamson S. Muula. 2008. "Availability of Supplies and Motivations for Accessing Voluntary HIV Counseling and Testing Services in Blantyre, Malawi." *BMC Health Services Research* 8 (1): 17.

Jindra, Michael, and Joël Noret. 2011. *Funerals in Africa: Explorations of a Social Phenomenon.* New York: Berghahn Books.

Johnson, Leigh F., et al. 2013. "Life Expectancies of South African Adults Starting Antiretroviral Treatment: Collaborative Analysis of Cohort Studies." *PLoS Medicine* 10 (4): e1001418.

Johnson-Hanks, Jennifer. 2004. "Uncertainty and the Second Space: Modern Birth Timing and the Dilemma of Education." *European Journal of Population / Revue européenne de Démographie* 20 (4): 351–73.

———. 2005. "When the Future Decides: Uncertainty and Intentional Action in Contemporary Cameroon." *Current Anthropology* 46 (3): 363–85.

———. 2006. *Uncertain Honor: Modern Motherhood in an African Crisis.* Chicago: University of Chicago Press.

———. 2014. "Waiting for the Start: Flexibility and the Question of Convergence." In *Ethnographies of Youth and Temporality: Time Objectified,* edited by Anne Line Dalsgard et al., 23–40. Philadelphia: Temple University Press.

———. 2018. "When the Wages of Sin Is Death: Sexual Stigma and Infant Mortality in Sub-Saharan Africa." In *International Handbook on Gender and Demographic Processes,* edited by Nancy E. Riley and Jan Brunson, 153–65. Dordrecht: Springer Netherlands.

———. Forthcoming. *How We Count.* Princeton, NJ: Princeton University Press.

Johnson-Hanks, Jennifer, et al. 2011. "The Theory of Conjunctural Action." In *Understanding Family Change and Variation,* 1–22. Dordrecht: Springer Netherlands.

Joint United Nations Programme on HIV/AIDS and World Health Organization. 2006. *Progress on Global Access to HIV Antiretroviral Therapy: A Report on "3 by 5" and Beyond.* Geneva: World Health Organization / UNAIDS.

Kahn, Kathleen, et al. 2012. "Profile: Agincourt Health and Socio-Demographic Surveillance System." *International Journal of Epidemiology* 41 (4): 988–1001.

Kahneman, Daniel. 2011. *Thinking, Fast and Slow.* New York: Farrar, Straus & Giroux.

Kahneman, Daniel, Edward Diener, and Norbert Schwarz, eds. 2003. *Well-Being: Foundations of Hedonic Psychology.* New York: Russell Sage Foundation.

Kaler, Amy, Nicole Angotti, and Astha Ramaiya. 2016. "'They Are Looking Just the Same': Antiretroviral Treatment as Social Danger in Rural Malawi." *Social Science & Medicine* 167: 71–78.

Kalindekafe, Leonard, et al. 2018. "Lightning Fatalities in Malawi: A Retrospective Study from 2010 to 2017." Paper presented at 34th International Conference on Lightning Protection (ICLP), Rzeszow, Poland, September 2–8.

Kalipeni, Ezekiel. 1992. "Political Development and Prospects for Democracy in Malawi." *Trans-Africa Forum* 9 (1): 27–40.

Kalwij, Adriaan, and Vesile Kutlu Koc. 2021. "Is the Accuracy of Individuals' Survival Beliefs Associated with Their Knowledge of Population Life Expectancy?" *Demographic Research* 45 (14): 453–468.

Kannisto, Väinö. 2000. "Measuring the Compression of Mortality." *Demographic Research* 3 (6): 1–24.

Karim, Salim S. Abdool, and Cheryl Baxter. 2019. "HIV Incidence Rates in Adolescent Girls and Young Women In Sub-Saharan Africa." *The Lancet Global Health* 7 (11): e1470–e1471.

Kay, John, and Mervyn King. 2020. *Radical Uncertainty: Decision-Making Beyond the Numbers.* New York: Norton.

Kennedy, Caitlin E, et al. 2022. "Self-Testing for Pregnancy: A Systematic Review and Meta-Analysis." *BMJ Open* 12 (2): e054120.

Kennedy, Pagan. 2012. "Who Made That Home Pregnancy Test?" *New York Times,* July 27. https://www.nytimes.com/2012/07/29/magazine/who-made-that-home-pregnancy-test.html.

Kennedy, Sheela, and Larry L. Bumpass. 2008. "Cohabitation and Children's Living Arrangements: New Estimates from the United States." *Demographic Research* 19 (47): 1663–692.

Kertzer, David I., and Tom Fricke. 1997. *Anthropological Demography: Toward a New Synthesis.* Chicago: University of Chicago Press.

Kerwin, Jason T., and Natalia Ordaz Reynoso. 2021. "You Know What I Know: Interviewer Knowledge Effects in Subjective Expectation Elicitation." *Demography* 58 (1): 1–29.

Keyfitz, Nathan. 1971. "Models." *Demography* 8 (4): 571–580.

———. 1980. "Population Appearances and Demographic Reality." *Population and Development Review* 6 (1): 47–64.

Keynes, John Maynard. 1921. *A Treatise on Probability*. New York: Macmillan.

Kieffer, Mary Pat, et al. 2014. "Lessons Learned from Early Implementation of Option B+: The Elizabeth Glaser Pediatric AIDS Foundation Experience in 11 African Countries." *Journal of Acquired Immune Deficiency Syndromes* 67 (S4): S188–S194.

Kilburn, Kelly, et al. 2018. "Paying for Happiness: Experimental Results from a Large Cash Transfer Program in Malawi." *Journal of Policy Analysis and Management* 37 (2): 331–56.

Kilonzo, Gad P., and Nora M. Hogan. 1999. "Traditional African Mourning Practices Are Abridged in Response to the AIDS Epidemic: Implications for Mental Health." *Transcultural Psychiatry* 36 (3): 259–83.

Kim, Hae-Young, et al. 2020. "HIV Seroconcordance among Heterosexual Couples in Rural KwaZulu-Natal, South Africa: A Population-Based Analysis." *Journal of the International AIDS Society* 23 (1): e25432.

Kim, Jae-Hyun, and Jang-Mook Kim. 2017. "Subjective Life Expectancy Is a Risk Factor for Perceived Health Status and Mortality." *Health and Quality of Life Outcomes* 15 (190): 1–7.

Kim, Sung Wook, et al. 2016. "Socio-Economic Inequity in HIV Testing in Malawi." *Global Health Action* 9 (31730): 1–15.

King, Brian. 2021. "HIV as Uncertain Life." *Geoforum* 123: 145–52.

King, Rosalind Berkowitz. 2005. "The Case of American Women: Globalization and the Transition to Adulthood in an Individualistic Regime." In *Globalization, Uncertainty and Youth in Society*, edited by Hans-Peter Blossfeld et al., 305–26. New York: Routledge.

Kiš, Adam D. 2007. "An Analysis of the Impact of AIDS on Funeral Culture in Malawi." *NAPA Bulletin* 27 (1): 129–40.

Klaits, Frederick. 2010. *Death in a Church of Life: Moral Passion during Botswana's Time of AIDS*. Oakland: University of California Press.

Knight, Frank H. 1921. *Risk, Uncertainty and Profit*. Cambridge, MA: Riverside Press.

Kodzi, Ivy A., David R. Johnson, and John B. Casterline. 2012. "To Have or Not to Have Another Child: Life Cycle, Health and Cost Considerations of Ghanaian Women." *Social Science & Medicine* 74 (7): 966–72.

Kohler, Hans-Peter, Francesco C. Billari, and José Antonio Ortega. 2002. "The Emergence of Lowest-Low Fertility in Europe during the 1990s." *Population and Development Review* 28 (4): 641–80.

Kohler, Hans-Peter, and Iliana V. Kohler. 2002. "Fertility Decline in Russia in the Early and Mid 1990s: The Role of Economic Uncertainty and Labour Market Crises." *European Journal of Population / Revue européenne de Démographie* 18 (3): 233–62.

Kohler, Hans-Peter, et al. 2014. "Cohort Profile: The Malawi Longitudinal Study of Families and Health (MLSFH)." *International Journal of Epidemiology* 44 (2): 394–404.

Kraehnert, Kati, et al. 2019. "The Effects of Conflict on Fertility: Evidence from the Genocide in Rwanda." *Demography* 56 (3): 935–68.

Kreager, Philip. 2009. "Darwin and Lotka: Two Concepts of Population." *Demographic Research* 21 (16): 469–502.

———. 2015. "Population Theory—A Long View." *Population Studies* 69 (S1): S29–S37.

Kumwenda, Newton, et al. 2006. "HIV Incidence among Women of Reproductive Age in Malawi and Zimbabwe." *Sexually Transmitted Diseases* 33 (11): 646–51.

Landis, Suzanne E., JoAnne L. Earp, and Gary G. Koch. 1992. "Impact of HIV Testing and Counseling on Subsequent Sexual Behavior." *AIDS Education and Prevention* 4 (1): 61–70.

Lee, Ronald D. 1987. "Population Dynamics of Humans and Other Animals." *Demography* 24 (4): 443–65.

LeRoy, Stephen F., and Larry D. Singell. 1987. "Knight on Risk and Uncertainty." *Journal of Political Economy* 95 (2): 394–406.

Lesthaeghe, Ron J. 1989. *Reproduction and Social Organization in Sub-Saharan Africa.* Oakland: University of California Press.

Levy, Jonathan. 2020. "Radical Uncertainty." *Critical Quarterly* 62 (1): 15–28.

Lexis, Wilhelm Hector Richard Albrecht. 1879. "Sur la durée normale de la vie humaine et sur la théorie de la stabilité des rapports statistiques." *Annales de démographie internationale* 2 (5): 447–60.

Li, Yu, et al. 2018. "Life Course Adversity and Prior Miscarriage in a Pregnancy Cohort." *Women's Health Issues* 28 (3): 232–38.

Lindberg, Laura D., et al. 2020. *Early Impacts of the COVID-19 Pandemic: Findings from the 2020 Guttmacher Survey of Reproductive Health Experiences.* New York: Guttmacher Institute.

Livi-Bacci, Massimo. 2015. "What We Can and Cannot Learn from the History of World Population." *Population Studies* 69 (S1): S21–S28.

Lopman, Ben, et al. 2008. "HIV Incidence in 3 Years of Follow-up of a Zimbabwe Cohort—1998–2000 to 2001–03: Contributions of Proximate and Underlying Determinants to Transmission." *International Journal of Epidemiology* 37 (1): 88–105.

Ludwig, A., and A. Zimper. 2013. "A Parsimonious Model of Subjective Life Expectancy." *Theory and Decision* 75 (4): 519–41.

Macamo, Elísio S. 2017. *The Taming of Fate: Approaching Risk from a Social Action Perspective Case Studies from Southern Mozambique.* Senegal: CODESRIA.

Mace, Ruth. 2014. "When Not to Have Another Baby: An Evolutionary Approach to Low Fertility." *Demographic Research* 30 (37): 1074–96.

Madise, Nyovani Janet, Zoë Matthews, and Barrie Margetts. 1999. "Heterogeneity of Child Nutritional Status between Households: A Comparison of Six Sub-Saharan African Countries." *Population Studies* 53 (3): 331–43.

Madise, Nyovani, Eliya Zulu, and James Ciera. 2007. "Is Poverty a Driver for Risky Sexual Behaviour? Evidence from National Surveys of Adolescents in Four African Countries." *African Journal of Reproductive Health* 11 (3): 83–98.

Magadi, Monica Akinyi. 2011. "Understanding the Gender Disparity in HIV Infection across Countries in Sub-Saharan Africa: Evidence from the Demographic and Health Surveys." *Sociology of Health & Illness* 33 (4): 522–39.

———. 2021. "HIV and Unintended Fertility in Sub-Saharan Africa: Multilevel Predictors of Mistimed and Unwanted Fertility among HIV-Positive Women." *Population Research and Policy Review* 40 (5): 987–1024.

Magruder, Jeremy R. 2011. "Marital Shopping and Epidemic AIDS." *Demography* 48 (4): 1401–28.

Magwira, Dr. Mcphail. 2016. *Malawi HIV Testing Services Guidelines.* Technical report. Lilongwe: Malawi Ministry of Health. https://www.medbox.org/pdf/5e148832db60a2044c2d38a6

Maiden, Emily. 2021. "Recite the Last Bylaw: Chiefs and Child Marriage Reform in Malawi." *Journal of Modern African Studies* 59 (1): 81–102.

Mair, Lucy P. 1951. "Marriage and Family in the Dedza District of Nyasaland." *Journal of the Royal Anthropological Institute of Great Britain and Ireland* 81 (1–2): 103–19.

Makofane, Keletso, et al. 2020. "From General to Specific: Moving Past the General Population in the HIV Response across Sub-Saharan Africa." *Journal of the International AIDS Society* 23 (S6): e25605.

"Malawi: 2nd Periodic Report on the African Charter on Human and People's Rights and the Maputo Protocol, 2015–2019." 2020. Technical report. African Commission on Human and Peoples' Rights, 66th Ordinary Session. https://www.achpr.org/public/Document/file/ English/Malawi%202nd%20Periodic%20Report,%202015-2019.pdf.

Manda, Griffin K. M. 1987. "Funeral Conduct in Nkhata-Bay." *Society of Malawi Journal* 40 (1): 30–36.

Manda, Mtafu A. Z. 2013. *Situation of Urbanisation in Malawi Report*. Technical Report. Mzuzu: Malawi Government Ministry of Lands and Housing.

Manning, Wendy D. 2020. "Young Adulthood Relationships in an Era of Uncertainty: A Case for Cohabitation." *Demography* 57 (3): 799–819.

Manski, Charles F. 2004. "Measuring Expectations." *Econometrica* 72 (5): 1329–76.

Manthalu, Gerald, et al. 2016. "The Effect of User Fee Exemption on the Utilization of Maternal Health Care at Mission Health Facilities in Malawi." *Health Policy and Planning* 31 (9): 1184–92.

Marston, M, et al. 2009. "Trends in Marriage and Time Spent Single in Sub-Saharan Africa: A Comparative Analysis of Six Population-Based Cohort Studies and Nine Demographic and Health Surveys." *Sexually Transmitted Infections* 85 (S1): i64–i71.

Marteleto, Leticia J., et al. 2020. "Live Births and Fertility amid the Zika Epidemic in Brazil." *Demography* 57 (3): 843–72.

Martorell, Reynaldo. 1999. "The Nature of Child Malnutrition and Its Long-Term Implications." *Food and Nutrition Bulletin* 20 (3): 288–92.

Maru, Natasha, et al. 2022. "Embracing Uncertainty: Rethinking Migration Policy through Pastoralists' Experiences." *Comparative Migration Studies* 10 (1): e5.

Maseko, Bertha, et al. 2020. "Perceptions of and Interest in HIV Pre-Exposure Prophylaxis Use among Adolescent Girls and Young Women in Lilongwe, Malawi." *PLoS ONE* 15 (1): e0226062.

Matovu, Joseph K. B., and Fredrick E. Makumbi. 2007. "Expanding Access to Voluntary HIV Counselling and Testing in Sub-Saharan Africa: Alternative Approaches for Improving Uptake, 2001–2007." *Tropical Medicine & International Health* 12 (11): 1315–22.

Matovu, Joseph K. B., et al. 2005. "Voluntary HIV Counseling and Testing Acceptance, Sexual Risk Behavior and HIV Incidence in Rakai, Uganda." *AIDS* 19 (5): 503–11.

McCracken, John. 1998. "Democracy and Nationalism in Historical Perspective: The Case of Malawi." *African Affairs* 97 (387): 231–49.

MDHS (Malawi Demographic and Health Survey). 2004. *Malawi Demographic and Health Survey*. Technical report. Washington, DC: ORC Macro, MEASURE DHS. https://dhsprogram .com/publications/publication-fr175-dhs-final-reports.cfm.

———. 2010. *Malawi Demographic and Health Survey*. Technical report. Washington, DC: ORC Macro, MEASURE DHS. https://dhsprogram.com/publications/publication-fr247-dhs -final-reports.cfm.

———. 2016. *Malawi Demographic and Health Survey*. Technical report. Washington, DC: ORC Macro, MEASURE DHS. https://dhsprogram.com/methodology/survey/survey-display -483.cfm.

Michelo, Charles, Ingvild Sandøy, and Knut Fylkesnes. 2008. "Antenatal Clinic HIV Data Found to Underestimate Actual Prevalence Declines: Evidence from Zambia." *Tropical Medicine & International Health* 13 (2): 171–79.

Mills, Melinda, Hans-Peter Blossfeld, and Erik Klijzing. 2005. "Becoming an Adult in Uncertain Times: A 14-Country Comparison of the Losers of Globalization." In *Globalization, Uncertainty and Youth in Society*, edited by Hans-Peter Blossfeld et al., 423–41. New York: Routledge.

Mische, Ann. 2009. "Projects and Possibilities: Researching Futures in Action." *Sociological Forum* 24 (3): 694–704.

Mishra, Vinod. 2006. "HIV Testing in National Population-Based Surveys: Experience from the Demographic and Health Surveys." *Bulletin of the World Health Organization* 84 (7): 537–45.

Mitchell, J. Clyde. 1956. *The Yao Village: A Study in the Social Structure of a Nyasaland Tribe*. Manchester: Manchester University Press.

Mkondiwa, Maxwell. 2019. "Games of Strategy in Culture and Economics Research." *Journal of Economic Methodology* 27 (2): 146–63.

———. 2020. "Mancala Board Games and Origins of Entrepreneurship in Africa." *PLoS ONE* 15 (10): e0240790.

Mojola, Sanyu A. 2015. *Love, Money, and HIV*. Oakland: University of California Press.

Mojola, Sanyu A., et al. 2015. "HIV after 40 in Rural South Africa: A Life Course Approach to HIV Vulnerability among Middle Aged and Older Adults." *Social Science & Medicine* 143: 204–12.

Mojola, Sanyu A., et al. 2021. "'A Nowadays Disease': HIV/AIDS and Social Change in a Rural South African Community." *American Journal of Sociology* 127 (3): 950–1000.

Montgomery, Mark R. 2000. "Perceiving Mortality Decline." *Population and Development Review* 26 (4): 795–819.

Montgomery, Mark R., and Barney Cohen, eds. 1998. *From Death to Birth: Mortality Decline and Reproductive Change*. Washington, DC: National Academies Press.

Moodley, Dhayendre, et al. 2009. "High HIV Incidence during Pregnancy: Compelling Reason for Repeat HIV Testing." *AIDS* 23 (10): 1255–59.

Moore, Ann M., Ann E. Biddlecom, and Eliya Msiyaphazi Zulu. 2007. "Prevalence and Meanings of Exchange of Money or Gifts for Sex in Unmarried Adolescent Sexual Relationships in Sub-Saharan Africa." *African Journal of Reproductive Health* 11 (3): 44–61.

Morgan, S. Philip. 1981. "Intention and Uncertainty at Later Stages of Childbearing: The United States 1965 and 1970." *Demography* 18 (3): 267–85.

———. 1982. "Parity-Specific Fertility Intentions and Uncertainty: The United States, 1970 to 1976." *Demography* 19 (3): 315–34.

Moyer, Eileen, and Anita Hardon. 2014. "A Disease Unlike Any Other? Why HIV Remains Exceptional in the Age of Treatment." *Medical Anthropology* 33 (4): 263–69.

Mpunga, Elizabeth, et al. 2021. "Readiness for Use of HIV Preexposure Prophylaxis among Men Who Have Sex with Men in Malawi: Qualitative Focus Group and Interview Study." *JMIR Public Health and Surveillance* 7 (10): e26177.

Mtika, Mike Mathambo, and Henry Victor Doctor. 2002. "Matriliny, Patriliny, and Wealth Flow Variations in Rural Malawi." *African Sociological Review* 6 (2): 71–97.

Muchabaiwa, Bob Libert, Tapiwa Kelvin Mutambirwa, and Nkandu Chilombo. 2020. *Investing in Quality Education: Breaking the Intergenerational Cycle of Poverty in Malawi*. Technical

report. Lilongwe: UNICEF Malawi. https://www.unicef.org/esa/media/6181/file/UNICEF
-Malawi-2019-2020-Education-Budget-Brief.pdf.

Mukherjee, Sudeshna, et al. 2013. "Risk of Miscarriage among Black Women and White Women
in a US Prospective Cohort Study." *American Journal of Epidemiology* 177 (11): 1271–78.

Mulder, Monique Borgerhoff, et al. 2012. "Remarkable Rates of Lightning Strike Mortality in
Malawi." *PLoS ONE* 7 (1): e29281.

Munthali, Alister C, Agnes Chimbiri, and Eliya Zulu. 2004. *Adolescent Sexual and Reproductive
Health in Malawi: A Synthesis of Research Evidence.* Occasional Report No. 15. New York:
Guttmacher Institute.

Muriaas, Ragnhild L., et al. 2019. "Why Campaigns to Stop Child Marriage Can Backfire." *CMI
Brief* no. 2019: 04. https://www.cmi.no/publications/6816-why-campaigns-to-stop-child
-marriage-can-backfire.

Musick, Kelly, et al. 2009. "Education Differences in Intended and Unintended Fertility." *Social
Forces* 88 (2): 543–72.

Mutsvairo, Bruce, and Massimo Ragnedda. 2019. *Mapping the Digital Divide in Africa: A Medi-
ated Analysis.* Amsterdam: Amsterdam University Press.

Muttarak, Raya. 2021. "Demographic Perspectives in Research on Global Environmental
Change." *Population Studies* 75 (Suppl.): 77–104.

Mutula, Stephen M. 2008. "Digital Divide and Economic Development: Case Study of Sub-
Saharan Africa." *Electronic Library* 26 (4): 468–89.

Muula, Adamson S. 2002. "HIV/AIDS Prevention Efforts in Malawi." *Malawi Medical Journal:
Journal of Medical Association of Malawi* 14 (2): 26–27.

———. 2008. "Language as Vehicle for Spread and Prevention of HIV in Malawi." *Croatian Medical Journal* 49 (6): 853–55.

Mwale, Macleod. 2005. "Infant and Child Mortality." In *Malawi Demographic and Health Survey 2004*, 123–32. Zomba / Calverton, MD: National Statistical Office (NSO) Malawi / ORC
Macro.

Mwambene, Lea. 2007. "Reconciling African Customary Law with Women's Rights to Malawi:
The Proposed Marriage, Divorce and Family Relations Bill Notes and Comments." *Malawi
Law Journal* 1 (1): 113–24.

Mweso, Clemence. 2014. "Legacy of One Party Dictatorship: Collective Memory and Contesta-
tion in Malawi 1994–2004." M.Phil., University of Cape Town.

National AIDS Commission. 2020. "Malawi National Strategic Plan for HIV and AIDS Sustaining
Gains and Accelerating Progress towards Epidemic Control 2020–2025." Technical report.

National Statistical Office. 1987. *Malawi Population And Housing Census, 1987: Preliminary Report.* Zomba, Malawi: National Statistical Office.

———. 2018. *Malawi Population and Housing Census Final Report.* Technical report. Lilongwe,
Malawi: National Statistical Office.

The Nation Online. 2021. "Lightning Kills 5 in Karonga." February 2. https://mwnation.com/
lightning-kills-5-in-karonga/.

Ní Bhrolcháin, Máire, and Éva Beaujouan. 2011. "Uncertainty in Fertility Intentions in Britain,
1979–2007." *Vienna Yearbook of Population Research* 9: 99–129.

———. 2019. "Do People Have Reproductive Goals? Constructive Preferences and the Discovery
of Desired Family Size." In *Analytical Family Demography*, edited by Robert Schoen, 47:27–
56. Springer Series on Demographic Methods and Population Analysis. Cham: Springer
International.

Nicholls, Nicky, and Alexander Zimper. 2015. "Subjective Life Expectancy." In *The Encyclopedia of Adulthood and Aging*, edited by Susan Krauss Whitbourne, 1–5. Hoboken, NJ: John Wiley & Sons.

Nishimura, Mikiko, et al. 2009. "A Comparative Analysis of Universal Primary Education Policy in Ghana, Kenya, Malawi, and Uganda." *Journal of International Cooperation in Education* 12 (1): 143–58.

Nnko, Soori, et al. 2004. "Secretive Females or Swaggering Males? An Assessment of the Quality of Sexual Partnership Reporting in Rural Tanzania." *Social Science & Medicine* 59 (2): 299–310.

Nobles, Jenna, Elizabeth Frankenberg, and Duncan Thomas. 2015. "The Effects of Mortality on Fertility: Population Dynamics after a Natural Disaster." *Demography* 52 (1): 15–38.

Notestein, Frank W. 1945. "Population—The Long View." In *Food for the World*, edited by Theodore W. Schulz, 36–57. Chicago: University of Chicago Press.

Nsanzimana, Sabin, et al. 2015. "Life Expectancy among HIV-Positive Patients in Rwanda: A Retrospective Observational Cohort Study." *The Lancet Global Health* 3 (3): e169–e177.

Nyasa Times. 2016. "Muluzi's Daughter Killed by Lightning Strike: Malawi Ex-President Left 'Devastated.'" December 12. https://www.nyasatimes.com/muluzis-daughter-killed-lightning-strike-malawi-ex-president-left-devastated/.

———. 2021. "Bizarre! Lilongwe Nsinja Candidate Struck by Lightning in His Sleep." March 22. https://www.nyasatimes.com/bizarre-lilongwe-nsinja-candidate-struck-by-lightning-in-his-sleep/.

Obare, Francis, et al. 2009. "Acceptance of Repeat Population-Based Voluntary Counselling and Testing for HIV in Rural Malawi." *Sexually Transmitted Infections* 85: 139–44.

Ochieng, Beverly Marion, et al. 2022. "Perspectives of Stakeholders of the Free Maternity Services for Mothers in Western Kenya: Lessons for Universal Health Coverage." *BMC Health Services Research* 22 (1): 226.

Oh, Jeong Hyun, Sara Yeatman, and Jenny Trinitapoli. 2019. "Data Collection as Disruption: Insights from a Longitudinal Study of Young Adulthood." *American Sociological Review* 84 (4): 634–63.

Osafo, Joseph, et al. 2021. "Factors Contributing to Divorce in Ghana: An Exploratory Analysis of Evidence from Court Suits." *Journal of Divorce & Remarriage* 62 (4): 312–26.

Palamuleni, Martin Enock. 1993. "Population Dynamics of Malawi: A Re-Examination of the Existing Demographic Data." PhD dissertation, London School of Economics and Political Science.

Parikh, Shanti. 2004. "Sex, Lies and Love Letters: Rethinking Condoms and Female Agency in Uganda." *Agenda: Empowering Women for Gender Equity* 62 (2, 1): 12–20.

———. 2015. *Regulating Romance: Youth Love Letters, Moral Anxiety, and Intervention in Uganda's Time of AIDS*. Nashville, TN: Vanderbilt University Press.

Patel, Pragna, et al. 2014. "Estimating per-Act HIV Transmission Risk: A Systematic Review." *AIDS* 28 (10): 1509–1519.

Perelli-Harris, Brienna. 2006. "The Influence of Informal Work and Subjective Well-Being on Childbearing in Post-Soviet Russia." *Population and Development Review* 32 (4): 729–53.

———. 2008. "Ukraine: On the Border between Old and New in Uncertain Times." *Demographic Research* S7 (29): 1145–78.

Pesando, Luca Maria, et al. 2021. "A Sequence-Analysis Approach to the Study of the Transition to Adulthood in Low- and Middle-Income Countries." *Population and Development Review* 47 (3): 719–47.

Petit, Véronique. 2013. *Counting Populations, Understanding Societies*. Dordrecht: Springer Netherlands.

Philbin, Morgan M., et al. 2022. "Long-Acting Injectable ART and PrEP among Women in Six Cities across the United States: A Qualitative Analysis of Who Would Benefit the Most." *AIDS and Behavior* 26 (4): 1260–69.

Pike, Isabel. 2021. "Men's Economic Status and Marriage Timing in Rural and Semi-Urban Malawi." *Social Forces* 100 (1): 113–36.

Pike, Isabel, Sanyu A. Mojola, and Caroline W. Kabiru. 2018. "Making Sense of Marriage: Gender and the Transition to Adulthood in Nairobi, Kenya." *Journal of Marriage and Family* 80 (5): 1298–1313.

Plummer, Mary Louisa, and Daniel Wight. 2013. *Young People's Lives and Sexual Relationships in Rural Africa: Findings from a Large Qualitative Study in Tanzania*. Lanham, MD: Lexington Books.

Pot, Hanneke, Bregje C. de Kok, and Gertrude Finyiza. 2018. "When Things Fall Apart: Local Responses to the Reintroduction of User-Fees for Maternal Health Services in Rural Malawi." *Reproductive Health Matters* 26 (54): 126–36.

Poulin, Michelle J. 2007. "Sex, Money, and Premarital Relationships in Southern Malawi." *Social Science & Medicine* 65 (11): 2383–93.

Preston-Whyte, Eleanor. 2003. "Contexts of Vulnerability: Sex, Secrecy and HIV/AIDS." *African Journal of AIDS Research* 2 (2): 89–94.

Preston-Whyte, Eleanor, et al. 2000. "Survival Sex and HIV/AIDS in an African City." In *Framing the Sexual Subject*, edited by Richard Parker, Regina Maria Barbosa, and Peter Aggleton, 165–90. Oakland: University of California Press.

Price, Alison J, et al. 2017. "Sustained 10-Year Gain in Adult Life Expectancy Following Antiretroviral Therapy Roll-Out in Rural Malawi: July 2005 to June 2014." *International Journal of Epidemiology* 46 (2): 479–91.

Ragnedda, Massimo, and Anna Gladkova, eds. 2020. *Digital Inequalities in the Global South*. New York: Palgrave Macmillan.

Rainie, Lee. 2017. "The Internet of Things and Future Shock: Too Much Change Too Fast?" Paper presented at the American Bar Association's Section of Science and Technology Law, Chicago, IL, May 10. https://www.pewresearch.org/internet/2017/05/22/the-internet-of-things-and-future-shock-too-much-change-too-fast/.

Randall, Sara. 1996. "Whose Reality? Local Perceptions of Fertility versus Demographic Analysis." *Population Studies* 50 (2): 221–34.

Ranganathan, Meghna, et al. 2018. "'It's because I like things . . . it's a status and he buys me airtime': Exploring the Role of Transactional Sex in Young Women's Consumption Patterns in Rural South Africa (Secondary Findings from HPTN 068)." *Reproductive Health* 15 (102): 1–21.

Rangel, Marcos A., Jenna Nobles, and Amar Hamoudi. 2020. "Brazil's Missing Infants: Zika Risk Changes Reproductive Behavior." *Demography* 57 (5): 1647–80.

Rau, Roland, et al. 2018. "The Lexis Diagram." In *Visualizing Mortality Dynamics in the Lexis Diagram*, edited by Roland Rau et al., 5–10. Cham: Springer International.

Raymo, James M., and Akihisa Shibata. 2017. "Unemployment, Non-Standard Employment, and Fertility: Insights from Japan's 'Lost 20 Years.'" *Demography* 54 (6): 2301–29.

Reniers, Georges. 2003. "Divorce and Remarriage in Rural Malawi." *Demographic Research* S1 (6): 175–206.

———. 2008. "Marital Strategies for Regulating Exposure to HIV." *Demography* 45 (2): 417–38.

Riffe, Tim, Jonas Schöley, and Francisco Villavicencio. 2017. "A Unified Framework of Demographic Time." *Genus* 73 (7): 1–24.

Rindfuss, Ronald R. 1991. "The Young Adult Years: Diversity, Structural Change, and Fertility." *Demography* 28 (4): 493–512.

Rishworth, Andrea, and Brian King. 2022. "Aging, (Un)Certainty and HIV Management in South Africa." *Population, Space and Place* 28 (4): e2552.

Rocca, Corinne, et al. 2010. "Measuring Pregnancy Planning." *Demographic Research* 23 (11): 293–334.

Root, Robin. 2010. "Situating Experiences of HIV-Related Stigma in Swaziland." *Global Public Health: An International Journal for Research, Policy and Practice* 5 (5): 523–38.

Rosenthal, Anat. 2017. *Health on Delivery: The Rollout of Antiretroviral Therapy in Malawi*. Oxford: Routledge.

Rublack, Ulinka. 1996. "Pregnancy, Childbirth and the Female Body in Early Modern Germany." *Past & Present* 150 (1): 84–110.

Ryder, Norman B. 1964. "Notes on the Concept of a Population." *American Journal of Sociology* 69 (5): 447–63.

———. 1965. "The Cohort as a Concept in the Study of Social Change." *American Sociological Review* 30 (6): 843–61.

———. 1973. "A Critique of the National Fertility Study." *Demography* 10 (4): 495–506.

Sandberg, John. 2006. "Infant Mortality, Social Networks, and Subsequent Fertility." *American Sociological Review* 71 (2): 288–309.

Sandberg, John, et al. 2012. "Social Learning about Levels of Perinatal and Infant Mortality in Niakhar, Senegal." *Social Networks* 34 (2): 264–74.

Sangala, Tom. 2018. "Lilongwe Muslims, Villagers Resolve Graveyard Row." *Times Malawi*, July 4. https://times.mw/lilongwe-muslims-villagers-resolve-graveyard-row/.

Santelli, John S., et al. 2015. "Trends in HIV acquisition, Risk Factors and Prevention Policies among Youth in Uganda, 1999–2011." *AIDS* 29 (2): 211–19.

Sasson, Isaac, and Alexander Weinreb. 2017. "Land Cover Change and Fertility in West-Central Africa: Rural Livelihoods and the Vicious Circle Model." *Population and Environment* 38 (4): 345–68.

Schaeffer, Nora Cate, and Elizabeth Thomson. 1992. "The Discovery of Grounded Uncertainty: Developing Standardized Questions about Strength of Fertility Motivation." *Sociological Methodology* 22: 37–82.

Scheper-Hughes, Nancy. 1993. *Death without Weeping: The Violence of Everyday Life in Brazil*. Berkeley: University of California Press.

Schneider, Daniel. 2015. "The Great Recession, Fertility, and Uncertainty: Evidence from the United States." *Journal of Marriage and Family* 77 (5): 1144–56.

Schneider, Jane, and Peter T. Schneider. 1996. *Festival of the Poor: Fertility Decline and the Ideology of Class in Sicily, 1860–1980*. Tucson: University of Arizona Press.

Schouten, Erik J., et al. 2011. "Prevention of Mother-to-Child Transmission of HIV and the Health-Related Millennium Development Goals: Time for a Public Health Approach." *The Lancet* 378 (9787): 282–84.

Schroder, Kerstin E. E., Michael P. Carey, and Peter A. Vanable. 2003. "Methodological Challenges in Research on Sexual Risk Behavior: II. Accuracy of Self-Reports." *Annals of Behavioral Medicine* 26 (2): 104–23.

Schwering, Markus. 2020. "Jürgen Habermas über Corona: So viel Wissen über unser Nichtwissen gab es noch nie." *Frankfurter Rundschau*, April 10.

Scott-Sheldon, Lori A. J., et al. 2010. "Subjective Life Expectancy and Health Behaviors among STD Clinic Patients." *American Journal of Health Behavior* 34 (3): 349–61.

Setel, Philip W. 2000. *A Plague of Paradoxes: AIDS, Culture, and Demography in Northern Tanzania*. Chicago: University of Chicago Press.

Shackle, G. L. S., Charles Frederick Carter, and J. L. Ford. 1972. *Uncertainty and Expectations in Economics: Essays in Honour of G. L. S. Shackle*. Oxford: Blackwell.

Sieber, Sam D. 1973. "The Integration of Fieldwork and Survey Methods." *American Journal of Sociology* 78 (6): 1335–59.

Sifuna, Peter, et al. 2014. "Health and Demographic Surveillance System Profile: The Kombewa Health and Demographic Surveillance System (Kombewa HDSS)." *International Journal of Epidemiology* 43 (4): 1097–1104.

Silver, Laura, et al. 2019. "Mobile Divides in Emerging Countries." Technical report. Pew Research, Washington, DC. https://www.pewresearch.org/internet/wp-content/uploads/sites/9/2019/11/PG_2019.11.20_Mobile-Divides-Emerging-Economies_FINAL.pdf.

Sironi, Maria, and Francesco C. Billari. 2020. "Leaving Home, Moving to College, and Returning Home: Economic Outcomes in the United States." *Population, Space and Place* 26 (4): e2302.

Smith, Adrian. 1995. "A Conversation with Dennis Lindley." *Statistical Science* 10 (3): 305–19.

Smith, Daniel Jordan. 2017. *To Be a Man Is Not a One-Day Job: Masculinity, Money, and Intimacy in Nigeria*. Chicago: University of Chicago Press.

———. 2020. "Masculinity, Money, and the Postponement of Parenthood in Nigeria." *Population and Development Review* 46 (1): 101–20.

Smith, Daniel Jordan, and Benjamin C. Mbakwem. 2010. "Antiretroviral Therapy and Reproductive Life Projects: Mitigating the Stigma of AIDS in Nigeria." *Social Science & Medicine* 71 (2): 345–52.

Smith, Daniel Scott. 1982. "A Perspective on Demographic Methods and Effects in Social History." *William and Mary Quarterly* 39 (3): 442–68.

Smith, Kirsten P., and Susan Cotts Watkins. 2005. "Perceptions of Risk and Strategies for Prevention: Responses to HIV/AIDS in Rural Malawi." *Social Science & Medicine* 60 (3): 649–60.

Smith-Greenaway, Emily. 2015. "Are Literacy Skills Associated with Young Adults' Health in Africa? Evidence from Malawi." Special Issue: Educational Attainment and Adult Health: Contextualizing Causality. *Social Science & Medicine* 127: 124–33.

Smith-Greenaway, Emily, and Jenny Trinitapoli. 2020. "Maternal Cumulative Prevalence Measures of Child Mortality Show Heavy Burden in Sub-Saharan Africa." *Proceedings of the National Academy of Sciences* 117 (8): 4027–33.

Smith-Greenaway, Emily, Sara Yeatman, and Abdallah Chilungo. 2022. "Life after Loss: A Prospective Analysis of Mortality Exposure and Unintended Fertility." *Demography* 59 (2): 563–85.

Sobotka, Tomáš, Vegard Skirbekk, and Dimiter Philipov. 2011. "Economic Recession and Fertility in the Developed World." *Population and Development Review* 37 (2): 267–306.

Sochas, Laura. 2021. "Challenging Categorical Thinking: A Mixed Methods Approach to Explaining Health Inequalities." *Social Science & Medicine* 283: e114192.

Solivetti, Luigi M. 1994. "Family, Marriage and Divorce in a Hausa Community: A Sociological Model." *Africa: Journal of the International African Institute* 64 (2): 252–71.

Spronk, Rachel. 2009. "Media and the Therapeutic Ethos of Romantic Love in Middle-Class

Nairobi." In *Love in Africa*, edited by Jennifer Cole and Lynn M. Thomas, 181–203. Chicago: University of Chicago Press.

Stigler, Stephen M. 1986. *The History of Statistics: The Measurement of Uncertainty before 1900*. Cambridge, MA: Belknap Press of Harvard University Press.

Stolzenberg, Ross M., and Howard Margolis. 2003. "Risk." In *Encyclopedia of Population*, edited by Paul Demney and Geoffrey McNicoll, 860–64. New York: Macmillan Reference.

Swidler, Ann. 1986. "Culture in Action: Symbols and Strategies." *American Sociological Review* 51 (2): 273–86.

———. 2001. *Talk of Love: How Culture Matters*. Chicago: University of Chicago Press.

Szwarcwald, Célia Landmann, et al. 2014. "Correction of Vital Statistics Based on a Proactive Search of Deaths and Live Births: Evidence from a Study of the North and Northeast Regions of Brazil." *Population Health Metrics* 12 (1): e16.

Tavory, Iddo, and Nina Eliasoph. 2013. "Coordinating Futures: Toward a Theory of Anticipation." *American Journal of Sociology* 118 (4): 908–42.

Tavory, Iddo, and Ann Swidler. 2009. "Condom Semiotics: Meaning and Condom Use in Rural Malawi." *American Sociological Review* 74 (2): 171–89.

Tawfik, Linda A. 2003. "Soap, Sweetness, and Revenge: Patterns of Sexual Onset and Partnerships amidst AIDS in Rural Southern Malawi." PhD dissertation, Johns Hopkins University.

Tawfik, Linda A., and Susan Cotts Watkins. 2007. "Sex in Geneva, Sex in Lilongwe, and Sex in Balaka." *Social Science & Medicine* 64 (5): 1090–1101.

Taylor, Darlene, et al. 2015. "Probability of a False-Negative HIV Antibody Test Result during the Window Period: A Tool for Pre- and Post-Test Counselling." *International Journal of STD & AIDS* 26 (4): 215–24.

Thomas, William Isaac, and Dorothy Swaine Thomas. 1938. *The Child in America: Behavior Problems and Programs*. New York: Knopf.

Thornton, Rebecca L. 2008. "The Demand for, and Impact of, Learning HIV Status." *American Economic Review* 98 (5): 1829–63.

Timæus, Ian M., and Tom A. Moultrie. 2008. "On Postponement and Birth Intervals." *Population and Development Review* 34 (3): 483–510.

Timberg, Craig. 2006. "How AIDS in Africa Was Overstated: Reliance on Data from Urban Prenatal Clinics Skewed Early Projections." *Washington Post*, April 6.

Timmermans, Stefan, and Mara Buchbinder. 2010. "Patients-in-Waiting: Living between Sickness and Health in the Genomics Era." *Journal of Health and Social Behavior* 51 (4): 408–23.

Tocchioni, Valentina, Marcantonio Caltabiano, and Silvia Meggiolaro. 2022. "Diverse Pathways in Young Italians' Entrance into Sexual Life: The Association with Gender and Birth Cohort." *Demographic Research* 46 (13): 355–96.

Toefy, Mogamat Yoesrie. 2002. "Divorce in the Muslim Community of the Western Cap: A Demographic Study of 600 Divorce Records at the Muslim Judicial Council and National Ulama Council between 1994 and 1999." MA thesis, University of Cape Town.

Trinitapoli, Jenny. 2006. "Religious Responses to AIDS in Sub-Saharan Africa: An Examination of Religious Congregations in Rural Malawi." *Review of Religious Research* 47 (3): 253–70.

———. 2015. "AIDS and Religious Life in Malawi: Rethinking How Population Dynamics Shape Culture." *Population-e* 70 (2): 245–72.

———. 2021. "Demography beyond the Foot." In *Covid-19 and the Global Demographic Research Agenda*, edited by Landis MacKellar and Rachel Friedman, 68–72. New York: Population Council.

Trinitapoli, Jenny, and Alexander A. Weinreb. 2012. *Religion and AIDS in Africa*. New York: Oxford University Press.

Trinitapoli, Jenny, and Sara Yeatman. 2011. "Uncertainty and Fertility in a Generalized AIDS Epidemic." *American Sociological Review* 76 (6): 935–54.

Turkle, Sherry. 2009. *Simulation and Its Discontents*. Cambridge, MA: MIT Press.

Tversky, Amos, and Daniel Kahneman. 1974. "Judgment under Uncertainty: Heuristics and Biases." *Science* 185 (4157): 1124–31.

UNAIDS. 2007. *Estimating National Adult Prevalence of HIV-1 in Generalized Epidemics*. Technical report. Geneva: Joint United Nations Programme on HIV/AIDS. https://data.unaids.org/pub/manual/2007/epp_concepi_2007_en.pdf.

———. 2014. "90-90-90: An Ambitious Treatment Target to Help End the AIDS Epidemic." Technical report. Joint United Nations Programme on HIV/AIDS, Geneva. https://www.unaids.org/sites/default/files/media_asset/90-90-90_en.pdf.

———. 2015. "2015 Progress Report on the Global Plan: Towards the Elimination of New HIV Infections among Children and Keeping Their Mothers Alive." Technical report. Joint United Nations Programme on HIV/AIDS, Geneva. https://www.unaids.org/en/resources/documents/2015/JC2774_2015ProgressReport_GlobalPlan.

———. 2016. "Methods for Deriving UNAIDS Estimates." Technical report. Joint United Nations Programme on HIV/AIDS, Geneva. https://www.unaids.org/sites/default/files/media_asset/2016_methods-for-deriving-UNAIDS-estimates_en.pdf.

UNICEF, ed. 2014. *Reimagine the Future: Innovation for Every Child*. New York: UNICEF. https://www.unicef.org/serbia/media/7116/file/Reimagine the future-innovation for every child.pdf.

United Nations. Department of Economic and Social Affairs, and Population Division. 2019. "World Population Prospects Highlights, 2019 Revision Highlights, 2019 Revision." Technical report. United Nations. https://population.un.org/wpp/publications/files/wpp2019_highlights.pdf.

Van Bavel, Jan, and David S. Reher. 2013. "The Baby Boom and Its Causes: What We Know and What We Need to Know." *Population and Development Review* 39 (2): 257–88.

Vance, Rupert B. 1952. "Is Theory for Demographers?" *Social Forces* 31 (1): 9–13.

van de Walle, Etienne. 1992. "Fertility Transition, Conscious Choice, and Numeracy." *Demography* 29 (4): 487–502.

Vandormael, Alain, et al. 2019. "Declines in HIV Incidence among Men and Women in a South African Population-Based Cohort." *Nature Communications* 10 (1): 5482.

Verheijen, Janneke. 2011. "Complexities of the 'Transactional Sex' Model: Non-Providing Men, Self-Providing Women, and HIV Risk in Rural Malawi." *Annals of Anthropological Practice* 35 (1): 116–31.

———. 2013. "Balancing Men, Morals and Money." PhD dissertation, Leiden University.

———. 2017. "The Gendered Micropolitics of Hiding and Disclosing: Assessing the Spread and Stagnation of Information on Two New EMTCT Policies in a Malawian Village." *Health Policy and Planning* 32 (9): 1309–15.

Véron, Jacques, and Jean-Marc Rohrbasser. 2003. "Wilhelm Lexis: The Normal Length of Life as an Expression of the 'Nature of Things.'" *Population-e* 58 (3): 303–22.

Vignoli, Daniele, et al. 2020. "Uncertainty and Narratives of the Future: A Theoretical Framework for Contemporary Fertility." In *Analyzing Contemporary Fertility*, edited by Robert Schoen, 51:25–47. Springer Series on Demographic Methods and Population Analysis. Cham: Springer International.

Vollmer, Sebastian, et al. 2017. "The HIV Epidemic in Sub-Saharan Africa Is Aging: Evidence from the Demographic and Health Surveys in Sub-Saharan Africa." *AIDS and Behavior* 21 (Suppl. 1): 101–13.

Waal, Alex de, and Alan Whiteside. 2003. "New Variant Famine: AIDS and Food Crisis in Southern Africa." *Lancet* 362 (9391): 1234–37.

Walters, Sarah. 2021. "African Population History: Contributions of Moral Demography." *Journal of African History* 62 (2): 183–200.

Wandeler, Gilles, Leigh F. Johnson, and Matthias Egger. 2016. "Trends in Life Expectancy of HIV-Positive Adults on ART across the Globe: Comparisons with General Population." *Current Opinion in HIV and AIDS* 11 (5): 492–500.

Wasserman, Herman. 2005. "Renaissance and Resistance: Using ICTs for Social Change in Africa." *African Studies* 64 (2): 177–99.

Watkins, Susan Cotts. 1990. "From Local to National Communities: The Transformation of Demographic Regimes in Western Europe, 1870–1960." *Population and Development Review* 16 (2): 241–72.

———. 1991. *From Provinces to Nations: Demographic Integration in Western Europe 1870–1960*. Princeton, NJ: Princeton University Press.

———. 1993. "If All We Knew about Women Was What We Read in Demography, What Would We Know?" *Demography* 30 (4): 551–77.

———. 2004. "Navigating the AIDS Epidemic in Rural Malawi." *Population and Development Review* 30 (4): 673–705.

Watkins, Susan Cotts, and Angela D. Danzi. 1995. "Women's Gossip and Social Change—Childbirth and Fertility-Control among Italian and Jewish Women in the United States, 1920–1940." *Gender & Society* 9 (4): 469–90.

Watkins, Susan Cotts, Ann Swidler, and Crystal Biruk. 2011. "Hearsay Ethnography: A Method for Learning about Responses to Health Interventions." In *Handbook of the Sociology of Health, Illness, and Healing: A Blueprint for the 21st Century*, edited by Bernice A. Pescosolido et al., 431–45. New York: Springer.

Watkins, Susan Cotts, et al. 2003. "Introduction to Social Interactions and HIV/AIDS in Rural Africa." *Demographic Research* S1 (1): 1–30.

Watkins-Hayes, Celeste. 2019. *Remaking a Life: How Women Living with HIV/AIDS Confront Inequality*. Oakland: University of California Press.

Wawer, Maria J, et al. 2005. "Rates of HIV-1 Transmission per Coital Act, by Stage of HIV-1 Infection, in Rakai, Uganda." *Journal of Infectious Diseases* 191 (9): 1403–9.

Weber, Max. [1905] 2001. *The Protestant Ethic and the Spirit of Capitalism*. London: Routledge.

Weinstein, Traci L., and Xiaoming Li. 2016. "The Relationship between Stress and Clinical Outcomes for Persons Living with HIV/AIDS: A Systematic Review of the Global Literature." *AIDS Care* 28 (2): 160–69.

Weitzman, Abigail, et al. 2021. "How Nearby Homicides Affect Young Women's Pregnancy Desires: Evidence from a Quasi-Experiment." *Demography* 58 (3): 927–50.

Wendland, Claire L. 2010. *A Heart for the Work: Journeys through an African Medical School*. Chicago: University of Chicago Press.

———. 2022. *Partial Stories: Maternal Death from Six Angles*. Chicago: University of Chicago Press.

WHO (World Health Organization). 2015. "Consolidated Guidelines on HIV Testing Services: 5Cs: Consent, Confidentiality, Counselling, Correct Results and Connection 2015." Technical report. https://apps.who.int/iris/handle/10665/179870?locale-attribute=en&.

Whyte, Susan Reynolds. 1998. *Questioning Misfortune: The Pragmatics of Uncertainty in Eastern Uganda*. New York: Cambridge University Press.

Williams, David R., et al. 2008. "Perceived Discrimination, Race and Health in South Africa." *Social Science & Medicine* 67 (3): 441–52.

Wilmoth, John. 2009. "The Lifetime Risk of Maternal Mortality: Concept and Measurement." *Bulletin of the World Health Organization* 87: 256–62.

Wilmoth, John R., and Shiro Horiuchi. 1999. "Rectangularization Revisited: Variability of Age at Death within Human Populations." *Demography* 36 (4): 475–95.

Wilson, Anika. 2013. *Folklore, Gender, and AIDS in Malawi: No Secret under the Sun*. Camden, UK: Palgrave Macmillan.

Wilson, Margot, and Martin Daly. 1997. "Life Expectancy, Economic Inequality, Homicide, and Reproductive Timing in Chicago Neighbourhoods." *British Medical Journal* 314 (7089): 1271–74.

Wood, Geof. 2001. "Desperately Seeking Security." *Journal of International Development* 13 (5): 523–34. https://onlinelibrary.wiley.com/doi/pdf/10.1002/jid.762.

———. 2003. "Staying Secure, Staying Poor: The 'Faustian Bargain.'" *World Development* 31 (3): 455–71.

Wu, Shang, Ralph Stevens, and Susan Thorp. 2013. *Die Young or Live Long: Modeling Subjective Survival Probabilities*. SSRN Scholarly Paper ID 2850220. Rochester, NY: Social Science Research Network.

Wyrod, Robert. 2016. *AIDS and Masculinity in the African City*. Oakland: University of California Press.

Yeatman, Sara. 2009a. "HIV Infection and Fertility Preferences in Rural Malawi." *Studies in Family Planning* 40 (4): 261–76.

———. 2009b. "The Impact of HIV Status and Perceived Status on Fertility Desires in Rural Malawi." *AIDS and Behavior* 13 (S1): S12–S19.

Yeatman, Sara, Stephanie Chamberlin, and Kathryn Dovel. 2018. "Women's (Health) Work: A Population-Based, Cross-Sectional Study of Gender Differences in Time Spent Seeking Health Care in Malawi." *PLoS ONE* 13 (12): e0209586.

Yeatman, Sara, and Emily Smith-Greenaway. 2018. "Birth Planning and Women's and Men's Health in Malawi." *Studies in Family Planning* 49 (3): 213–35.

Yeatman, Sara, and Jenny Trinitapoli. 2011. "Best-Friend Reports: A Tool for Measuring the Prevalence of Sensitive Behaviors." *American Journal of Public Health* 101 (9): 1666–67.

———. 2013. "'I Will Give Birth But Not Too Much': HIV-Positive Childbearing in Rural Malawi." In *Women, Motherhood and Living with HIV/AIDS*, edited by Pranee Liamputtong, 93–109. Dordrecht: Springer Netherlands.

Yeatman, Sara, Jenny Trinitapoli, and Sarah Garver. 2020. "The Enduring Case for Fertility Desires." *Demography* 57 (6): 2047–56.

Yeatman, Sara, et al. 2013. "HIV Treatment Optimism and Its Predictors among Young Adults in Southern Malawi." *AIDS Care* 25 (8): 1018–25.

Yeatman, Sara, et al. 2015. "Health-Seeking Behavior and Symptoms Associated with Early HIV Infection: Results from a Population-Based Cohort in Southern Malawi." *Journal of Acquired Immune Deficiency Syndromes* 69 (1): 126–30.

Zaba, Basia, and Simon Gregson. 1998. "Measuring the Impact of HIV on Fertility in Africa." *AIDS* 12 (1 Suppl.): 41–50.

Zhou, Amy. 2016. "The Uncertainty of Treatment: Women's Use of HIV Treatment as Prevention in Malawi." *Social Science & Medicine* 158: 52–60.

Zimba, Chifundo, et al. 2019. "The Landscape for HIV Pre-Exposure Prophylaxis during Pregnancy and Breastfeeding in Malawi and Zambia: A Qualitative Study." *PLoS ONE* 14 (10): e0223487.

Zimmermann, Okka, and Dirk Konietzka. 2018. "Social Disparities in Destandardization—Changing Family Life Course Patterns in Seven European Countries." *European Sociological Review* 34 (1): 64–78.

Zulu, Eliya Msiyaphazi, and Gloria Chepngeno. 2003. "Spousal Communication about the Risk of Contracting HIV/AIDS in Rural Malawi." *Demographic Research* 1 (8): 247–78.

Zureick, Sarah Marie. 2010. "Certainty in Timing of Death: A New Analysis of Shifting Mortality and Life Span Disparity." PhD dissertation, University of California, Berkeley.

Index